The Stains of Culture

Raphael Patai Series in Jewish Folklore and Anthropology

*A complete listing of the books in this series
can be found online at http://wsupress.wayne.edu*

General Editor
Dan Ben-Amos
University of Pennsylvania

Advisory Editors
Jane S. Gerber
City University of New York

Barbara Kirshenblatt-Gimblett
New York University

Aliza Shenhar
University of Haifa

Amnon Shiloah
Hebrew University

Harvey E. Goldberg
Hebrew University

Samuel G. Armistead
University of California, Davis

The Stains of Culture
An Ethno-Reading of Karaite Jewish Women

RUTH TSOFFAR

Wayne State University Press   Detroit

© 2006 by Wayne State University Press, Detroit, Michigan 48201.
All rights reserved. No part of this book may be reproduced without formal permission.

10 09 08 07 06   5 4 3 2 1

Library of Congress Cataloging-in-Publication Data

Tsoffar, Ruth.
The stains of culture : an ethno-reading of Karaite Jewish women / Ruth Tsoffar.
    p. cm. — (Raphael Patai series in Jewish folklore and anthropology)
Includes bibliographical references and index.
ISBN 0-8143-3223-4 (pbk. : alk. paper)
1. Purity, Ritual—Karaites. 2. Karaite women—Religious life. 3. Menstruation.
I. Title. II. Series.
BM185.T76 2006
296.8'1—dc22
2005017431

∞ The paper used in this publication meets the minimum requirements of the American National Standard for Information Sciences—Permanence of Paper for Printed Library Materials, ANSI Z39.48-1984.

CONTENTS

Preface: Words and Cinnamon, Reading and Fire   vii
Acknowledgments   xiii

Introduction   1

1. Karaite History, Historiography, and the Subject of Truth   25
2. Shabbat, Purity, and Making Love   51
3. Talking Menstruation: The Language of Blood   75
4. Mother-Daughter Teaching   89
5. "Please, No Handshaking": Quantifying the Arbitrary Body   105
6. The Site of Impurity   125
7. Resolution from Within: The Encounter between *Niddah* and *Yoledah*   159
8. Beyond Binarism: Mother's Milk and Karaite Dietary Law   175

Conclusion   193

Notes   199
Bibliography   219
Index   235

PREFACE:
WORDS AND CINNAMON,
READING AND FIRE

> To the incendiary we have granted the right to set fire.
> Edmond Jabès, *The Book of Margins*

There is silence and then there is another silence. Silence that is concealed by another silence. White over white, a blank page over another blank page. And yet if silence has motivated this work, it is because within minority cultures, and within female Karaite culture in particular, silence, over time, has become safe. If a scream is too loud, or colors are too noisy, then difference is disturbing. Yet their words lay coiled under accumulated layers of neglect and immobilized patterns.

To some extent, the eminent medieval Karaite poet and physician Moses Ben Abraham Darʻi resisted this silence. A prolific writer, he wrote interpretations of the Bible, hymns, praise, prayers, and elegies. Like many of his religious and philosophical contemporaries in the Muslim world, he also wrote both holiness poems and secular poems that addressed subjects such as love, separation from friends, marriage, and his existential pain in everyday life. The following poem tells us about some of the force behind his writing:

חָכָם מַחֲרִישׁ לֹא יִוָּדַע/ אִם הוּא חָכָם אוֹ נִבְעָר;
כַּקִּנָּמוֹן, שֶׁכָּל רוֹאָיו/ חָשְׁבוּ עֵץ עַד בָּאֵשׁ נִבְעָר,
נוֹדַע; וּדְבַר אִישׁ מַכִּירוֹ/ אִם מֵבִין אוֹ מִבִּין נִבְעָר.[1]

A wise man, when silent, cannot be known/
Whether he is wise or stupid.
Like cinnamon, which is thought to be ordinary wood/
By all who see it, until it is burned with fire,
Then it is recognized. So also a man's word reveals him and shows/
Whether he is a person of understanding, or one bereft of it. (Weinberger 2000, 421–22)[2]

Dar'i's poem, typical of Andalusian poetry, is written in the quantitative meter of a *qasida*. In it, Dar'i plays with the two meanings of the Hebrew adjective *niv'ar:* as an adjective it means "dumb," "ignorant," or "stupid"; as a derivative passive form of the verb *ba'ar*, it means "burnt" or "consumed."[3] By juxtaposing the two meanings, Dar'i makes a lucid statement about the problematics of representation: a quiet man might be considered ignorant by those who see him, for what appears to the eye is trustworthy—after all, silence does not articulate difference. But Dar'i's dilemma is not about the inability to differentiate between the wise man and the fool so much as it is about our inability to distinguish between one silence and another.

As such, the poem struggles with the popular prevailing realism of representation and knowledge. In the case of the cinnamon, it is fire that can breathe life into its material and burst its fragrance to be released. Fire reveals identities; it tells the material from its performance. And for the poet? Clearly, Dar'i's desire is for the words to act like fire and "speak him" and "speak the poet's essence," as if to allow it to be "born" from within the fire, assuming that such fire (words, ideas) can, indeed, tell what or who the poet is. Yet, at the same time that Dar'i discloses to his reader this philosophical key to distinction, he invites us to identify him, the author, through the reading of his poem. It is as if he says: "Read my words and you will recognize me, my flavor. Burn with me. Or rather burn me; be my fire. Read me."

Those who write have always wrestled with the question of how they are being read—the process of writing itself forces them to anticipate and negotiate between potential readers. Addressing the implied reader can be an incendiary issue among those who read and are marked as Others. Women, minorities, and Third World writers have long sought to speak from this position of difference, constantly attentive to the possibility of being misread. Lacking an authoritative voice and having to invent themselves through the process of writing, they are at the mercy of their readers and often, too, their own perception of their readership. In that sense, Dar'i's poem does not necessarily highlight his knowledge so he may intentionally brag about himself; rather, it speaks for a self-consciousness in readability. Dar'i writes from the limited, imprisoning space from which the reading subject perceives itself-being-perceived, or the to-be-looked-at-ness of the poet's self-representation in a cross-cultural milieu (Mulvey 1988, 93). Burdened to control his representation, Dar'i is engaged in an allegorical discursive exchange with those who control him. From the constraints of that excluded space, writing is an act that exposes the deeper, less visible condition of otherness.

If we take into account some of the poem's political dynamics and the historical framework in which it was written, writing and reading become a careful dance of stratagems, maneuvers of loaded ideological acts of differentiating authenticities. To the degree that writing and reading are words, they are, as Foucault said, the "very object of man's conflict" (Foucault 1972, 216), because they have the potential to liberate. In the case of Darʻi, fire is an alternate practice of reading said to release identity, to liberate it. More than any other practice, and more than any other Jewish group, Karaite reading best exemplifies how the Otherness of Judaism is articulated, and, more significantly, what this otherness within Judaism means.

Karaite historiography contends that Karaism emerged out of its rejection of the Talmudic authority of Rabbanite Judaism in Babylon in the eighth century of the Common Era; taking a divergent path toward strict biblical-textual observance, it has maintained a separate identity ever since.[4] Karaite ethnography articulates a theory of ethnological practice regarding "reading" and "translation" that marks a territory as distinct from Foucault, for words are fire; more than potentiates for liberation, they are signs of a complete break. They constitute separate and silenced historiography along another minority historiography. In other words, within the Rabbinate and within an extremely powerful western tradition of reading, writing, interpretation, and hermeneutics, Karaites present their own exegetical methods through language and body.

In fact, it is hard to imagine a more contested group within Judaism that has been both a subject and an object of such (mis)reading and (mis)recognition.[5] Nevertheless, to the extent that Karaite culture endured throughout history and in different diasporas, its unique position has fostered an immense burden on self-representation, with the additional unique distinction of inner force of pride. As a physician patriarch of the upper class, Darʻi was privileged within the power hierarchies of Karaite culture, and thus was able to gain his voice. His poem, nevertheless, serves as an allegory of the way contemporary Karaites invite us to read their culture and make distinctions.

Even now, I read this poem with the same urgency that Karaite women communicated to me from the very beginning of my study. I had read widely in Karaite culture, and through the teaching of Karaite women, nearly immediately, I was asked to read differently.

From the very outset of this project I was aware of the need to take into account my position as a non-Karaite. This forced me to question what I could contribute to an accurate representation of Karaite culture. I also considered the extent to which my outsider status would hinder this contribution. True, I share with the Karaites the critical experience of being an excluded minority, whether as a woman, Mizrahi and Sephardi, or Israeli and Jewish.

I, like many of the Karaite women, am also a stranger in my native (Hebrew and Arabic) and second (English) languages. Like them, I speak and write from a position of difference, and this difference has, to some extent, motivated and informed my scholarly explorations. More specifically, my work on minority cultures, ethnicities, feminism, and colonialism has prompted me to challenge my own taken-for-granted assumptions and to rethink my theoretical and political positions. At the same time, throughout the process of researching and writing this book, I was reminded of my advantages as an anthropologist and a writer of culture, and of my privileged position as a Jew (Rabbanite) of Israeli-Sabra upbringing.

In the winter of 1989, I spent my first few months with the community in the Bay Area of California. Later that year, in Jerusalem, I met with several members of the Israeli Karaites. Their approach to culture might surprise the Western-trained ethnographer. Over tea and cookies I spoke with one of the rabbis, Joseph,[6] and his wife Deborah, both committed and involved scholars of Karaite halakhah and history. Our conversation turned to my research topic, Karaite Passover and the contemporary exodus, the emigration of the Egyptian Karaite community in the latter half of the twentieth century. There, in their modest living room, in a newly built neighborhood, they both seemed perplexed. "Don't study Passover. You should study the *niddah*," Deborah advised. And so it was, early in the ethnographic process, that I was encouraged to study instead the *niddah*, the menstruating woman and the relevant laws in Leviticus.[7]

I was surprised. Would these women, whom I had known for only a few months, talk with me about the intimate experience of their bodies from the perspective of *niddah*? Would they even have a language to articulate it? The *niddah* seemed the most inaccessible of Karaite subjects. The stories of the menstruating woman have been mostly absent from Karaite culture precisely because the appropriate location of the contaminated and contaminating is construed as outside the social order. Did not Karaite law intend to cover up menstrual blood by making the menstruating woman invisible? And Deborah did not strike me as a person who would talk about the intimacy of *niddah* and other issues of sexuality. But if Deborah appeared reserved and discreet, she still seemed committed to the topic. Actually, Deborah had been "reading." *She* certainly directed me to the right page, knowing the markers of her culture like a good ethnographer who has already written a verisimilar book. If there was any remaining doubt in my mind, it was laid to rest when I returned to the Bay Area. There, Sophia, the acting rabbi's wife, and herself one of the leading

Karaite women, responded with excitement, "If for the Rabbanite Jews *the* issue today is the question of dietary laws, for us, the Karaites, no doubt, it is the question of the *niddah*." Sophia not only squarely placed the issue of *niddah* at the center of contemporary Karaite life but also set it in juxtaposition to Rabbanite culture.

In retrospect, the Karaite women (*Kara'iyot,* singular *Kara'it*) themselves were aware of the profound significance of their practices, the subject whose reading signified their place in the world. Issues of purity and impurity, I came to learn, structure Karaite women's lives. It was through this intimate discourse that I would be initiated into the community, not only as an ethnographer studying and writing about the subject but also as a woman who was invited to be part of their world, and thus is subject to the same codes of purity.[8] The Karaite *niddah* uncovers another deep site of silence. It is, however, the primary site from which to speak for Karaites' legitimacy in a contemporary politics within the overall Jewish community. A combined oral and textual reading, it is therefore a conscious effort on behalf of the women to bring out and articulate that which was ambiguously kept in silence. This book is about the Karaites, the way they read, and the way they want us to read them. But first, who are the Karaites? What do I mean by "reading"? And who is the Karaite *niddah*?

ACKNOWLEDGMENTS

This book is about ways of reading and of being read, but writing it proved to be a personal journey over paved and bumpy roads; a continuous process of writing, erasing, and rewriting; an intimate process demanding my commitment to words and their meanings in multiple languages and dialects.

Many people helped in the creation of this book. I owe heartfelt thanks to the San Francisco Karaite community, and especially to the Karaite women for sharing their stories with me. Special thanks are due to Remy and Joe Pessah, Marcelle Lisha, Murād al-Qudsī, the Dabbah family, Edna Farag, and Hayim Halevi.

I wish to give loving thanks to my Israeli family—my mother Julet (Violet), the wisest of us all; my late father, Naji Saffar, who passed away before I started my academic career; and my late maternal grandmother, Toya (Victoria) Kor—all of whom introduced me to the intricate dynamics of closeness and distance, voice and silence. I am blessed with sisters and brothers (and their families)—Laila Shem Tov, Shoshi Sharabani, Tikva Cohen, Zamir Nehushtan, Yehudit England, Sefer Nehushtan, and Irit Sterenson—all of whom continue to share with me their excitement about life and ideas.

There are many friends and colleagues whose assistance, expertise, and generosity greatly facilitated both my research and this manuscript at various stages. At Berkeley, I owe special thanks to William Brinner, who introduced me to the Karaite community, and also to Chana Kronfeld, Daniel Boyarin, Stanely Brandes, Rutie Stronach, Rondi Gilbert, Nancy Scheper-Hughes, and Dona Goldstein. An early incarnation of this book was my doctoral dissertation, and I benefited from the collective wisdom and support of the three writing groups of which I was a member during my "Berkeley days." For their friendship and support I am indebted to Gil

xiv   Acknowledgments

Anidjar, Rivka Ben Daniel, Karyn Berger, Sumi Colligan, Marci Epstein, Homa Firouzbakhch, Tory Griffith, Rosi Hayes, Avi Hoffer, Harris Lenowitz, Orly Lubin, Felicia McCarren, Debora Porter, Stephen Sheehi, Johanna (Shoshana) Sholl, Ella Shohat, Peter Sluglett, Kathy Wyer, and Yael Zerubavel.

I would like to thank those friends and colleagues in Ann Arbor who enriched the context in which this book came to fruition, including Kathryn Babayan, Carol Bardenstein, Gary Beckman, Ruth Behar, Celeste Brusati, Elliot Ginsburg, Arlene Keizer, Deb Labelle, Anita Norich, Rachel Persico, Marianetta Porter, Janet Richards, Anton Shammas, Stefanie Siegmund, Lucia Suarez, and Terry Wilfong.

I would like to extend heartfelt thanks to the late Professor Alan Dundes, my teacher and mentor, who taught me not just how to approach major disciplines and fields of study with ease but also how to generate great excitement from small details; to Dan Ben-Amos, the general editor of the series, for his encouragement and friendship; and to Jennifer Robertson, for her intellectual companionship and dear friendship. And finally, to Francesc Burgos, thanks for your daily inspiration in our life together, your art, and your cooking. The book is dedicated to our son, Oriol, whose humor and wit never cease to amaze me.

Finally, I owe grateful thanks to Kathryn Wildfong and Carrie Downes for their patient and expert editing, to Eric Schramm for his thorough copyediting, and to the anonymous reviewers of this manuscript who provided thoughtful and helpful suggestions.

I presented work related to the subject of this book at the World Congress of Jewish Studies, Jerusalem; the American Academy of Religion/Society of Biblical Literature, Salt Lake City; the Western Jewish Studies Association; the Association of Jewish Studies; the American Folklore Society; the American Anthropological Association; "Boundaries in Question," University of California, Berkeley; the California Folklore Society; Duke University; Oberlin College; and the University of Michigan, Ann Arbor.

Fieldwork and archival research in California and Israel were funded by the following institutions, fellowships, and grants: the Foreign Language and Area Studies Academic Year (1988–89); the Koret Foundation Fellowship in Jewish Studies (1989–90); the Friedberg Fellowship in Jewish Studies, University of California, Berkeley (1990); the Chancellor's Dissertation Year Fellowship, University of California, Berkeley, (1991); the Newhouse Fund, University of California, Berkeley (1992); a Faculty Summer Research Grant, University of Utah (1995); a Research Assignment, Humanities, University of Utah (1996); the Faculty Fellow Award,

University of Utah (1997); the Frankel Center of Jewish Studies Travel Grant, University of Michigan (2001); and the Office of Vice President for Research and College of Literature, Science and the Arts, University of Michigan (2005).

Chapters 2, 3, and 7 are significantly reworked and expanded versions of my articles, "Reading *it*, Naming *it*, and Talking *it:* The Karaite *Niddah*, *'Ada* and the Language of Menstruation," in *Folklore Interpreted: Essays in Honor of Alan Dundes*, edited by Regina Bendix and Rosemary Levi Zumwalt; "Ethnography, Ethno-reading and the Disclosure of the Karaite Female Body," in *Shofar*, a special issue on *Women in Jewish Life and Culture*, edited by Esther Fuchs; and "The Body as a Storyteller: Karaite Women's Experience of Blood and Milk," in the *Journal of American Folklore*, respectively.

Introduction

> It took twenty years for a community of a thousand years to dissolve. The ice melted as slowly as possible, but it is now sitting in boiling water.
> An American male Karaite scholar

Karaite culture is a reading community: first was the Bible, and then came the sect; *first* was reading and *then* came identity. Given their historical formation, *Kara'im* are *kor'im,* that is, "Karaites read" or "Karaites are readers."[1] True to their cosmopolitan Egyptian origin, contemporary Karaites are well versed in French, Arabic, Italian, Turkish, and English, converse among themselves in Egyptian Arabic, and read in Hebrew. Women also read, and the gender-specific term *Kara'iyot* designates women readers. Within Karaite culture, reading is the prism through which Karaites perceive themselves. As the sect's marker of difference, reading expresses the distinctiveness of the group from its early ideological formation. As such, reading is an act that produces body and text; it produces the Karaite way of life. Methodologically, reading becomes the paradigm for understanding, representing, and articulating the community today.

"Reading" in this study designates a wide continuum, an active engagement with the text, from oral recitation to an awareness that is informed by the historical relations of the community with the Bible. The act of reading, therefore, extends beyond the dichotomy of reading/writing and beyond its immediate connection to a culture of writing (D. Boyarin 1992). Throughout history, the Karaites' mode of reading has insisted on fidelity to the word of God, and to its textual authority that is unmediated by post-biblical oral tradition. Such reading demands an unyielding commitment to the text even before one starts to interpret its meaning. As an ideology (see Street 1984; Fabian 1992), reading encompasses a set of tactics that enables Karaites to preserve their unique identity while continually adapt-

2   Introduction

ing and changing, to keep the extraordinary balance between "formation and differentiation" (Ben-Sasson 1950).

I study Karaite women as the markers of their community, its history, and its distinct identity as an ethnicity. Their methods of prioritizing *niddah* and other stains represent the innovation of "reading" against the blank page but not necessarily in the context of the conventional historiography of ethnology. Indeed, only toward the final stage of the ethnography did I realize that the subject of the *niddah* extends beyond the subject of the menstruating woman to issues such as the confinement of women after birth, the immense significance of breast milk and ways to protect it, and even beyond women's culture, to the dietary laws around milk and meat. More than that, conversations with individual Karaites and my observation of the general community sent me from the field back to the Bible, an indication that this ethnographic focus could and did help me better understand wider popular issues, such as the Karaite interpretation of the biblical prohibition "Do not cook a kid in its mother's milk." Once I discerned aspects of Karaite female consciousness and its internal logic, I was better able to "read as a Karaite" and bring this knowledge of ethnography back to the Bible and Karaite commentaries on the subject. I conceptualized the more theoretical aspect of this process in the concept of "ethno-reading" and "reading as a Karaite." In what follows, I elaborate on the two aspects of reading as a Karaite: the one particular to a community of readers, and the other inspired by feminist work on "reading as a woman." I then develop the idea of "ethno-reading" and discuss its broader implications.

Karaites in the Bay Area

Most members of the San Francisco Karaite community were among the last Jews to leave Cairo between 1956 and 1973. Their departure was the last phase of the twentieth-century Karaite exodus, which mainly comprised the upper middle class of the remaining community. Many Karaites, after hearing discouraging stories of maltreatment in Israel, reluctantly decided that better opportunities awaited them in Europe and the United States. After temporary residence in Italy and France, they found refuge in North America.[2] The Karaites who settled in the Bay Area were attracted to the multicultural environment and mild climate of Northern California, as well as the economic opportunities that it provided, particularly in the high-tech sector. There are currently 700 families scattered throughout the peninsula, forming the largest Karaite community outside Israel. The demographic and cultural diversity of greater San Francisco further enhances the diasporic Jewish community, known for its tolerance of al-

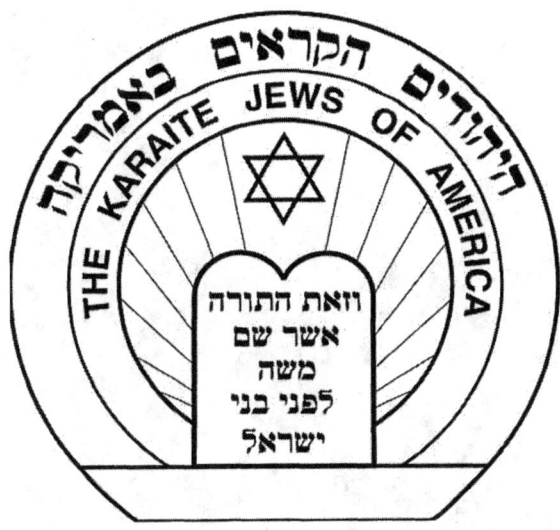

The logo of the Karaite Jews of America. (*KJA Bulletin* 1991)

ternative Jewish lifestyles and religious practices. This comfortable social milieu afforded Karaites the space and resources to redefine their identity according to their needs. They still perceive themselves as Zionists, supporting Israel and looking to Jerusalem as the city that encompasses their sentiments and aspirations.

In September 1982, the newly arrived Karaites established their legal status as a voluntary organization under the name of the Karaite Jews of America (KJA). Once they filed the appropriate documents for incorporation, articulated their by-laws, and were granted non-profit status, they organized the first KJA board as well as monthly Shabbat meetings in Foster City (Pessah 1994, 3). It was in a conservative synagogue there that they also held monthly Shabbat services and where I conducted the majority of my fieldwork. Since then, the Bay Area Karaite community has built its own synagogue and begun publication of a monthly newsletter, the *KJA Bulletin*. The October 1994 issue, for example, included the names of board members and their contact information, an editorial by and interview with the new KJA president, Maurice Pessah, a short overview of the history of the Karaites, an advisory titled "International Karaites, Interfaith Spouses (Registration, Preservation & Genealogy Office)," announcements of weddings, bnei mitzvah, graduations, births, and obituaries, information on a summer camp, pictures of a Purim party, brief instructions on how "to grow a gigantic fava bean," a poem titled "How to Be Happy," and an invitation to use the new matchmaking service, "Super

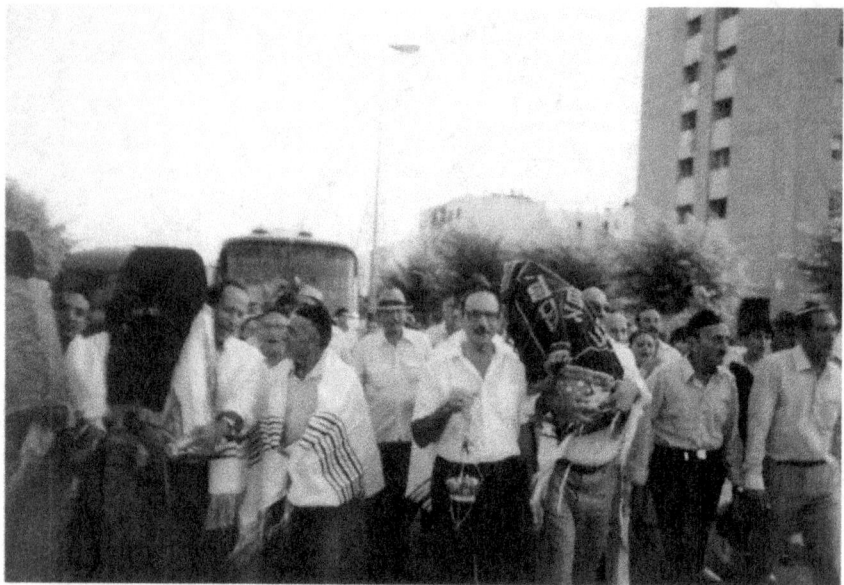

Transferring the Torah scrolls to the newly constructed synagogue in San Francisco, 1992. (Photo courtesy of Remy Pessah)

Match." The community's board of directors consists of a president, acting rabbi, vice president, secretary, and treasurer. The KJA board has seven associates and continues to make efforts to include women in their number (see also Hirshberg 1987, 1994).

The Karaites have adjusted rapidly to the working environment of California, and most are comfortably well off. Nevertheless, what defines a Karaite as a member of this group in daily life is subtle. The question is even more critical for Karaites in the Bay Area because the resources and aspirations that tie them together are limited and the cultural identity of the group is rapidly eroding. In theory, a strict adherence to the biblical text should guarantee their continuity as a people, but the receding memory of their Egyptian past and the allures of an American lifestyle threaten the Karaites' collective memory and sense of their own history. The meetings at the synagogue succeed in bringing together scattered individuals and defining them as a community. The majority of Karaites in the Bay Area, however, attend few such gatherings and are more likely to intermarry or assimilate, which redefines the boundaries of Karaite exclusivity. In addition, the absence of a formally trained religious or spiritual leader exacerbates the lack of direction within the community.[3]

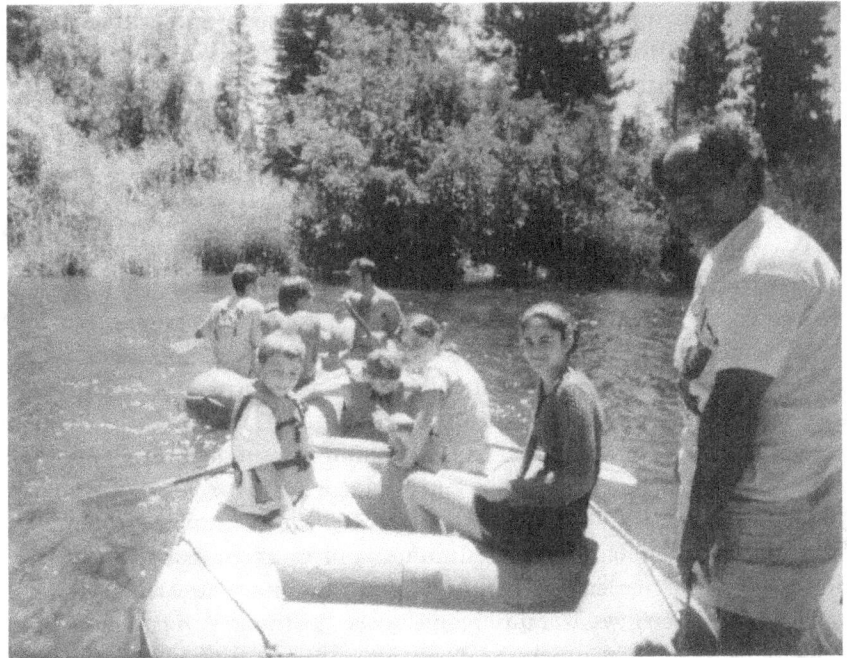

American-born Karaite teenagers and children on a rafting trip on a Northern California river. (Photo courtesy of Remy Pessah)

Nevertheless, whereas the older generation is engaged in synagogue life, and tries to attract families with children to the synagogue, the younger generation—particularly women—is making Herculean efforts to regenerate and revitalize the community. In short, the community is active in its attempts to solidify its culture. Videotapes are sent from the Israeli Karaites along with other printed materials in order to preserve the melodies of text recitation, and the former Karaite Chief Rabbi of Israel was invited to San Francisco for six months to teach and educate adults and children. Even summer camps are organized to bring Karaite children together. The Karaites' efforts to teach both girls and boys to read and sing the Hebrew prayers is yet another response to such concerns. For example, Simchat Torah is becoming the most important holiday of incorporation, initiating children into Karaism by reciting biblical verses out loud in a festival of dance and food (Hirshberg 1987).

Karaite Jewish women bear the responsibility within the community to impart laws and tradition of menstruation, birth, holidays, home life, and the living experience of the oral Torah. My interest in the Bay Area

Karaite women was inspired by women like Deborah and Sophia, who were committed to making their culture accessible and legible. Also significant was their role in the evolving Karaite community's negotiation of the multicultural American experience.

Reading as a Karaite

The extreme marginal position of Karaites provides an excellent opportunity to study a textual culture within the broader power structure and hierarchies of other reading communities and their ideological war on "true" reading. A critique of power and cultural domination lends itself to a critique of ethnography, as it addresses some of the same underlying assumptions.

Contemporary Karaite self-representation is a product of a long history that has anchored their existence (and experience) in the primary "discursive authority" of the Bible (Briggs 1996). Even today, contemporary Karaites imagine themselves through a form of coexistence with the Bible; as one of the leading figures in the community attested, "As long as the Bible exists, we, Karaite people, exist." Although the Bible is not indigenous to Karaites, it gained its significance and authority within the polemic climate of the sect's political development. Like the *Shari'ah* for the Muslims, it has become a "total discourse" (Messick 1993). Such a discourse constitutes different constructs of meaning, giving rise to religious, legal, moral, and political systems. Beyond religious authority, the Bible provides the framework for Karaites' articulation of resistance with their unique national, genealogical, and historical identity. As a "total discourse," the Bible has been appropriated to play a formative historical role in constructing Karaite historiography and collective consciousness.

My claim that reading as a Karaite constitutes a unique approach to texts is based on the two aspects of Karaite identity: the first is their cultural emphasis on reading together with their intimate and organic relationship with the Bible, to the point of naming themselves "*Bnei Mikra*" (the children of the Torah), as if symbolically they had been conceived by the Torah. The second is the Karaites' specific minority position within the dominant culture, especially the Rabbanite culture, but also the wider Muslim, Ottoman, or Christian cultures. Together, these dominant hegemonies shaped Karaites' general position as readers and helped to negotiate their strategies of self-representation. In the realm of Karaite women's culture, however, cultural reading differences are not only a matter of gender but also point to their significance in understanding the permanency of reading in the description of the entire Karaite culture.

These two aspects of reading as a Karaite are not separated. Within the embedded context of other reading societies who valorized sacred texts, including the Rabbanite "'am ha-sefer," people of the book, and the Muslim "'ahl el-kitab," Karaites represent an intensified, extremist position; as part of the wider history of a minority culture, Karaites' practices around texts articulate their position as an allegory of resistance. As Deleuze and Guattari assert in their study of Kafka and Jewish literary minorities, the language of minor literature is always political, always collective, and always deterritorialized. Therefore, to read as a Karaite is to accept as allegorical the obstructed position of reading from a minority position (Deleuze & Guttari 1986, 16–27). In other words, these two aspects work together to emphasize both actual reading and engagement around the Bible, and allegorical, sociopolitical meaning attached to the act of reading.

The Karaite corpus of legal codes, *Sevel ha-yerushah* (literally the endurance of tradition) and *Ha'ataka Mishtalshelet* (the chain [literally, duplication] of transmission),[4] conforms to a limited set of rules of interpretation instituted by Karaite sages. These sages provided specific methodological instructions for reading the Bible and throughout history attempted to reinforce their approach through oral teaching, published manuals, and guidebooks. To read the Bible and interpret its law, therefore, is to a large extent to apply directly the interpretive methods of reading instructed by the Karaite scholars. Although the Bible is closed and defined, it is continuous and eternal, generating possibilities of historically situated reading. Unlike interpretations that encourage extratextual explorations and the application of a metaphoric imagination, Karaites seek to travel back to the disputed place of origin that gave them birth. In his book of Karaite legal codes, *Sefer ha-mitzvot* (The Book of Precepts), Anan ben David, the founder of the Karaites, advocated leaving a space for personal interpretation of the Bible: "'*Chapsu be-'Orita shafir ve-'al tisha'anu 'al da'ati*" (search diligently in the Torah and do not rely on my opinion).[5] This principle permitted individual readings beyond the conventional Karaite principles, and is often used, even by the Bay Area community, to refute the claim that Karaite exegesis is dogmatically imposed. The main premise here is that the truth of the text can be communicated through its accessible language.

Over time, *Sevel ha-yerushah*, however, came to stand for an interpretive principle in itself, consistent with the other two main principles, *katuv* or *pshat* (literal interpretation) and *hekesh* (analogy). The Karaites' desire to imagine themselves embodied by the Bible is especially evident in their literalness, which is their main method of interpretation. Literal interpretation derives meaning from the words as they appear in the Bible, highlighting the linguistic competency of the reader and advocating concrete meaning. In contrast, the *hekesh*, or analogy, operates on the notion of sameness. Analogy works by comparing the unfamiliar against the familiar, thereby defining the space of the signifier and framing the range of referentiality. Unlike metaphors, analogy corresponds to an underlying set of given assumptions that while limiting its application, draws in immediate associations to the target domain by seeing it in terms of the source domain (Holyoak and Thagard 1995; Indurkhya 1992). Over time, analogies articulate a solid referential system or a "cognitive model" such that its consistency within the culture feeds the interpretive process. At the same time, this referentiality reintroduces the subject within a different contextual framework. These three principles of interpretation are applied to the Bible, and determine the interpretive parameters of reading. They restrict the space of dialogic reading from within, thus keeping the semiotic gap between signified and signifier to a minimum (Semi 1984).

This work joins recent studies of the interpretive paradigm of power and discipline around texts and reading practices in Middle Eastern cultures. In *The Calligraphic State: Textual Domination and History in a Muslim Society,* Brinkley Messick examines relations between writing and authority in Muslim society. For him, Yemen's textual practice is a "manuscript culture" within a "calligraphic state"—which is both a political entity and a discursive condition (1993, 1). "Textual domination," he writes, "entails the interlocking of a polity, a social order, and a discursive formation." Drawing the attention to the way this domination plays in authoritative institutions, he ties the production of literary texts to the process of authority that they acquire. "To investigate the role of texts in a specific state, however, requires a view of writing that stresses its cultural and historical variability rather than its universal characteristic, and its implication in relation to domination rather than its neutrality or transparency as a medium" (ibid., 1–2). In contrast to Yemenite culture, Karaite textuality for the ethnographer, literary theorist, and feminist compels a strikingly innovative and interdisciplinary position among various authorities in times of cultural transition.

Textuality as writing, for Messick, is analogous to textuality as reading in the Jewish (Karaite) tradition, and reminds us that *niddah* is more than just another discursive formation of interlocking social order, issues of power, and politics of reading. Reading in Karaite culture, as the name of the sect implies, is socially embedded: it is through collective practices that this reading shaped the Karaite self-identity and ideology. Unlike contemporary authority of Muslim documents, manuals, and court judgments, contemporary Karaite authority keeps inventing new practices around the reading of the Torah: meetings on Saturday mornings and holidays, teaching the Hebrew language and melodies to Karaite children, and importing teaching material from Israel. The Karaite library is remarkable in its adaptation to new reading formats for their own cultural and religious education, as seen in a range of books, newsletters, visual and audio material, and even database and Web material.

The other aspect of reading as a Karaite acknowledges the specific cultural history of Karaites as a cultural Jewish minority. More precisely, it is a poststructuralist approach to Karaite culture as a gendered, ethnic, religious minority, assuming that different cultural locations result from different readings. Reading as a Karaite is reading a canonical text from the highly hierarchical underprivileged margins as a model of reading that questions the normative, canonic power (cf. Lubin 2003). Karaite reading, accordingly, is informed by the Karaite experience as an excluded minority, asserting that prevailing social and political forces are being brought back into the text and to the process of reading (cf. Culler 1982, 46). Indeed, since "difference is produced by differing" (ibid., 50), reading as a Karaite highlights their strategic position of difference around texts and the politics of reading. Since such a reading goes beyond a historical and stereotypical construct of Karaites as a heretical group, for Jews in particular, it might ease anxieties about religious and ethnic difference and expand the limits of tolerance within Jewish culture. It pays attention to the politics of reading sacred texts within Judaism as much as within the wider context of different Muslim sectarian traditions that evolved around the Koran. Such a reading is attentive to Karaite history of exclusion and inclusion, a proactive response to their debased position as blasphemers and heretics. At the same time, being nonmonolithic, and situated in different geographical settings, Karaite reading is a strategy to critique, resist, and subvert authority. As an act of resistance, Karaite reading led to the emergence of a whole system of legal conducts and practices, giving rise to a Karaite calendar marked with days of fasting, sexual abstinence, dietary restrictions, and celebrations.

If to read as a woman is "to avoid reading as a man, to identify the specific defenses and distortions of male readings and provide correctives" (Culler 1982, 54), then to read as a Karaite is to avoid reading as a Rabbanite, to insist that one revisit and refute the charges of Karaite heresy, and to reassert their legitimacy within Judaism. However, this contrastive, binary formula oversimplifies both women's and Karaites' initiatives in creating new discursive spaces of autonomy and self-determination. Yet, whereas reading as a woman highlights differences of sex and gender, reading as a Karaite is a construct that makes manifest religious and ethnic differences; one especially salient religious difference is that of reading. In this connection, Brian Stock claims that the "act of reading is part of a model of society, which assumes that differences between communities can be reduced, or even eliminated, by a common experience of the text" (Stock 1992, 271). However, whereas Stock refers to textual traditions of Muslim communities, aiming to reduce ethnic, national, and religious differences to the experience of the Koran, understanding "reading as a Karaite" acknowledges the exclusive experience of Hebrew texts as a way to mark differences between cultures and genders.

Indeed, throughout history, Karaite identity, so tightly connected to the Bible, was shaped by the inner logic of Karaite historiography and ideology in conjunction with a dialectical interaction with Rabbanite Judaism. Ironically, Rabbanite culture spurred among Karaites the study of the Bible and encouraged their identification with the biblical text.[6] Murād al-Qudsī, a contemporary Karaite historian, sums up their textual identification: "Without [the Rabbanites], the Torah would have been lost, because the Talmud [read by Rabbanites] has reinforced the learning of the Torah [by Karaites]." In that sense, reading in Karaite culture was, from its early days, a political force for instituting, differentiating, and consolidating a unique identity, and for developing a counterhegemonic tradition.

As the hegemonic voice of text interpretation, Rabbanite authority has been undoubtedly a mobilizing force in Karaite hermeneutics. Amos Funkenstein articulated their shared history as such: if Karaites originated as a political movement that challenged Rabbanite authority, then Karaites can be defined only in close proximity to their point of reference—the Rabbanites—because the Karaites' anti-Rabbanite history is the essence of their collective memory.[7] Memory constitutes self-consciousness, and collective memory is, in part, analogous to language, in the Saussurian sense, being a system of signs, symbols, and conventions. But more than language, collective memory is mostly direct and unmediated, and, like Nietzsche's concept of "monumental history," it is oblivious to the specificity of history, reducing historical events, people, and institutions to a topocentric construct (Funkenstein 1993, 13–19).

Whereas Funkenstein contends that one's consciousness cannot escape the grasp of collective memory (ibid., 11–34), Michel de Certeau asserts that one's body cannot escape the grasp of the law: "From birth to mourning after death, law 'takes hold of' bodies in order to make them its text" (1984, 139). Yet it is possible to bring both together and make a strong case for inscription of text as embodied memory. As this study shows, a certain offshoot tradition, largely concerning body praxis, has developed among Karaites, particularly among the *Kara'iyot*. This tradition is, in itself, an interpretive extension arising from the *Kara'iyot*'s own understanding and development of their texts and reading. It appears in the women's representation of the ritual around the purity of the body, in relation to the sacred Torah and the way the code of purity was read in order to guarantee cleanliness. Considering the implication of textual authority among the "clean" and "unclean," women's narratives around the code of purity result in telling the informal, unofficial story that is used to legitimize Karaite reading today. This is where text and body meet.

Thus, the ethnography of the body enables us to study Karaite self-representation without making strong ties or comparisons with the Rabbanite culture. A pivotal question in this search for a Karaite system, however, is *What does it mean to read as Kara'it, both as a woman and as a Karaite?* If the Karaite desire is to maintain an unmediated relationship with the text, how then is the body incorporated into this ideology of reading? Such an approach reaffirms the presupposition that the text inscribes its meaning on the body, translating verbal language into the language of practice. The transition from Karaite textual teaching to the body, therefore, is an attempt to introduce the body as unmediated, subject to the same cultural treatment as the text: if it can be read, it also can read. The historical framework gives the body immense symbolic responsibility of purification by extending beyond its biological roles and by including the mother and her maternal position in the overall production of pure Karaite culture. Sophia and Deborah, therefore, did not direct me to compare their culture to that of the Rabbanites, but rather to develop the fuller narrative of women's participation in the culture.

Within the Karaite method of reading, the body has a special configuration as a discursive agent, constituting a site of Karaite interiority in culture. It infuses its meaning into a presence, a certain mobility and relatedness. It accommodates history and geography while being attentive to the ideological nuances of power and authority, renewal and preservation. Text communicates identity through the body that reads. The body can read and can also be read, because the referential mechanism from the body to the text and from the text to the body is dynamic, serving the different strategies employed by the culture to preserve itself and negotiate its invented tradition. Moving away from the text to its livable chapter, I address next how this literal approach is translated by Karaites into the body: Can we talk about a literal body? To what extent?

Reading, Ethno-Reading, the Literate, and the Literal

Rather than claiming that reading is merely a linguistic act or an interpretive process, I would like to elaborate on the idea of ethnography as a project of translation; reading, in the way it has been represented in Karaite culture, is a multilayered and complex act of cultural translation. Such an act is constitutive of Karaite identity; it points to internal Karaite methods of interpretation, their cultural differences, and the wider politics of reading. The representation of culture through the trope of reading and its embodied memories goes hand in hand with the accumulated memory of "being read" and the history of becoming the object of memory.

But more than that, if reading constitutes identity, then to read as a Karaite means to *become* a Karaite. This is where the connection between the method of reading and the subject of research converges, illustrating that theory is not separate from the specific subject of research and the methods of interpretation (Chow 1995, 180). Indeed, my own reading of Karaite practices brings to the forefront issues of meaning and interpretation essential not only for understanding Karaite culture, but also for probing the parameters of "ethnography" as a practice of "writing culture" (Clifford 1984). Can we argue for a case of "ethno-reading," focusing on "reading culture," as an important aspect of the poetics and politics of cultural production?

Rey Chow, among other scholars, addressed the crisis of ethnography by deconstructing the classic epistemological foundations of visual culture in ethnography and anthropology (1995, 173–202). Ethnography, according to this critique, is a modernist discourse of domination and control that translates cultures asymmetrically from the ethnographer's privileged position, producing a Western monologue (ibid., 1995, 175; Derrida 1978; Asad 1973, 1984; Niranjana 1992). Inevitably, cultures are translated into established discourse, enhancing existing hegemonies of power and language (Asad 1984). In spite of the fact that ethnography, or ethnology, advocated cultural relativism and humanism, it nonetheless resulted in the assumption of a "totalizing, teleological concept of a universal history" (Niranjana 1992, 71).

It is not surprising that within such an imposed epistemological paradigm, the subaltern subject of ethnography, as Tejaswini Miranjana asserts, "exists only 'in translation,' always already cathected by colonial domination" (ibid., 43). In the context of Middle Eastern cultures and representation, a Eurocentric, Orientalist approach has dominated the field, making obvious that translation of culture is overdetermined by ideological and national or religious discourses (ibid., 21). Especially in the case of the Karaites, and of the women's practices in particular, translation of culture highlights the complexity of a cross-cultural "reading" of a minority within a minority, within a colonized culture.[8] As opposed to ethnography, ethno-reading acknowledges the heterogeneity of culture (and texts) in constructing both "reality" and "subject"; it challenges the transparency of language and alerts readers to the role of history and historicity in the configuration of power and representation (Miranjana 1992, 85–86). Indeed, at the heart of ethno-reading is the situated reading—or "reading as a Karaite, woman, etc."—which is inherently interdisciplinary and thus attentive to the multiple positions of reading.

At the same time, and especially in the context of Karaite culture, ethno-reading cannot be separated from the historical Karaite memory of reading and from the ideological valorization of the textual tradition of Karaite sages. Internal Karaite methods of reading elucidate modes of halakhic interpretation that duplicate and modulate regimes of truth, to the point of blurring the distinctions between the subject and its representation. Karaite halakhah is the end result of the concern with God's truth. *Ha'atakah mishtalshelet* (duplicated transmission), therefore, is the careful transmission of culture that is controlled by the "copy-rights" (of Karaite sages) within the limited permitted space for change and elaboration. Karaite reading always strives to keep close to the biblical texts and narratives as religious authority in order to maintain their "subjective origins." Reading in this regard is a preserving institution, as it keeps Karaite culture close to its constitutive text, building less on the Bible's potentiality than on its origins. Focusing on Karaite reading reveals that textuality is a force that grounds, preserves, and strengthens ties and links to the Karaite past and in particular to the Karaites' and Rabbanites' split origin as a point of departure and reference. To some degree, considering Karaite reading as the ultimate difference within the asymmetric Karaite/Rabbanite power relationship legitimates the literal economy of the text, as it fills and empties the epistemic space of reading ethnicity with the meaning of resistance (Mahler 1949). Such space determines the discursive movement from the text into Karaite life and back again into the text, a cultural location that marks the limits of historical memory. The ethno-reading presented by Karaite women further emphasizes that even in the context of migration and travel, within the historical ruptures of exile and exodus, reading provides the conditions for and means of connectedness.

Rather than exploring solely the "to-be-looked-at-ness" (Mulvey 1988; Chow 1995, chap. 3), Karaite ethno-reading allows us to move from the conventional observation of culture via the observant gaze to attempt an interpretive approach to textual traditions as a new possibility for reading a culture. Reading as a Jewish minority, reading as a Kara'it, and reading as a *niddah* all mean that we not only acknowledge the specific cultural position of the subjects of ethnography, but also that we understand the contribution of Kara'iot's textual tradition by exposing the multilayered cultural construct that embeds its interpretation. Still, ethno-reading approaches culture from the position of its discursive authority, arguing that reading as a Karaite is a political, ideological act that, with its emphasis on the literal meaning of the Bible, encapsulates the very core of Karaite coexistence with text. It inevitably takes into consideration the way that Karaites perceive themselves being read through the eyes of the others. By alluding to different levels and practices of objectification, ethno-reading helps legitimize the linguistic and political choices of a minority culture.

Moreover, ethno-reading highlights the distortion of ethnography as a mode of representation that privileges writing culture and builds on the modes of representation that Karaites themselves employ: even while ethno-reading privileges textuality, it combines sites of reading with the position of being read. If interpretation is at the core of Karaite descriptive practices, then definition through reading becomes an alternative way to represent or critique culture, a way that ties together the Karaites' cultural aspiration and my methodology of describing culture, namely, ethno-reading.

For Walter Benjamin, "a real translation is transparent: it does not cover the original, does not block its light, but allows the pure language, as though reinforced by its own medium, to shine upon the original all the more fully" (Benjamin 1968, 79). The literal, for Benjamin, is a condition for real translation whose main purpose is to release "that which seeks to represent, to produce itself in the evolving of language," in order to reveal the original intention of the text. To liberate the language imprisoned in a work is the translator's re-creation of that original work. Rather than a fixed truth, literal reading produces meaning through "mobility, proximity, and approximation"; rather than being considered simplistic, naive, or lacking in sophistication, literal reading is a "supplement for truth," or rather complementary (ibid., 80).

In this sense, translation uncovers the meaning hidden in the text. Rather than loading the signifiers with accumulated layers of meaning, Karaite reading seeks to remain simple and plain. As *pshat*, the name of the interpretive reading method in Hebrew, conveys ambiguously, meaning should remain uncovered and undressed. While the native Hebrew speaker may not immediately make the etymological connection between *pshat*, as a simple reading of the text, with *lehafshit*, to undress, the semantic connection between the two is nevertheless apparent. A "naked reading," accordingly, is a reading that is neither concealed nor concealing.

Aiming to remain faithful to the original, authentic meaning of the word, it seeks to keep the text exposed and its meaning always accessible. The fact that the Hebrew word *bagad,* betrayed, is etymologically connected to *begged,* a piece of clothing, may suggest that dressing up, within the reading ideology of fidelity and infidelity (Chow 1995, 182–89), is an act of deception that covers authentic bodies and, in the realm of text, words and signifiers.[9] The episteme is ambiguous while the truth is conserved through literal reading. It emphasizes that true meaning can be exposed as long as signifiers remain bare and exposed. More germane to the Karaites, the Bible is depicted as a living body: the metaphor of text as body, dressed and undressed, naked or concealed, narrows the distinction between the body that reads and the body (the book) that is being read.[10] Unlike Rabbanites, Karaites resisted accumulated and layered meanings of the Bible. Anan's evocation to access the language of the Bible "*chapsu be-'Orita, shafir*" is not anarchistic, as scholars of Karaism presumed, but is consistent with the whole concept of this literal reading. It presupposes that the interpretive trajectory of reading can be easily approximated by the true accessibility of the Torah's literal language. "Naked reading" corresponds with the Karaite notion of history: like the wine made out of raisins for Passover, history is kept unfermented yet preserved.

Even if we do not problematize the literal and take Karaites' self-representation literally, it is clear that from the outset the body played an important role in conveying the Karaite position as longtime mourners of the destruction of the Temple. The *'Ananim* changed the locus of the ritual and highlighted the metonymic body/Temple relations as a trope of identity. The "mourning body" not only preserved in its posture the loss of the religious center, it also replicated the Temple as it shifted the cultic site of purity and impurity to the human body (see "The Mourners of Zion" in Mahler 1949). In general, this aspect of Karaite ritual is emphasized already in Anan's *Book of Precepts,* in which Anan elevated the status of the priests to teachers in order to crystallize the enduring cultic orientation of the sect (Ben-Sasson 1950). Whereas Rabbanites eventually used prayer as an alternative to cultic ritual, Karaite sages initially imposed stricter prohibitions, such as adding more fasting days to the calendar, prohibiting sexual intercourse on Shabbat and holidays, and prohibiting the eating of meat (outside of Israel) and the drinking of wine.

Until the 1940s, descriptions of Karaites (in Europe, Jerusalem, or Turkey) sitting in their cold, dark homes during Shabbat was a common theme in travelers' accounts (Deinarda 1880, 77; Fahn 1928; Goitein 1964, 402–4), even though Karaites had introduced the lighting of Shabbat candles, after long internal debate, in the fifteenth century (Ankori 1959,

265–69). A certain melancholic undertone still dominates Karaite demeanor. "We are a very serious people," Susana told me. A radiant woman in her late forties, her sparkling eyes full of humor and warmth contrasted sharply with the somber analysis of her community. "We take things more seriously, much more seriously. We are not a relaxed tribe."

The Karaite *Niddah*

Was it possible, I thought at the beginning of this study, that the discourse of Karaite menstruation might indeed set fire to the cold ream of Karaite silence? There is a totality, a harshness and severity in the semantic field of the term *niddah*. Chapter 3 addresses in detail the term and its usage, establishing that *niddah* corresponds to Douglas's (1966, 1975) notion of anomaly and its treatment, going back to Leviticus: "And if a man shall lie with a woman having her sickness, and shall uncover her nakedness; he hath discovered her fountain: and she hath uncovered the fountain of her blood: and both of them shall be cut off from among their people" (Lev. 20:18).[11] The harshness of "cutting off," or *karet*, finds its way to the Karaite halakhic vocabulary of legislation. Anan Ben David, contrary to his usual strict ruling with regard to halakhic innovations, replaced the biblical death penalty with *nidduy 'olam*, a life sentence (Ben-Sasson 1950, 49 n. 60). *Nidduy 'olam* and *niddah* are derived from the same root, *ndh*, alluding to the strict uncompromising verdict of ostracization and/or expulsion. The man sentenced to *nidduy 'olam* was excommunicated and cut off from any social/religious life whatsoever. Thus, this etymological proximity overloads the semantics of the concept of *niddah* and its implication.

In fact, the different traditions of *niddah* make clear that menstrual taboos are culturally constructed. This study follows the anthropological, sociological, and psychological body of knowledge on menstrual blood—including the groundbreaking works of Mary Douglas's *Purity and Danger* (1966) and Julia Kristeva's *Powers of Horror* (1982). I depart, however, from their claims on menstrual universalism, while adding to the already established scholarship on menstruation from a specific cultural perspective. As Buckley and Gottleib argue, "Above all, menstrual taboos are cultural constructions and must first be approached as such—symbolic, arbitrary, contextualized, and potentially multivalent whose meanings emerge only within the contexts of the fields of representations in which they exist" (1988, 24).

Both Karaites as well as Rabbanites read the verses of Leviticus concerning *niddah*. Yet to say that each community simply developed its own code of conduct that adheres to internal methods of interpretation and philosophy would not be accurate in the case of the Karaites. For even the severity of Leviticus, with its penalty of *karet*, and the seriousness with which the Karaites interpreted and enforced it, did not gain the Rabbanites' validation of their practice. Rabbanites have read Leviticus and codified the *niddah* laws, dedicating an entire tractate of the Talmud to the discussion of menstruation with a myriad of detailed instructions, including how to interpret colors and stains, when to start counting the unclean days, and when to go to the *mikveh* (Biale 1984; Wasserfall 1999; Fonrobert 2000).

The differing traditions that emerged around Leviticus are not simply variant versions of reading (Fonrobert 2000). Rather, they point to *niddah* as a contested site that articulates and highlights differences, founding distinct interpretations, practices, and identities. More than any other site, *niddah* encapsulates the power struggle between the Karaites and the Rabbanites over who controls the text and how it is being controlled. In other words, it determines who has the right to speak and who is relegated to silence. In their attempts to legitimize self and delegitimize the other, historical Rabbanite accusations that Karaites are not "pure" stem mainly from the fact that a husband and wife resume marital relations following menstruation (*niddah*) after only seven or eight days (whereas Rabbanites count at least twelve) and that the women do not immerse in a *mikvah* (ritual bath). Thus traditional Rabbanites have characterized Karaite men as *"bo'alei niddot"* (those who have sexual intercourse with menstruating women) (Asaf 1936, 214).[12] This disparaging sixteenth-century formulation has the effect of "staining" the entire Karaite community, and men in particular, as both contaminated and as effeminized by menstruating women. The articulation of Karaite culture as contaminated and therefore contaminating is at the core of hegemonic Rabbanite cultural politics toward the Karaite minority. It clearly condemns Karaite conduct as illegal and alludes to innumerable unlawful ramifications of the Karaite legal system. This context largely explains that the Karaite halakhic record is not free of historical accusations and that being "clean" and "unstained" have developed into the central features of Karaite self-representation.

Moreover, until the sixteenth century, each Karaite was halakhically marked as *"safek mamzer,"* an illegitimate child unless otherwise proven. This was the position held by both Sephardic and Ashkenazi rabbis. For instance, Rabbi Hayim Hezkeyah Medini, a Sephardic sage from the nineteenth century, quotes a commonly held approach toward Karaites that is summarized in Rabbi Moshe Suzin's expression of the mid-nineteenth century: *"Kara'im 'einam mit'achim le-'olam"* (Karaites can never be stitched together, or cannot be mended [with a passive or reflexive verb]) (cf. Zohar 1987, 22). The fact that the verb *mit'achim*, from the root *'achah*, is etymologically related to the noun *'ach* (brother or kinsmen) further enhances the ironic depth of this statement, alluding to the finality of the rupture between Rabbanite and Karaites. The rupture is not only national and religious: the word *'ach* implies an explicit understanding of the rupture within the collective Jewish body.

In the historical politics of pure and impure, the term *bo'alei niddot* has become an offensive stain on the Karaite body. It encapsulates the impossible location of Karaites and the impossibility for Karaites to read from a place that is not informed by this discrimination. Even more problematic than Dar'i's cinnamon—after all, the aroma of the cinnamon can be perceived even before it is burned—is the demand to be studied through the *niddah*. Menstrual practices have also been a silencing force within Karaite culture. Menstruation shapes women's ability to articulate their way of disciplining the contaminated blood, and forces them to focus vigilantly on their bodies, whose inappropriateness is always already marked and marking.

Studying Karaite menstrual blood is problematic because it easily challenges the reader's own comfort level with regard to women, body, and blood.[13] In Israeli discourse, talking about dirt makes the speaker dirty. This is especially true for women, and perhaps even more so for those from the Middle East. Implicit in the association of menstruation with dirt is the presumption of a lower standard of living, undeveloped aesthetics, and unhygienic bodily practices. These presumptions, moreover, are an essential aspect of Israeli identity politics, where the hegemonic class tends to consider itself tainted by the inclusion of Mizrahim, who are marked as Arabs, partaking of Arabic culture and with a Third World status. Even within the legal discussion surrounding *niddah* in Jewish law, where the rabbis attempt to define every single aspect of *niddah* precisely, the discussion clearly resorts to a language of analogy and metaphor, effectively objectifying and silencing women (D. Boyarin 1993). In other words, menstrual blood constitutes intimacy; it signifies the interiority of the domestic sphere. Its blood flows in the deepest chambers of a woman's being. And blood, like intimacy, is silent.

When they asked me to write about the *niddah*, the Karaite women were aware of the narrativity of their bodily experience. Obviously, they had a clear idea that their practice could generate a story (Bal 1985). But more than that, to follow Dari's words, telling is part of the practice; thus, narrating the *niddah* is purifying. It completes the practice. The ethnography of *niddah*, then, was for me already a poetic discussion of the utterance and nonutterance of their contemporary and conflicted Karaite culture. If as the Egyptian Jewish poet Edmond Jabès observed, "exile is unavoidable and chronic" (Jabès 1993, x), then what the Karaites produce are "wounded words," if not the very "material of writing" itself. The Karaite women's verbal attention to their bodies revealed their persistent desire to construct a narrative, which, like the cinnamon wood, tell the Karaite history of purity.

Niddah, therefore, is not a personal story but rather a collective one. The individual *niddah* tells a collective experience, through which individual women speak about a private calendar, space, and experience, weaving together the ongoing story of their mothers and daughters. This collective holds together by virtue of Karaite historical memory and the imagined self that it conjures, endorsed by the authority of the texts. Modes of reading are neither univocal nor static, even if presented as part of female plurality. And ethnography, in this case, witnesses the testimony of contemporary Karaites.

Moreover, this book raises important methodological questions about the possibility of writing history or ethnography as an autonomous discourse, an especially pressing issue for subalterns, including women in both a feminist and colonial context. Is it possible to avoid the comparative paradigm that inherently preserves the hierarchy between Karaites and Rabbanites? More crucially, can the Karaites themselves, escape the comparative paradigms that have shaped their identity? The historical interhalakhic relationships between the two were not, and are not, manifested only on theoretical, theological levels. Because of the proximity of the law to everyday life, in every case of intermarriage, and in every attempt to cross the boundaries between the two, questions of legitimacy regarding every aspect of daily life arose. These questions had an immediate bearing of existential significance with immediate implications on identity and its future development.

It is precisely within the comparative paradigm of Rabbanites-Karaites that Karaites represent themselves. Not surprisingly, Karaites, especially those in the Middle East and North America, have continually negotiated their standards of cleanliness within the Jewish interhalakhic, interethnic textual relationship. The Rabbanite/Karaite framework determines the way the Karaites see themselves: always in reference to the dominant Rabbanite, always in that distorted mirror that warps their interpretation. In the wider sense, therefore, *The Stains of Culture* is not only the study of the female Karaite body but also a study of the complementary relationship between hegemonic and marginal cultures.

As seen throughout the book, Karaite women still long for self-cleaning and purification, or koshering, through their story of *niddah*. Through this practice the body is positioned in its "proper" cultural location. Koshering through the stains of culture primarily reasserts the authority of Leviticus and its role in constituting Karaite consciousness.[14] The subject of *niddah* allows the bodily fluids of blood, milk, and urine to tell another story in which orality and textuality are juxtaposed. The women's speech ties together fragmented oral recollections referring them to their bodies and then to the Torah. Purity in this context is not only a practice but also an immense cultural mechanism that slowly developed over time and that in each Karaite woman marks her engagement and commitment to text and body in everyday life.

Karaites are readers, and precisely for that reason "the book" has a meaning for them that is embodied in the practices of purity and impurity enacted by women. Koshering the female body, it becomes clear, is not remote from the cultural mechanism behind the reading of the dietary laws. This is where the appropriation of the maternal body takes on its human appearance in the women's narrative of purity. The *niddah*, the value of milk and breastfeeding, the fluids of the body, mother-daughter teaching—all constitute the vocabulary of the discourse of maintaining the social kosher body and the mechanism of its reproduction.

I situate this work in the field of cultural studies: its interdisciplinary approach to Karaite culture integrates scholarship in ethnography, literary criticism, feminism, and minority studies. I worked with a relatively small sample of individuals who represented diverse class, education, and age groups, as well as varying levels of tradition, political positions, and awareness of the operations of the sex/gender system. My interviews elicited a wide range of biographies, a multivocality that in spite of variations preserves a distinct female Karaite voice. My role during the interviews was active. I asked and answered questions, reformulated them, moved from English to Egyptian Arabic, Hebrew, and back. When I sensed that a woman struggled between the conventions of her community and her own ideas, I asked the same question in a different, gentler way. Although the tone of my questions and the level of personal engagement differed from one occasion to another, the overall process was informal and congenial.

In order to be able to read as a minority (within a minority), and particularly to read as a literate minority, chapter 1 develops a situated and contextualized framework of Karaite history. While it takes into consideration the historically contested and distorted record of their representation, it also constructs an alternative paradigm for telling Karaite history from within. Using a variety of Karaite and Rabbanite sources, I provide such an overview of Karaite history, its demographic and migratory changes under different empires and nations, and the dynamics of Karaites' double minority status in the overall cultural climate of their time.

In chapter 2, I introduce readers to the Karaite community through a description of a Saturday morning service in Foster City. This monthly event gathers the scattered members in the Bay Area together as a community, and was the vehicle through which I was initiated into the community at large. I review the cultural principles that contemporary Karaites follow in their attempt to reproduce the standards of pure Torah, pure blood, and pure body. I conclude with an excerpt from a discussion with the women about Saturday night, when married couples resume sexual relations, having abstained from sex during the Shabbat in order to respect the purity of the Torah. Women at different ages argue about and reflect on purity, sexuality, and on the tenacity of tradition.

Chapter 3 focuses on the contemporary language of women in referring to *niddah*, asking how the secrecy of the body and its pollution is encoded in language. I look at the extent to which Kara'iyot still refer to menstruation in the language of the biblical text (*niddah* means to remove, expel, and ostracize), and the aspects of the biblical lexicon and rules they have internalized. By examining the rhetorical clues in Karaite women's discourse, I aim to find the nuances of their self-perception as females belonging to a group defined by a cultural norm shaped by gender ideology.

Chapter 4 focuses on the mother-daughter teaching of cleanliness. Their mothers' teaching is best reflected in women's narratives about their first menstrual period. In these stories Karaite mothers emerge collectively as a discursive authority who make clear that female reproduction is inseparable from the female conception of knowledge. Careful, everyday teaching of verbal and nonverbal instructions concerning the sites of blood, sanitary napkins, and washing, as well as physical distancing, timing, and counting, constitute an alphabet for reading the "textual body." Together they compose a unique method of disciplining the blood as it appears on the pads—a blank page of informing textuality. This discourse not only mobilizes the tradition of reproduction of "pure" Karaite bodies but also further pushes the limits of reading to include the obvious, though less acknowledged, schooling of the mother.

Chapter 5 examines the measures of women's impurity. It examines the units of measurement, who counts, and using what scales. I emphasize the specific discourse that the counting of impurity generates and how it constitutes a specific reality not only for the Kara'iyot but for the whole community. The numerical discourse of the Karaite body is expressed in terms of the bodily calendar in female personal life. But counting and quantifying also generate narratives. I thus follow the Kara'iyot's commentary on Leviticus (12:1–7), according to which a woman is impure for forty days after the delivery of a son and eighty days after that of a daughter. Ways of rationalizing counting and calendars can explain how text and body function as mutually referential sources. If the counting of days is a personal, intimate discourse of the woman, it regulates her public appearance and disappearance, providing standards for marked biography and mapped geography.

Chapter 6 presents the ultimate site of Karaite ethno-reading: the "impure body." Here I describe the physical relationship between pure and impure, and between the menstruating woman and the rest of the community. Since the conception of menstruation as uncontained impurity is repeatedly enforced in the culture, the key questions address where the female body begins and where it ends. I answer these questions by describing the physical taboos of impurity and the dynamics of distancing the female body. For Karaites, even the shadow of the female body is contaminating. Understanding the meaning of gender difference and its structuration inevitably results in an account of the experiences generated in the space of impurity and of the strategies women have developed over time. I conclude with a short analysis of Passover as the point of departure for Karaites' twentieth-century exodus and communal reemergence in the Bay Area.

The female body is a locus of the social forces of purity and impurity in the Karaite body politics. Issues of purity and impurity structure the Karaite woman's life within a unique hierarchy of female bodily functions. For example, a breastfeeding mother becomes vulnerable in the presence of a menstruating woman, who is more polluting, because Karaites believe that the flow of breast milk will stop. In chapter 7, I examine two descriptions of such hierarchical encounters, with special attention to the valorization of mother's milk within a discourse of bodily fluids (blood, milk, and urine). I turn to the representation of the body as divided, demeaned, and reduced to its fluids, and discuss the resolution that the women provide for this drama of the open body.

The purifying quality of women's rituals (and narratives) of the body is capable of legitimizing other contested areas in Karaite life, such as feeding and dietary habits. The ethnographic accounts of cleansing allow us to go back to the Bible and reread as a Karaite woman the prohibition "Do not cook [seethe] a kid [goat] in its mother's milk." Karaites' treatment of this law, as I show in chapter 8, can be better understood in relation to the maternal body, within its wider context of maternity, motherhood, and lactation. For Karaites, this prohibition highlights the junction of togetherness and separation, affirming that the mother-kid bond is inseparable.

Karaites conclude that an animal should not be slaughtered if pregnant or during the first seven days after birth. As a metaphor of age and time, within the maternal bond, the milk humanizes the offspring before it is recognized as meat. Karaites do not maintain a dietary separation between milk and meat (in contrast to the Rabbanites). Ethnography, supplemented by Karaite commentaries, helps us understand that breast milk and nursing constitute an event that binds maternity to the next generation and that the mother-child bond is therefore intrinsically inseparable. Karaites understand maternal bonds as always indelible, prompting inedibility. Demystifying purification involving women, bodies, and blood offers an analogy for those of us in scholarly communities seeking a critically balanced reading of ourselves within globalized cultures.

I

Karaite History, Historiography, and the Subject of Truth

> It cannot be said that the Karaites reject the whole body of Rabbinic tradition—they reject only a certain part of it, and the Sages have never stated which part of tradition is so fundamental that denial of it constitutes heresy.
>
> A Karaite's response to a Rabbanite charge

History from Within

Sometime in the summer of 1984, Murād al-Qudsī (or el-Kodsi) sent an urgent letter to Joe Abel, the president of the Karaite Jews of America. The letter asked Abel to respond to al-Qudsī's claim that a recently published book about the Karaite Jews of Egypt by Yosef Algamil—an Israeli Karaite rabbi and author of two volumes of Karaite history—was "almost identical" to his manuscript. After two years and numerous threats of legal action, a committee of the Karaite council in Israel mediated an agreement between al-Qudsī and Algamil that both men—the only active Karaite historians in the United States and Israel today—accepted. Nevertheless, sixteen years later, al-Qudsī included in his 2002 book, *Just for the Record in the History of the Karaite Jews in Egypt in Modern Times*,[1] both photocopies of the documents that led to the claim against Algamil as well as corrections of Algamil's work. Al-Qudsī argues that Algamil "tried to cover his action by changing some parts. In so doing, he made many mistakes. These mistakes must be corrected, otherwise the history of the Karaite Jews in Egypt in modern times will be forever distorted" (al-Qudsī 2002, 97). Their dispute is thus about more than just facts of publication; it is at heart a dispute about history-making and even history itself.[2]

Indeed, Karaite history has been problematic for several reasons. To start with, it is difficult to differentiate between Jewish history at large and Karaite history in particular. Often, Karaites have viewed their history alongside the wider record of Judaism, while at other times they have chosen to separate themselves, or to align their origin with other minorities or national and ethnic groups, as in the case of the Eastern European Karaites. Part of the difficulty lies in the paucity of manuscripts and other artifacts, few of which are attested by the extant documents. But without a doubt, one of the main factors in establishing Karaite history is the politics of representing a minority culture. Being a minority within a minority constrains Karaite representation; that is, the representational paradigm of the Jews as a minority culture within the different diasporas has been superimposed on, or transposed to, the Karaite-Rabbanite relationship.

The record of Karaite history can be easily divided into two distinct sources, Rabbanite and Karaite, whose differences call for (re)consideration of the practices of writing history from within a paradigm of power and domination. Such a paradigm tends to distort the Karaite historical record, leaving the door wide open for non-Karaite historians to create Karaite history based on nothing more than their misunderstanding, biases, and imagination (al-Qudsī 2002, 1). This situation not only objectifies Karaites, but it also contributes to their silence and disappearance from the whole of Jewish history. By the same token, Karaites themselves have used the making of history at different junctures in space and time to negotiate their claims to a specific position within a broader identity politics, as made apparent throughout this book. Karaite history, its uses and abuses, bears the burden of its representation; in this sense history (or historiography) is productively viewed as a staging ground for their social and cultural visibility.

The paradigmatic differences, evident in Karaite and Rabbanite history making, alert us to the knotty theoretical problems in Jewish history and collective memory in particular. Yerushalmi and Funkenstien have emphasized the unique typology that characterizes traditional Jewish history, at least until the nineteenth century, with its direct relation to the biblical narratological patterns (Yerushalmi 1989; Funkenstein 1991). Yael Zerubavel builds on their notion of a Jewish collective consciousness in emphasizing history as a cultural construct. In her study of Israeli national historiography, she meticulously points to the complex and dynamic mechanism of writing history and to the arbitrary nature of historiography and its periodization. Writing history, she concludes, is compromised by the interpretive process, the way and order in which events are selectively recounted, and the narratological framework of their representation (Zerubavel 1995, 3–12). As I elaborate in various contexts, the writing of Karaite history is no less compromised.

Hayden White further expounds on the complex issues occasioning and informing the writing of history. For White, to write history means primarily to perform a "*poetic* act" that "*pre*figures" or stages the very ground of the discipline, thereby creating a field for the deployment of theories to explain "what was *really* happening" or happened (White 1973, x). If the poetic act constitutes historical consciousness and imagination, the question remains: What kind of sensibility is a prerequisite in order to better understand and appreciate the "poetics" of Karaite history? Equally important is how this understanding of the "poetics of history" can elucidate what it means to read as a Karaite.

In general, the project of writing history, Michel de Certeau warns, is deceiving because it aims "to establish the law in the name of the real" (de Certeau 1988, xxvii). Like other cultural practices of representation, history writing attempts to depict itself as scientific: it appears as referential and grounded, refusing mysticism or folkloric genres that are associated with superstition and irrationality (ibid., 86). Moreover, history establishes a well-determined place for readers by redistributing the space of symbolic references and thus impressing a "lesson" upon them; "it is didactic and magisterial" (ibid., 87). In its attempt to transform "the space of the Other into a field of expansion for a system of production," history becomes "*writing that conquers*" (ibid., xxvi). Within the discursive practices of colonial (or colonizing) forms of representation, Karaite history falls into the modes of Europeanist (Ashkenazi) approaches to the history of religious minorities and Middle Eastern (Sephardic and Mizrahi) Jews.

Whereas White highlights modes of historiography as "formalizations of poetic insights" and de Certeau exposes the "scientific" veneer of history writing, Greg Dening helps us to better understand how "poetics" figures in history's anthropology, or the anthropology of history:[3] "History is the texted past for which we have a cultural poetic. It is in that sense not all experience, but that part of it which is transformed into texts." Within specific social and cultural typologies and systems, history and historiography are nothing but a performance or staged theater, a "very vernacular ... everyday, every moment act" (Dening 1995, 14–15). History is, accordingly, gossip, a diary, a birth certificate, a monument or inscription; it is a crafted, self conscious, poetic act. History's anthropology—the writing of its experience—is an inevitable part of history. As Dening proclaims, "History is both a metaphor of the past and a metonymy of the present" (ibid., 13–15). In this book, I join Dening in calling for an "anthro-historical" approach to culture that engages the politics of knowledge and the double vision of cross-cultural reading and writing. The cross-cultural reading of the history of minority "strangers" entails a critical competence in deciphering their internal poetics, or their "signs of intimacy" (ibid., 14).

Truth, and its underlying relationships to God and the Torah, is at the crux of Karaites' ideology of reading and writing history. Consequently, the matter of how to achieve "scientific truth" through history-making is of great relevance to Karaite writing. Writing history as truth furthers their claims to legitimacy and legitimization, and presents those claims as grounded and referential. Perhaps ironically, however, even as this approach to writing history critically shapes Karaites' textual, halakhic, social, and cultural position, it simultaneously provides only a rigid and constricted space for cultural expression and self-representation, permitting but a few possibilities for moving beyond the polarized, fixed binary of Karaite versus Rabbanite.

Recent Karaite scholarship conveys the depth of anguish Karaite writers undergo as they struggle to write their own history. For historians such as Algamil and al-Qudsī, history, and the process of writing it, has become an emotionally taxing endeavor. As their history has been infused by the distorted record of the past, they are motivated to write "all the truth and nothing but the truth" as history's only testimony. In fact, the more writing history as "truth" informs Karaite approach to their history, the more it becomes their premise for an "objective," "rational," accurate representation. This creates a vexing dilemma: their preoccupation with the subject of truth to such a degree turns history—their history—into a story about consistent misrepresentation and the anxiety associated with the inability to escape it. As White strongly suggests,

> For subordinate, emergent, or resisting social groups, . . . this recommendation—that they view history with a kind of "objectivity," "modesty," "realism," and "social responsibility," . . . can only appear as another aspect of the ideology they are indentured to oppose. They cannot effectively oppose such an ideology while only offering their own version . . . of this "objectivity" and so forth that the established discipline claims. (White 1987, 81)

Indeed, Karaites and Rabbanites reveal themselves through the practice of making history. The silencing power of Rabbanite hegemony is manifested in the historical record of Karaites. It is not surprising, therefore, to find that not only do Rabbanites hold the monopoly of writing Karaite history, but also that this history is ambivalent and confused. In many ways, Karaites have been a product of Rabbanite imagination, misgivings, and apprehensions. At the same time that it is motivated by fascination and commitment to the field of Karaism and to the rhetorical ethics of "scientific" chronology—culminating in compendiums of research and study—

this literature is also full of rejection, alluding to the inferior ability of the Karaites to write their own history.[4]

Late nineteenth- and early twentieth-century Rabbanite scholarship of Karaites is characterized by ambivalence and double standards. At the risk of oversimplification, we can identify three main trends in Karaite historiography as written by Rabbanites. The work of scholars such as Heinrich Graetz, Abraham Geiger, Samuel Holdheim, Simhah Pinsker, Samuel Abraham Poznanski, Simon Dubnow, and Leopold Zunz collectively constitutes what one might call the first wave of modern Karaite scholarship. Their approach is consistent with the writing of the Wissenschaft des Judentums (Mendes-Flohr 1995; Meyer 1987), constructing the Jewish grand narrative that connects the dots from antiquity to the present in a chronological, linear manner.[5] Whereas these scholars saw themselves as the organic inheritors of Rabbinic Judaism, their position reflected some of the common trends of the Western European Age of Reason, in which history emerges as Eurocentric and ethnocentric; for the most part they either ignored or absorbed minority cultures into their grand narrative. These scholars perceived and established Karaism as a deviation from what they considered to be normative Judaism (Mahler 1949, 11). "According to Graetz, Samuel Poznanski and almost all of the historians of Karaites," Raphael Mahler, a Marxist scholar of Karaites, suggested, "Karaites' clinging to the Scriptures sealed their fate. Once Karaism had severed its roots from the historical soil of Jewish history, once it positioned itself in opposition to the very life dynamics that could have delayed or prevented its action, the sect withered away, leading to its ultimate petrifaction" (ibid., 40).[6]

Building on the historical foundation of this scholarship was the cornerstone of the second wave of Karaite research, represented by scholars such as Jacob Mann, Abraham Harkavy, Salomon Schechter, Raphael Mahler, Leon Nemoy, Salo Baron, and Zvi Ankori, who were active in the mid-twentieth century. As in other fields of study, they sought to expand the field by incorporating additional documentation that was previously unavailable or ignored. With painstaking attention to minute philological details, Mann, for instance, carefully studied and compared legal aspects of Karaites' law and texts. Using the wealth of material from the Cairo Genizah, Goitein compiled an extensive history of medieval Karaites' and Rabbanites' everyday life. Nemoy and Ankori, two of the leading doyens of Karaite studies, strove to integrate Karaite literary and legal texts and commentaries in order to provide a specific historical description of Karaites over time.

Leon Nemoy's classic anthology of translated Karaite manuscripts not only reinforced their marginal location, it stifled with the weight of its scholarly acceptance any possible Karaite response that would undermine its position. Indirectly, however, even Nemoy's negative evaluation of Karaite scholarship and poetic contribution that he injected systematically throughout the book has been left self-evident. There are many examples. Salmon Ben Jeroham is a "schismatic," his work is characterized as "violent," "belligerent" with "savage force." In general, according to Nemoy, Karaite commentators, philosophers, poets, and theologians are lacking a "genuine poetic gift" (Nemoy 1952, 71, 84, 133, 237–38).[7]

Over the past two decades, there has been a burgeoning scholarship on Karaism that draws from research based on the documents from the Cairo Genizah and, more recently, from materials and sources housed in the Firkovitch Collection in St. Petersburg. Most of this scholarship explores the historical vicissitudes of Karaite philosophy through a linguistic, philological, literary, and historical approach to Karaite texts. Scholars such as Haggai Ben-Shamai, Daniel Lasker, Geoffrey Khan, Daniel Frank, and Rina Drori have written extensively on both medieval Karaite commentaries and Karaism's unique halakhic, legal, philosophical, and historical position. Other historians, such as Nathan Schur, Dan Shapira, Philip Miller, and Mikhail Kizilov, have mostly focused on European-Karaite history, although some, like William Brinner, specialized in the social history of Karaites in Islamic regions.[8] Ethnomusicologist Jehoash Hirshberg focuses on sociocultural aspects of Karaite music and liturgy. Meira Polliack's edited volume of Karaite studies (2003), Fred Astren's recent (2004) book on the evolution of Karaite historical expression, and the commitment of the Izhak Ben Zvi Institute in Jerusalem to compile, catalogue, and translate Karaite documents (headed by Haggai Ben-Shamai) are examples of current undertakings in the field of Karaite studies.

The E. J. Brill book series Études sur le Judaïsme Médiéval has been instrumental in providing a home for some of this new scholarship, with its general emphasis on compilation, annotation, translation, and analysis of historical Karaite documents and manuscripts. Among the publications in the series are Judith Olszowy-Schlanger's historical and philological study of Karaite marriage documents from the Cairo Genizah (1998), Polliack's study of Karaite traditions of Arabic bible translation (1997), and Leon Weinberger's collection of the poetry of Moses Dar'i (2000).

The corpus of Karaite scholarship and the visibility of Karaites within Jewish history has grown with the availability of historical materials and a huge volume of key documents in different languages. However, what remains consistently overlooked or unacknowledged in this scholarship is both the operations of the sex-gender system and the roles of women in constructing genealogies of Karaite cultural history. In fact, however varied, the relatively narrow methodological premises and conservative theoretical orientations of Karaite scholarship to date not only preclude the possibility of a feminist, gendered-based study of Karaism, but also "disappear" the centrality of Karaite women in reproducing, physically and symbolically, Karaite culture itself.

Both Rabbanism and Karaism are premised on androcentric ideologies. But whereas Rabbanite Judaism developed strategies of halakhic contemporarization through a long genealogy of ongoing rabbinical commentaries, the Karaites have professed their fidelity to the Bible in an ortho-linear and literal way and, for the most part, have eschewed commentary as a viable strategy. Paradoxically, Karaite textual practices leave significant space for women's performance and situated interpretation. For Karaites, the female is responsible for purity, while the Karaite male embodies a strict, inflexible, or "pure" linearity. As I elaborate over the course of this book, the enigma that is the cultural construct "Karaite-woman" is precisely her embodiment of ambivalence: she is both absolutely biologically essential to the physical reproduction of the Karaite people, while at the same time, according to Karaite ideology, her female physiology engenders her status of impurity. Through the processes of purification, the Karaite-woman enables her community as a whole to claim both bodily and textual purity.

As I am able to show through ethnographic fieldwork, each generation of Karaite women creates an interstitial discursive space in which to negotiate and renegotiate the terms of their embodied impurity together with methods of purification. Moreover, the nature of that space is inflected and shaped by the historical, geographical, and sociocultural environment inhabited by each diasporic situation of women (Egypt vs. Israel vs. Europe vs. the Bay Area). The women, therefore, keep Karaism relevant and contemporary in every generation even as they consent to the general terms of their impure female condition upon which claims of and for the Karaite pure body, pure blood, and pure Torah are premised. Female-centered purification processes and mother-daughter teaching are key to the transmission of the Karaite praxis of purity, as they contain the possibility of subverting ideological linearity. Cognizant of their crucial role as cultural reproducers, females negotiate and offer commentary on the general Karaite rituals on a trajectory parallel to and "below" that of the ortho-linear track of androcentric biblical fidelity.

Purification practices around female pollution are far more central to the integrity of Karaite culture than publicly performed religious music per se, as Jehoash Hirshberg maintains (1987). What my ethnography highlights is this informal, gynocentric history of commentary on Karaite

Judaism. I hope to introduce here a new approach to the study of Karaites, women, and minorities that can yield a more accurate and complete understanding of how groups and cultures that on the surface appear unchanging and unchangeable are actually undergoing critical structural transformations. It is precisely their focus on the female body as a cultural repository of purity and impurity that allows Karaites, women and men alike, to remain conscious of the need to both reproduce and contemporize "pure" Karaite culture through a dynamic process of reading and its interpretation. The continual negotiation of Karaite culture within different diasporic locations emphasizes the flexibility of what might appear to be a rigid preoccupation with textual orthodoxy.

In light of the patronizing, canonic historical record produced by Rabbanites, Karaite historiography, as written by Karaites, emerges as a "history from below," attempting to rescue and emancipate its position from its historical marginalization. More important, being aware of history's significance in constructing both collective knowledge of the past and the articulation of the present, "history from below" tells us about the way Karaites imagine and position themselves through time (Thompson 1968 [1963]). Perhaps it is even more accurate to argue for Karaite history as "history from within," a position that enables us to strip away accreted layers of projected history that, over time, have covered up the social Karaite body and its story. For Karaites, writing history is more than composing a story about truth. It is an act of belonging and social incorporation that is a critical counterdiscourse about their strategy of self-representation, always vigilant toward issues of reception and legitimacy. In that sense, the Karaite record of history serves multiple purposes, questioning and correcting the established record, as well as reintroducing Karaite history with its unique "signs of intimacy" from within. If, as Dening elaborates, history is the anthropology of strangers, it is important to read Karaite historiography as an attempt to write themselves as the subject of their own narrative, as the authentic native.[9]

I have situated my ethnography of women's experience in the interstices of historical representations of Karaite culture. Ethnography as an aspect of history allows us to move away from the paradigmatic axioms of the Rabbanite-Karaite interrelationship and to focus on internal and intimate—to the extent possible—life parameters of culture. As mentioned, studying women's experience of *niddah* as a collective ethno-reading can elucidate an alternative authentic site of cultural performance. Even more, the cultural burden on the woman's body—at the junction of male patriarchal texts and communal constraints of purity and reproduction—articulates Karaites' unique moment of moving away from a multilayered metaphoric overload to what we might call the transparency of culture.

Writing Karaite History

Within the Karaite narrative of history, the record of origin plays an important part in defining Karaite identity and in establishing the group's reference to their authenticity and legitimacy. The story of origin resets the very narrative of Karaites' formation, and for that reason, it does not refer to the time of the split between Rabbanites and Karaites but goes back to the very time of creation. Karaites imagine themselves within the people of Israel as the people of Israel. Hence, as maintained on one Karaite Web site, "The Karaite Korner" (www.karaite-korner.org), "Karaism has been around since God gave his laws to the Jewish people.... At first there was no reason to label the righteous as a separate sect because there was only the one sect which consisted of the whole Jewish people" (Gordon 2004, 1). Alternatively, Karaites date their origin to a major schism in Jewish history, when Jeroboam, the son of Nebat, divided Solomon's kingdom (al-Qirqisani, in Nemoy 1952, 45–49). Such a timeframe indicates that Karaites, like other societies, understand that the more ancient their origin, the more revered they are (Funkenstein 1991, 31). But, just as important, the act of revisiting this chapter in Jewish history is tantamount to a sensible self-positioning within internal Jewish history, making the schism of Karaites and Rabbanites, and Karaites' subsequent emergence, a predetermined act of God.[10]

And yet, Karaism as a movement actually began in another diaspora. Although the extent to which Karaites are a product of Jewish and Muslim experiences is debatable, scholars generally agree that their emergence as one people took place in Babylon, at the second half of the eighth century. Even though the Karaite "fathers"—'Anan ben David and Benjamin al-Nahawandi—lived in the East during the formative period of Islam, the Karaite legacy spread throughout the East and West, coexisting with Jewish, Arabic, Byzantine, Andalusian, Tatar, and Slavic traditions (Ankori 1959, 3; Mahler 1949; Nemoy 1952; Frank 1990, 16).

Karaite writers highlight the fact that resistance to rabbinic authority, which culminated with the canonization of the Talmud, was not exclusively Karaite, and that as early as the Second Temple period different groups such as the Boethusians and the Essenes (the "Dead Sea Sect") contested this authority. Some historians believe that the split between the Sadducees (Zadokites) who adhered to the Torah of Moses (and cultic sac-

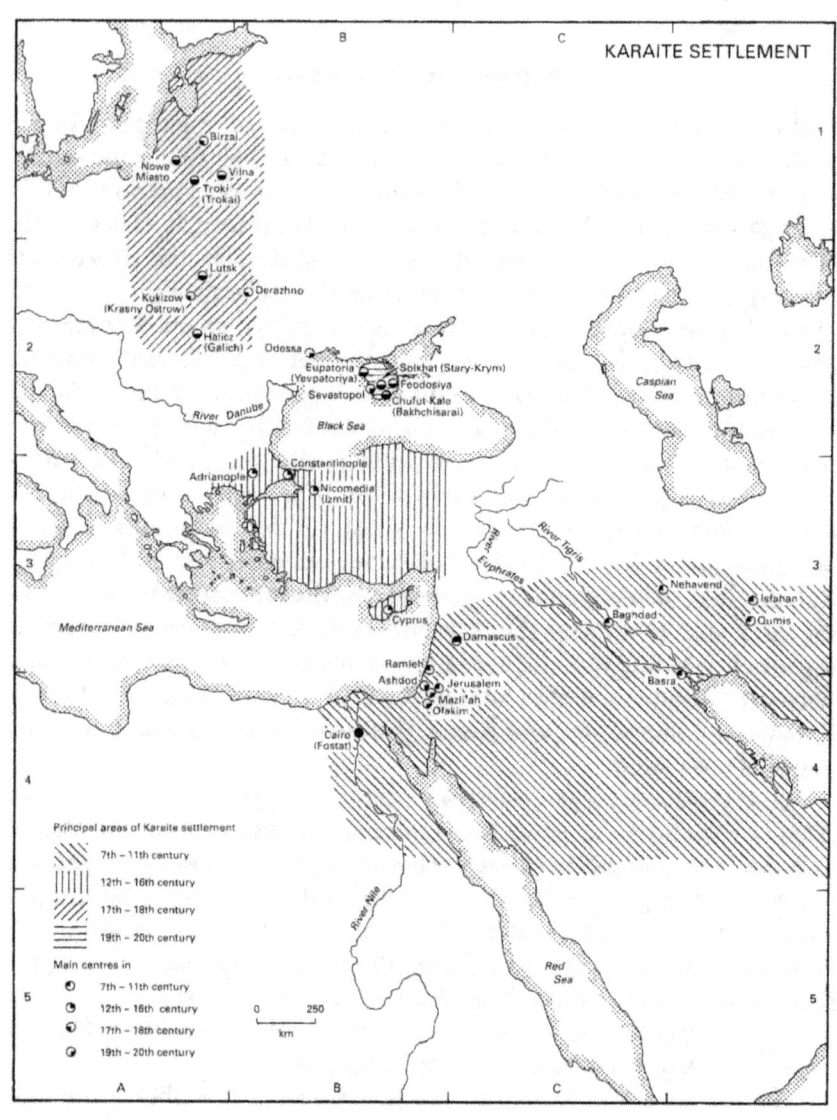

Karaite settlements, seventh to twentieth centuries. (http://www.routledge.com/textbooks/0415236614/resources/maps/map28.jpg)

rificial practices) and the Pharisees preceded the emergence of the movement (Nemoy 1971, 763). It is plausible that the intensified production of Jewish interpretative practices and knowledge gave rise to competing ideas and movements that responded to the emerging hegemonic authority of the Talmudic rabbis (Mahler 1949). Indeed, in a period in which religion controlled all aspects of private and public life, "the ideological aspects of opposition could manifest themselves only in religious nonconformity" (Ankori 1959, 5). In the same way, different social and political groups were challenged to articulate their platform as a "new religious program," resulting in their collective opposition to the Talmud that lasted many years after the time of the Talmud and the Geonim, as evident in the Genizah's documents (Mahler 1949, 12).

The Babylonian Talmud accentuated religious differences between competing groups, extending far beyond the immediate controversies of dietary, calendrical, and other daily practices. It made inevitable the class struggle between the literate and the unlearned, poor population, for whom Talmudic rabbinic scholarship offered no redemptive and messianic possibilities. At the same time, the ruling system of the academies in Babylon extended itself throughout the Middle East, imposing the Jewish law of the Talmud on all Jews. In fact, Karaism may have arisen out of a desire to provide the Jewish masses at the outskirts of the empire some relief from the heavy taxes and punitive measures of the legal system imposed by the emerging religious aristocracy of the rabbis and Geonim (Mahler 1949, 88–123; Ankori 1959, 3–25). Their unique, autonomous system of economic and scholastic hierarchy helped to support the religious institutions, headed by the exilarch.[11] Karaite historiography emphasizes that resistance to the Talmud began in the eastern part of the Persian Empire with Abu Isa al-Isfahani, who led an armed insurrection against the caliph 'Abd al-Malik (685–705) (Gordon 2004; Mahler 1949, 105–11; al-Qirqisani, in Nemoy 1952, 51).

The Ananite period began in 750 with 'Anan ben David, a leader of Davidic lineage who was denied the position of exilarch. In response, he organized scattered resistance groups and unified them into a single movement, later named the Ananites. Anan's teaching reflected an ex post facto reading of the Bible that justified the sectarians' already prevailing practices, advocating an ascetic life style that conformed to strict halakhah (Ankori 1959, 17; Ben-Sasson 1950, 45). His book, *Sefer ha-Mitzvot* (The Book of Precepts), was written in Aramaic and is considered the first Karaite code of reading of various halakhic issues concerning moral observances.[12] As noted earlier, it emphasized the ritualistic pragmatic aspect of Karaite law, the principles of reading the Bible (i.e., *hekesh*, or analogy), and individual interpretation, following his dictum that one should "search diligently in the Torah and not rely on my opinion" (Ankori 1959; Nemoy 1952; Ben-Sasson 1950, 42–50).

Only a generation later, in Benjamin al-Nahawandi's book, we first find the collective term *Kara'im* (Corinaldi 1984, 251), possibly alluding to other anti-Talmudic groups known as "Followers of the Bible" or, in Hebrew, *Bnei Mikra'* and later "Kara'im." Al-Nahawandi was active in the northeastern Persian area of the Abbasid Caliphate and later immigrated to Palestine, and he was the first Karaite scholar to write his commentaries and legal codes in Hebrew (Nemoy 1971, 767; Nemoy 1952, 21–22); his followers were known as the Benjaminites (810-50). Some scholars argue that al-Nahawandi was the founder of the Karaites, who were first inspired by Anan.[13]

Early on, Anan's efforts to establish Karaite ideological doctrine around Galuthocentric nationalism, with its relation to the Temple, its destruction, and the city Jerusalem, resulted in a "Diasporic Asceticism" (Ankori 1957, 16–17). Jerusalem remained at the center of the nationalistic diasporic community, an enduring allusion that evokes Karaite historical origins and future aspirations. In general, the Karaites' strong attachment toward Israel helped to strengthen the opposition toward the authority of Babylonian exilarchy. The endorsement of the Bible as a complete deliverance of God's truth by Moses reinforced Karaites' opposition: closed and sealed, the words of the Bible could never be supplemented (Mahler 1949). Together, an attachment to the land of Israel, especially to Jerusalem, and a specific reading of the Bible were at the core of Karaite national ideology and ethos.

Initially, the Karaites' primary mission was to restore memories of the destroyed Temple in the hope for redemption. Early Karaite leaders emphasized the sacred geographical center, whose "territorial restoration," once destroyed, was replaced by the synagogue, the Temple in miniature (*mikdash me'at*) (Ankori 1957, 16). As Ankori's historical account reveals, "A detailed set of rules was established with the objective of imbuing the synagogue service with the closest resemblance to the ancient Temple rite." At the same time, physical abstinence, fasting, a restricted calendar for sexual relations, and an emphasis on bodily purity replaced the cultic sacrifice, enhancing the Karaites' corporeal posture of the mourner. During the tenth century, a group of Palestinocentric nationalist Karaites named *Avelei Zion* (the Mourners of Zion), like other extreme movements at the time, incorporated the body and its daily reality into a cycle of ritual as an expression of the loss and as a means of obtaining redemption.

The tenth and eleventh centuries are regarded as the golden age of

Karaite literature. Jerusalem was the main intellectual and cultural center for the production of Karaite knowledge, teaching, translation into Arabic, and publication of biblical commentary, and thus attracted many Karaite scholars from Iraq and Persia. Earlier, around 880, Daniel al-Kumisi, a native of the Iranian province of Kumis, made a significant contribution toward the solidification of the national Karaite movement by persuading Karaites and followers of other religious groups in Persia and Babylon to immigrate to Jerusalem (Schur 1995b; Nemoy 1971, 768). Al-Kumisi wrote a Hebrew commentary to the Bible and identified the three main principles of Karaite identity: rejection of the Rabbanite oral tradition and Talmud and engagement in the study of the Bible and the individual pursuit of its meaning; return to Palestine; and pursuit of an ascetic lifestyle (Polliack 1997, 26).[14]

Palestine provided the culturally dynamic and productive environment that encouraged interaction among intellectuals from different religions and regions, as illustrated by the work of Abu Yusuf Ya'qub al-Qirqisani, the greatest Karaite philosopher of the tenth century.[15] Al-Qirqisani wrote extensively on issues of theology, philosophy, science, and liturgy, as well as on the art of translation.

Karaite writing extends beyond religious treatises and includes poetry and polemical writings involving theological disputes with Rabbanite scholars who condemned Karaism. Saadia ben Joseph al-Fayyumi of the Sura Academy in Iraq, known as Saadia Gaon, was considered a scholar of vast knowledge, an intellectual giant who reshaped Jewish history and opened a new era in Jewish epistemology. As the Karaite's staunchest opponent, Saadia took a radical position in articulating the polemic against Karaites, vehemently attacking Karaite doctrine. His treaties ultimately led to the complete rupture of Karaism from mainstream Judaism, to the point that some Karaites contend that their emergence occurred only as a result of Saadia's action. Saadia was engaged in refuting—and by default, also acknowledging—Karaism, which indirectly led him to reintroduce literary innovations to Rabbinic Judaism. In fact, it can be effectively argued that by shattering Karaite heresy, Saadia also barred the door against any possibility of Karaites' inclusion within normative Judaism. His strategy articulated the circumscribed location of a dependent minority upon another dominant minority, constructing the relational paradigm between Karaites and Rabbanites for generations, as it became the representative, prototypical voice in Jewish canon.[16]

Salmon ben Jeroham, a charismatic Karaite scholar who was the subject of numerous legends regarding his influence on Rabbanites and Karaites and well known for his harsh criticism of Saadia Gaon and his exegesis, was active in the geographical area between Egypt and Syria.[17] Continuing ben Jeroham's tradition, Japhet ben 'Eli, a native of Basra and a prolific writer, translated the entire Bible into Arabic, along with extensive commentary and theological and polemical treatises. Among the many other prolific writers were Sahl ben Masliah[18] and Jeshuah ben Judah, both unrelenting opponents of Saadia Gaon. Jeshuah ben Judah also translated the Pentateuch into Arabic and wrote a major philosophical and exegetical treatise on incest, *Sefer ha-Yetser* (The Book of Desire). The work was translated into Hebrew during Jeshuah's lifetime (Nemoy 1952, 124).

During this period, Karaism entered the realm of the academy with the assimilation of the Mu'tazilite school of Basra and the writing of 'Abd al-Jabbar (d. 1025) and its influence on Karaite contemporaries in the rational theology of divine unity and justice (Frank 1988, 1). Many Karaite grammarians and linguists helped to develop the first Hebrew lexicons and the now standardized approach to translating the Bible into Arabic. One of the most prominent, Abu Yaakub Yusuf ibn Nuh, lived in Palestine and founded a college in Jerusalem with some seventy Karaite scholars. He wrote a grammar that addressed issues of language structure and morphology (Polliack 1997, 14–16). As we have seen, the wide range of literary production underscores the rich and wide cross-cultural Karaite encounter with Arabic literature, the Koran, rabbinic and midrashic works, and the New Testament. In total, scholars of this period were multilingual, reading and writing Hebrew in addition to Aramaic, Arabic, Spanish, and Latin.

Two hundred years of Karaite activity in Palestine came to an abrupt end when Jerusalem was captured by the crusaders in 1099, leading to the dispersion of the Karaites to Egypt and Byzantium (Schur 1995; Nemoy 1971, 769). The Karaites first arrived in Constantinople (Istanbul) sometime around 1077 (Ankori 1959, 147) and continued to immigrate to Byzantium from the twelfth through sixteenth centuries, when many Karaites dispersed from Iraq and Persia (Corinaldi 1984, 252). Karaite culture in Asia Minor flourished during this time; the scope of Karaite literature increased with the translation into Hebrew of classical Arabic texts in the Jerusalem Academy.

Several important Karaite sages were active in transforming Asia Minor into another productive scholastic environment for Karaism. Prominent in this list are scholars such as Judah ben Elijah Hadassi, "the Mourner," from Edessa, in Turkey (near the Syrian border), a member of the movement *Avelei Zion,* and author of *Eshkol ha-Kofer* (The Cluster of Heresy), an encyclopedic volume of Karaite teaching (Nemoy 1952, 377). The books authored by Aaron ben Elijah of Nicomedia are a remarkable addition to the Karaite library, especially because they integrated the entire

Karaite system of meaning into a coherent whole.[19] Eliyahu ben Moses Bashyazi (b. 1420) worked in Constantinople and his correspondence had a far-reaching impact that was felt beyond Turkey and as far away as the Karaite community in Poland. His book *Aderet Eliyahu* (The Mantle of Eliyahu), on which he worked for thirty years, and which was continued by his brother-in-law Caleb ben Eliyahu Afendopolo, became the standard manual of Karaite code and law. Both he and his brother-in-law wrote about theology, philosophy, astronomy, and poetry.

Karaites in Europe

Karaites in Istanbul started migrating to the Crimean Peninsula and the southern Ukrainian plains after the big fire in the Jewish quarter in 1203, opening the northern route in Karaite life. This itinerary corresponded, in part, to the slave trade of Kipchak-Turkish pagans, who had migrated from East Mongolia, which was also active along the axis of Egypt, Istanbul, and Crimea (Shapira 2003, 2–3). Indeed, Zajaczkowski (a Karaite scholar in Poland) reiterates that the ethnic origin of Karaim (or Qaraim) in Crimea goes back to the seminomadic Kipchak-Turkic tribes of Middle Asian origin, who invaded the region in the early period of the Khazars and adopted the Karaite religion during the end of the eighth century (Zajaczkowski 1961, 38–39). By the time the Tatars invaded Europe and Anatolia in the middle of the thirteenth century, Karaites had already moved from Crimea to Troki, Vilna, Halicz, and Kiev (Nemoy 1971, 772; Shapira 2003, 1–3). The Judeo-Tatar dialect, along with the Kipchak-Turkic language "Karaim" or "Qaraim" that was associated with the Karaites of Tatar origin, replaced the Judeo-Greek language of the Byzantine Empire.

Karaite life as an ethnic and religious minority in Europe was often disruptive. From the turn of the fourteenth century until the twentieth century, famine, plagues, wars, the rise and fall of empires, and ethnic and national treaties shook Karaite communities, resulting in expulsions and transfers within and across the region. In approximately 1392 the Grand Duke Witold of Lithuania resettled 330 Karaite families in Troki; a century later, in 1495, Grand Duke Alexander expelled the Karaites (and Rabbanites) of Lithuania.[20] A different version of events relates that even earlier, at the end of the eleventh century, the Crusader Baldwin I transferred 250 Karaite families from Jerusalem to Crimea. The history of the forced relocation of the Karaites continued during and after World War I. The German High Command transferred the Karaites of Troki to the Crimea, permitting them to return only after the German surrender in 1918. Shortly after, the Soviets resettled thousands of Karaite refugees from the Crimea and elsewhere in Troki.

The Ottoman conquest of the Byzantine Empire also increased the flux of immigrants from Istanbul to Crimea until the middle of the eighteenth century.[21] Along with their influential community in Lithuania (around 1750), Karaites began developing their own intellectual center in Crimea, led by Simhah Isaac ben Moses. Crimea remained a flourishing Karaite region until the nineteenth century. One of the most notable contributors to Karaite literature and exegesis in this period was Isaac ben Abraham Troki (1533–94), who published the anti-Christian treatise *Hizzuk Emunah*. His pupils continued his work and published numerous books on subjects such as the Karaite calendar, science, and mathematics. Over the years, Karaites in Crimea maintained close contact with Karaites in Egypt and Turkey, exchanging religious materials, spiritual leadership, and providing financial support to the dwindling community in Istanbul (Shapira 2003, 4–5).

Many Karaites living in the Crimea and Lithuania were brought under Russian rule in the late eighteenth century. Over the course of the century, they gradually gained civil recognition, a process that significantly differentiated them from Rabbanite Jews as much as it affected their own internal development. Karaites also lived in Lvov, in what is now Poland, in the quarter that was until 1457 outside the city walls; although they had a synagogue of their own, they shared the cemetery with the Rabbanites. Until 1795, Karaites and Rabbanites had the same legal status under Tatar and Turkish rule. This changed with Empress Catherine II, who exempted the Karaites in Crimea from certain tax payments and permitted them to purchase land. In 1827, the Crimean Karaite leader, Hakham Simhah Babovitch, persuaded the Russian government to excuse the Karaites from military service, which was otherwise required of all Jews. Some years later the Karaites acquired a new status as an autonomous church. Similar to the Muslims, Karaites were permitted to establish their own religious institutions and autonomous society. By 1863 the Karaites were granted equal rights, giving them the same status as the native Russian population (Nemoy 1971, 774). These radical changes contributed to the Karaites' sense of ease and belonging, prompting them to move to major cities such as Vilna and St. Petersburg and to improve their economic status, which significantly distinguished them from the Rabbanites.

Abraham ben Samuel Firkovitch (1786–1874), the Karaite scholar also known as Even Reshef, wrote extensively and traveled throughout Crimea, the Caucasus, Syro-Palestine, and Egypt as he archived the invaluable collection of Karaite books and manuscripts at the Leningrad Public Library.[22] Recent scholars have defined Karaites' attempts to differentiate themselves from Rabbanite Jews as "dejudaization," attributing this to Babovitch and Firkovitch, and especially to the latter's efforts to represent Karaites as ethnic Turks rather than of Jewish origin (Freund 1991). This question of Karaite origins had important implications during the Second World War, when the Nazis attempted to define Karaites along racial, linguistic, and religious lines. In fact, historical documents and testimonies show that the Nazis were not consistent in the way they categorized the Karaites. Some accounts attest that Karaites, for the most part, were not considered Jewish, and were spared from the death camps. Other Karaites fought in the Wehrmacht Waffen SS and Tartar Legion in Crimea in 1944. But there are also documents that provide evidence that several hundred Karaites were killed and interred in the mass grave of Babi Yar (Russia) alone in 1941 (Spector 1986, 93; Friedman 1960).[23]

Nevertheless, the Second World War devastated the Karaite community, reducing its number and reshaping their demographics. Between the world wars there were approximately 9,000 Karaites (of which 6,500 lived in Crimea), but by 1986 there were only 600 remaining in Poland, mostly around Warsaw, Gdansk, Varcelova, and Pele (Spector 1986). In 1991 there was a small community in Moscow and St. Petersburg and in Ukraine. There were also small groups of Karaites in Italy, Germany, and France by this time. Spector suggests that a slow process of assimilation occurred among Karaites in this period (1986, 90).

Karaites in Egypt

Karaites count twenty-seven generations of Egyptian Karaite *nesi'im*, or chief rabbis, beginning in the eighth century with Anan's arrival in Cairo, until the twentieth century, a genealogy reinforcing the claims of the Egyptian Karaite community that theirs is the oldest in existence (Algamil 1988, 513). This historical genealogy is a cogent symbol of Karaite legitimacy and continuity linking them to the ancient land of Egypt. Nevertheless, it articulates a dynamic society with strong ties, described below, to other Karaite communities in cities such as Jerusalem, Damascus, Baghdad, or Isfahan in the east, Constantinople, the region of Crimea, Lutsk, or Troki in the north, and in the west as far as Andalusia, Morocco, and various North African cities. In addition to maintaining relationships via migration and visits, Karaite scholars corresponded regularly with each other regarding halakhic (legal) queries, family announcements, educational materials, and monetary appeals, and also participated in rabbinic exchanges (Algamil 1988, 513–23).

On this cultural map, Cairo was a vital junction of Karaite life and history between Europe and the Middle East. It was in Cairo where contested political solidarities and affiliations were mediated and reconfigured at different moments in history. Several historical forces contributed to a rich environment in which conflicting political and social interests played a role, forcing Karaites to shift loyalties and realign themselves along different identity politics. Whereas their daily contact with Muslims and the Arab tradition highlighted Karaites' shared affinity with their local culture, their intimately shared minority status with Rabbanite Jews, as a protected minority (*dhimmī*) under Islamic law, often emphasized their commonalities and their Jewishness. In fact, for this reason, Middle Eastern Karaites aligned themselves much closer to Judaism than did their European counterparts (Brinner 1989). As a matter of fact, as early as the middle of the nineteenth century, European and Middle Eastern Karaites developed strongly divergent opinions regarding their identity as Jews, their Judaism, and their attitudes toward the land of Israel (ibid., 4). At the same time, Eastern European Karaite authority kept a watchful paternal eye on Egyptian Karaites, making sure to maintain their common alliances based on their collective history and memory and their shared ethnic identity. To a certain extent, Karaites responded to the different political forces by emphasizing different aspects of their identity through changing their names.[24] But, as Brinner suggests, "the differing presentation of Karaite identity and loyalty is due more to the attitudes and values of the surrounding majority religion to which Karaism was forced to adapt itself, than to indigenous Karaite religious beliefs and principles" (ibid., 69). The increasingly fundamentalist Islamic movement at the end of the Second World War, especially among the Muslim Brotherhood, affected Jews and other non-Muslim minorities (Algamil 1987, 40–59). The parallel rise of modern Zionism and pan-Arab nationalism introduced an overwhelming variable with regard to Karaites identity politics: by overstating their identification with the Zionist cause, Egyptian authorities called into question Karaites' long historical Egyptian loyalty to their nation. As such, it introduced new challenges to Karaites, forcing them to carefully position their identity, while at the same time to chart new routes in their twentieth-century map of exodus.

Karaite life in Ḥarat al-Yahūd al-Kara'iyim, the Karaite neighborhood next to Ḥarat al-Yahūd al-Rabbaniyin, the Rabbanite area—both located in the al-Gamaliyah district in Cairo, and in Fustat, the Islamic capitol from the seventh through tenth centuries—is often referred to in marriage contracts, giving us a fascinating, albeit partial perspective of the cross-cultural interaction between the two communities (Olszowy-Schlanger 1998). Although what intermarriage reveals of intercommunal relationships is questionable (Asaf 1936, 209–11), within Jewish historiography at least, it is seen as an important indicator of the official position that the rabbis and the Karaite *hakhamim* took toward this issue, and their imagined perception of each other. Based on the Genizah's documents between the tenth and twelfth centuries, intermarriage between Karaites and Rabbanites for the most part involved male Rabbanites and female Karaites who were allowed to follow their own halakhic practices. "Inter-communal marriages were considered socially and halakhically possible and legitimate. No party was required to abandon their faith and life style, but rather able to co-exist in spite of the differences between them" (Zohar 1987, 21). Although references to such social interaction are alluded to as if taken for granted, halakhically they were discouraged. Indeed, from the thirteenth century onward, Rabbanite authorities prohibited intermarriage. Up until the sixteenth century Karaite and Rabbanite scholars debated the terms of conversion and the limits of tolerance. After that time, the subject became nonnegotiable, culminating in the consensual position of excommunicating Karaites from the Rabbanite community (ibid., 22).

During the rule of Salah al-Din and the Ayyubid dynasty in Egypt (1171–1250), Karaites enjoyed a less stringent enforcement of tax collection and greater mobility under the pact of Omar, and they also benefited from their protective *dhimmī* status under Quranic law.[25] Many other Karaites from Christian countries, especially scholars, immigrated to Egypt (Algamil 1988, 514). The status of the Karaites and other non-Muslim minorities changed drastically, however, with the rise of the Mamluks (1250–1517), who imposed heavy taxes and limited their autonomy. Still, the Karaite and Rabbanite neighborhoods in Cairo and Fustat allowed a certain degree of autonomy (al-Qudsī 2002, 7). According to the Genizah documents, in 1481 there were 150 Karaite families in Cairo, in a community of 850 Jewish families (Algamil 1988, 514).[26] Not long after this date and into the middle of the sixteenth century, a large influx of Jews from Spain and Portugal settled in Egypt and strengthened the pulse of Jewish life. Japheth al-Barqamani wrote polemical treatises and medical works in Arabic. Japheth ibn Saghir was a theologian and jurist who wrote in Arabic, and Samuel ben Moses al-Maghribi was a physician who in 1434 wrote the legal codex *al-Murshid* (The Guide) in Arabic.

The rise of the Ottoman Empire (1517–1914) brought some improvement in the situation of non-Muslim religious minorities, which continued until 1805, when Muhammad Ali's advent as governor put a permanent end to resurgent Mamluk rule. In spite of Ali's reputation as a ruthless leader, this period is viewed as a major turning point in the history of Egyptian minorities, marked by economic growth that followed on the heels of governmental reforms in the industrial, agricultural, health, and

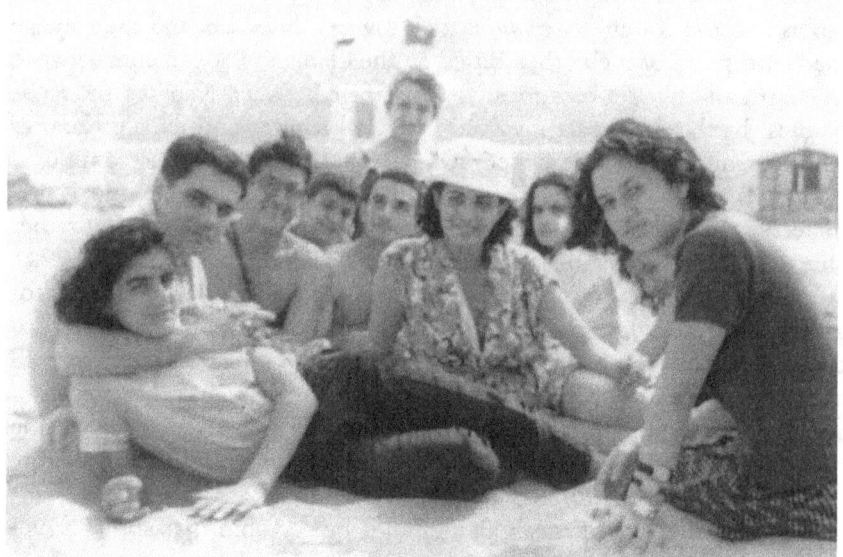

Karaite teenagers in Kanatar, Egypt, ca. 1950, embodying secularization and Europeanization. (Photo courtesy of Remy Pessah)

educational sectors. The decline of the Ottoman Empire brought with it increasing colonialism from European powers in Egypt and throughout the Middle East, culminating in British occupation in 1882. In general, British and French Mandates in North Africa accelerated the processes of urbanization and secularization. According the al-Qudsī, the status of minorities continued to improve during the British protectorate, granting equal standing to both Muslims and non-Muslims under the law, and enabling both Karaites and Rabbanites to enter educational institutions (al-Qudsī 1987, 8).

At the turn of the century, the demographic map of the Karaites extended from Tripoli in North Africa to Egypt and Jerusalem, to Italy and Turkey, all the way to northern Iraq, while Karaites contributed to the formation of what Shelomoh Dov Goitein referred to as "a Mediterranean society" (see also Shamir 1987). At the same time, Egyptian Karaites were also well integrated into the surrounding Muslim culture, as illustrated by the prolific literature of Murad Faraj Lisha' (1867–1956), a leading Karaite intellectual and prolific writer who was active in shaping the liberal Karaite lifestyle (al-Qudsī 1987, 244–57; Somekh 1987; Beinin 1998). Western lifestyle and other demographic, economic, or educational reforms increased the generation gap between the conservative (mostly elder) and progressive (mostly younger) Karaites. He advocated a more relaxed approach toward Karaite halakhic stringency in favor of more solidarity with the wider Egyptian society, especially Rabbanites. According to Sasson Somekh, Faraj was the only active Jewish writer who was engaged in both Arabic culture and modern Arabic poetry, and biblical and Karaite halakhic literature (Somekh 1987, 130–40).

If Faraj was among the liberal Karaites, Tubiah Simhah Levi Babovitch represents the more orthodox version of twentieth-century Karaism, advocating a certain degree of separatism from Rabbanite Jews and Zionism (Colligan 1980; Beinin 1998). Chief Hakham Babovitch (1879–1956) arrived in Egypt from Crimea in 1934 and, as Algamil and al-Qudsī report, emerged as the overarching authority of Karaite knowledge and dogma. He published two books and numerous halakhic articles in Russian, Polish, Arabic, and Hebrew. As the Chief Hakham for twenty-two years, he especially opposed legal reforms with regard to religious family law (divorce and marriage), which brought him resistance from those who wanted more individual freedom. Babovitch gained community respect through his exemplary dedication of time and money, although as a representative of more conservative views, he often opposed many of the local customs, with little success (Algamil 1987, 1997a, 1997b; al-Qudsī 1987).

Overall, Middle Eastern Karaites constitute a subgroup within the larger community of Jews, including Rabbanites, Karaites, and Samaritans, and since all three were recognized under Quranic law as "people of the book" ('*ahl el-kitab*)—a significantly better position than other minorities—Egyptian Karaites perceived themselves as an integral part of Judaism. Karaites themselves assert that "until [we] left Egypt in large numbers, the large majority of Egyptians, Muslims, Christians and Jews, felt just that, Egyptians; [their] Arab identity was not strong at all" (al-Qudsī 2002, 203).[27]

With the establishment of the State of Israel, the Karaites' strong pro-Zionist position would tie Karaites' and Rabbanites' future together. For example, Dr. Moshe Marzuq was a Karaite member of He-Halutz, the Zionist underground in Egypt, and was executed for his involvement in a potentially violent espionage campaign (Beinin 1998, 43–44). Karaites in Egypt were persecuted in 1948 as a result of the war in Palestine, and through immigration to Israel their number dropped by 60 percent to about 2,000 by 1956 (ibid., 71). The Six Day War in 1967 also had a tremendous impact on the Karaites remaining in Egypt, for it further redefined them as a national minority that supported the enemy. Karaites as well as Egyptian Jews in general could leave Egypt, but they were subject to several restrictions, introduced in 1958. Not only were they forced to obtain tax certificates, the Egyptian government also ruled that those who intended to leave must have Egyptian passports instead of a "laissez-passer" document (Laskier 1992, 284–85). Further, upon departure, they were to be stripped of their citizenship and thus lose their property and economic benefits. Karaite men with Egyptian citizenship were arbitrarily imprisoned, by virtue of being Jewish, at Abu Zaabal and Tora prison camps for periods of two and three years. In the absence of fathers, husbands, brothers, and sons, women, often the younger ones, took the initiative in preparing exit documents and activating diplomatic connections with different agencies and organizations (see also chapter 6 of this volume). They left even though the men remained imprisoned in Egypt. The Jewish organization HIAS was instrumental in facilitating the departure of Egyptian Jews; they also helped with their adjustment in Israel and elsewhere for the first few months, for example placing the children in schools and providing financial assistance. With the help of the Red Cross and other agencies, HIAS continued to help the imprisoned men in Egypt, assisting their release and departure to Israel and in some cases to Europe and the United States.

Al-Qudsī and Algamil have updated the record of Karaite publications by republishing original manuscripts and expanding the Karaite manuscripts library. Algamil's several volumes of history of Egyptian Karaites (1979, 1981, 1985) constitute an important narrative of the daily life of the community. His later works on Rabbi Simhah Babovitch, for example, document not only the fascinating relationship between Karaites in Crimea and Cairo but also the internal dynamics of Babovitch's leadership and the way he negotiated with Rabbanites, Christians, and Muslims during the first half of the twentieth century in Cairo (Algamil 1987, 1997a, 1997b). Al-Qudsī, who arrived in New York in 1959, is an important scholar, teacher, and writer of Karaite matters and one of the most active intellectuals in the United States. His books *The Karaite Jews of Egypt 1882–1986* (1987) and *The Karaite Communities in Poland, Lithuania, Russia and Crimea* (1993) are good sources of historical documents and photographs, as well as important accounts of Karaite historical institutions, figures, and communal events.

Israeli Karaites

The rise of Israeli nationalism and the escalating conflict between Egypt and Israel occasioned the first and second waves of Karaite immigrants to Israel (1949–50 and 1955–56) who joined the Egyptian Rabbanites in the

History, Historiography, and the Subject of Truth

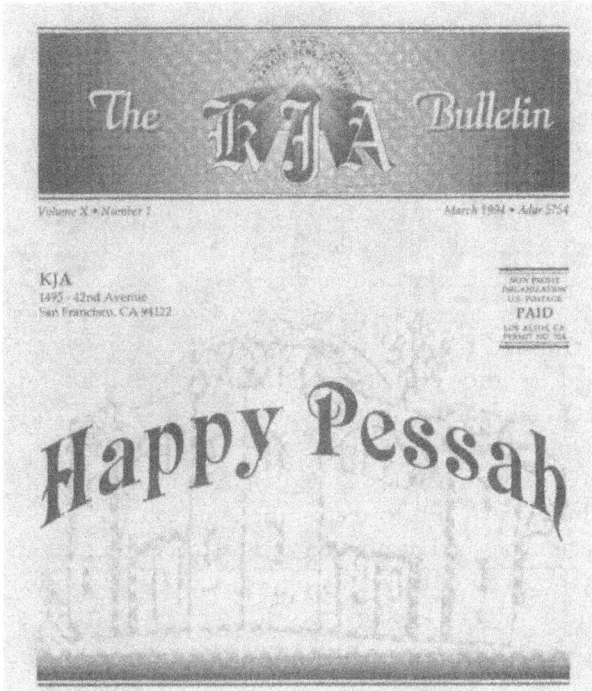

The cover of Passover 1994 issue of the *KJA Bulletin*.

Zionist enterprise. Given the increasingly bitter hostility between the two countries, the Karaites' complete exodus from Egypt became inevitable. There are around 30,000 Karaites in Israel today, with the Karaite administrative center and main synagogue in Ramleh and two exclusive Karaite *moshavim*, Masliach and Renan. Karaites have formed other small communities, in cities such Ofakim, Lod, Ashdod, and Jersualem. Ramleh houses the Karaite Bet Din, a major synagogue and seat of the Karaite council, as well as other religious institutions such as the burial society. Most of the books on Karaites were first published by the Karaite society *Chevrat Hatslachah Li-vnei Mikra'*, which was instituted in 1957–58 through contributions to the community. Later the National Karaite Council in Ramleh began to publish new and old manuscripts, guide books, a Passover haggadah, and other religious materials. Karaites also publish the periodical *Dover Bnei Mikra'*, a continuation of the Egyptian *Al Kalim*. In general, Israeli Karaites exert tremendous efforts to increase the volume of published educational material. Halevi's *Ma'ayan Hayyim* (in Hebrew, 1988b) is a good example of a halakhic text for young adults.

According to Israeli law, Karaites can neither convert to Rabbanite Judaism nor be given the status of another denomination of Judaism (Colligan 1980; Kashani 1978, 74–75). The Ministry of Religion initially assigned them to the Department of Muslims and Druze (in 1958). The Karaites were later moved to the jurisdiction of the *Nidchei Yisrael,* which administers the affairs of isolated communities of Jews (Colligan 1980, 81) who are categorized as "*mi'utim,*" or minorities. As a community, therefore, the Karaites are trapped within the Israeli legal system, whose apparatus dictates that Karaites are neither Jewish nor non-Jewish (ibid., 77, 82). Even though government officials such as David Ben-Gurion and Golda Meir recognized and affirmed the Jewishness of Karaites, their general legal position continued to enforce their second-class position, limiting the secular government's ability to rectify this status. As late as 1980, they were still not granted equal standing with Rabbanite Jews, unlike the case of Ethiopian Jews, who, although never excluded, were formally acknowledged as Rabbinates in 1975. A bill to rectify the situation was subsequently introduced to the Knesset, but it failed and has never been resurrected (ibid., 89). Still, the Karaite Bet Din (Court of Law) is responsible for all issues that pertain to internal halakhic jurisdiction such as marriage, divorce, and paternity. Otherwise, legal jurisprudence falls to the general Israeli civil court.

The Karaites' religious status has been often challenged, which has led to them being denied funds for various educational, economic, and religious programs (ibid., 82). But if Karaites' official personal status is problematic, the politics of ethnicity complicate their status even more: they considered themselves to be culturally closer to the Sephardic/Mizrahi (Middle Eastern or North African) community than to those Israelis of Ashkenazic (European) origin. Status affects the lives of Karaites in many aspects, including their ability to function as an independent religious community and to function as private citizens with full access to all the civil rights that citizenship in Israel theoretically entails (ibid., 296).

The Israeli Karaite community has been the subject of few ethnographies. Sumi Colligan's work focused on the anomalous minority position of Karaites in Israel, demonstrating that because Israeli Rabbanite and Karaite ideologies share overlapping symbols, institutions, and meanings, Karaites are able to assert multiple identities. Sometimes they distinguish themselves from the Rabbanite majority and other times they "pass" as Rabbanites when they choose (ibid., 2001). The anthropological historian Emanuela Trevisan Semi researched the unique status of Karaites in Masliah as both an ethnic and a religious minority (1984). In general, Semi's work addresses the social and ethnohistorical practices of Karaites in Egypt and Israel, such as endogamy and exogamy, rituals of mourning, and Passover. She also has published numerous articles in English (1990 and 1991) on the sociological aspects of Eastern European Karaite lifeways.

Jehoash Hirshberg, an ethnomusicologist at the Hebrew University of Jerusalem, studies the Karaite musical tradition in prayers and its role in forming identity and cohesiveness among contemporary Karaites, especially in the San Francisco community (Hirshberg 1986). Hirshberg integrates ethnography with history, asking what is the Karaites' "distinct mode associated with the affect of mourning" and what are the development and special changes of this music. For Hirshberg, Karaites' musical heritage continues to suffer from the prolonged displacement of the community. As a result, different modes and melodic formulas are used simultaneously, to the point that no authoritative version emerges.

Karaites travel; even after different diasporic experiences, they perennially revisit their place of origin. Therefore it behooves us to accompany them on their historiographical journey. I have situated the idea of Karaite ethno-reading in the context of historiography and writing history in order to foreground modes of Karaite history-making as they are performed in everyday life. As I have argued, for Karaites, writing history is more than composing a story about truth; it is a primary method of achieving legitimacy and authenticity within the Jewish nation. Karaite history, being a history from within, strips away the metaphoric veneer of projected history so that Karaites may reveal themselves as the authors and subjects of their own narrative. Similarly, and to some extent subversively, in the following chapters I show how an ethno-reading of the *niddah* designates the Karaite woman, and her body, as an alternative site for the narration and reading of Karaite history.

2

Shabbat, Purity, and Making Love

> As a matter of fact, there was far less of a distinction between the Karaites and the Rabbanites of that time than there is nowadays between the Orthodox and the Reformed factions of Jewry, and yet would it never occur to anyone to attempt the exclusion of the latter from the ranks of Jewry, the reason being that we are living in a more liberal age than did the rabbis of the 8th and 9th centuries.
>
> Zvi Cahn, *The Rise of the Karaite Sect*

Saturday Morning in Foster City

Foster City in 1990 is mostly concrete, gas stations, and nondescript condominiums. The lazy traffic on the 580 freeway early Saturday morning makes the drive from Berkeley a relatively easy forty minutes. As soon as I cross the San Mateo Bridge, I feel relieved—only two more exits to go. Even now, when I reflect back, I realize how symbolic was the bay in my transition from one world around the university to the small island of the Karaite Jews in the midst of Northern California. As I exit the freeway, turn right, and drive toward the synagogue that they share with the Conservative Jewish community, I think about some of the incongruencies of this situation: I, a secular, Mizrahi, Israeli Jew who rarely went to synagogue as a child now find myself frequently attending and participating in the Shabbat services of the Karaite community—and enjoying the experience.

I slip off my shoes and leave them with the other pairs clustered at the entrance, quietly open the door, and step into the Hebrew classroom that has been transformed into a Karaite prayer room. Karaites always remove their shoes before entering a prayer room to avoid polluting (symbolically) the purity of that space. While sinking into the Persian rug, I respond to the welcoming faces.[1] Smiles, nods, friendly touches. I look around; there are around sixty people, including fifteen children. It is still early; more people will arrive later. We are facing east, where a beautiful crafted ark, or *'aron*, is placed against the wall. The *'aron*, made of oak and decorated with the golden Star of David, contains the Torah scrolls. Both men and some women, for reasons of convenience, wear a generic *kippah* (skullcap), usually made of shiny black or dark blue satin. I also take a *kippah* and a prayer book from the large cardboard box at the corner of the room and go to the back of the room, standing among the women.

Shabbat is obviously important here. Most people are dressed elegantly: the men sport dark tailored suits with ties, and the women wear silk jewel-toned dresses, simple make-up, and are well coiffed. Even the kids are dressed up: Dalia runs around in a frilly pink and white dress, and Daniel wears a white button-down shirt that makes him look older than his ten years. Families continue arriving throughout the morning. Once they enter the room they prostrate themselves, softly intoning a prayer of transition from outside to inside, after which they stand or sit on the rugs.

During the prayer, men stand in uneven rows near the front of the room. Most of the women sit in the back of the room on folded chairs, although several younger women sit directly on the rugs. During the rest of the month the synagogue uses this room for religious school. There is a blackboard on the wall, along with children's artwork. But once a month, at the beginning of each service, the men carefully unfurl the relatively new, colorful Persian rugs on top of white sheets to separate the floor and the rugs. The prayer area reaches toward the middle of the room and is not strictly defined. Men and women share a common space; it is understood that men stand apart from the women. Most often, it is the children who impatiently, if joyfully, move in and out of the room and from the men's area to the women's area. For now, all present hold their prayer books open and follow the reading. A father holds a child by his side, helping her, pointing with his finger so that she can follow the words.

The choice of Foster City seems arbitrary as the location for the synagogue that became a beacon attracting Karaite families to the southern part of the peninsula. Actually, the choice was based not on centrality, but where they were offered space. Over the last ten years, many families bought houses in the southern part of the Bay, in San Mateo or Redwood City, forming a closer community around Foster City. Other Karaites commute from as far away as Davis, Berkeley, Richmond, and Walnut Creek in the north. Those who do not drive depend on others for transportation: Daisy, who lives in the heart of San Francisco, most often rides with her sister. Occasionally, she rides with me. Nadia lives much farther away and can only come to the service when her son-in-law or, less frequently, her son takes her. As it happens, the elders' insistence on participating in the services indirectly involves the younger generations in these gatherings. The difficulty of assembling themselves is most evident in cases of birth or death, where often the place of gathering is another Karaite house, not necessarily in Foster City.[2]

I was amazed at how comfortable and welcome I felt—and was made to feel—during my initial visits. Men and women alike were gentle and mild mannered. Their warmth was familiar and reminded me of my own family; moreover, their codes of interaction and body language helped me feel at home. Karaite music and their style of praying also took me back to my childhood, bridging the distances between Cairo, Baghdad, Israel, and California. Simply standing shoeless in the informal prayer room put me at ease. I keep to the women's area, close to the window, and open my prayer book. Lailah, on my left, winks at me, half smiling, and points to the page from which we are reading. I join the reading, my voice blending easily with the others.

Lailah's voice rises above the dominant blend of men's voices. A fluent Hebrew speaker who is typically shy and reserved outside the prayer room, Lailah pronounces the Hebrew prayers confidently. She even corrects someone who mispronounces a word. Indeed, the pleasure of seeing friends and family compels those present to act spontaneously, despite the ritual decorum. Everyone is excited about the monthly meeting—especially the women and children who are louder and less inhibited than the men. The women can hardly wait until the end of the service to chat among themselves. The children fidget impatiently, preferring to play with friends whom they do not see very often.

The Hebrew reading from the Karaite prayer book opens and closes the service.[3] After nearly three hours of praying, and before reading from the Torah, there is a short break. David, a board member, makes the announcements. People acknowledge and greet each other: shaking hands, kissing both cheeks in the French manner, and saying "Shabbat Shalom" (a peaceful Shabbat), to each other. The acting rabbi gives a brief summary of both the preceding chapters and *parashat ha-shavu'a*,[4] the weekly reading, especially informative in light of the three-week gap between services. Sometimes, during an intermission, the rabbi engages the children, asking them questions to encourage them to participate in a discussion. Before reading the *parashah* people have an opportunity to select by bidding the prayers that will be recited the following month, an innovative fund-raising procedure for raising money to build a Karaite synagogue. Jacob, the treasurer, stands in front and calls out the name of each prayer, waiting for members to bid. Typically the bidding begins at around ten dollars.

Some prayers, not surprisingly, are worth more than others. On holidays and other festive occasions, a prayer can fetch up to one hundred and fifty dollars.

For the most part, men make the bids, although often a woman urges her husband or child to acquire the privilege of reciting a specific prayer. Building a synagogue is a slow, long-term investment that requires significant commitment and capital. Not only does bidding provide a social stage upon which one may demonstrate generosity, but it also provides a means for everyone to have a share in the selection of prayers and the reading of the Torah. The Karaites realize that their future as a community depends on being organized around a religious-cultural center.[5] Their lack of a center emphasizes their transition from the intimate local Karaite Jewish neighborhoods of Ḥarat al-Yahūd al-Kara'iyim and 'Abbāsiyyah to California, reinforcing a sense of isolation among a thriving Rabbanite Jewish population in a new American reality. Yet it is precisely this new reality—scattered yet interdependent—that compels them to make use of an available, if not ideal, meeting place.

Finally the bidding is finished. All conversations cease. The women who were outside preparing the table for the meal now enter the room, with the exception of menstruating women, who must remain outside throughout the entire prayer. The men open the *'aron*, take out the Torah, and parade it around the room. The silver ornaments clink on the metallic case, adding a kind of musical accompaniment to their a capella signing of an uplifting melody. Na'imah and Lailah kiss their hands and then touch the Torah. Rachel and Daisy touch the Torah, kiss their finger, and place them over their closed eyes. Everyone crowds around the Torah, touching it gently.

Once the circuit is completed and the scroll returned to the front of the room, the reading of *parashat ha-shavu'a* begins. Several men, including occasional visitors, are granted the honor of reading the text. The formula that introduces each reader of the *parashah* is recited first. Based on a call and response, the Kohen (considered a descendant of the ancient Temple priesthood who still maintains particular symbolic ritual functions) calls out and the *'edah* (community) calls back. There are seven readers corresponding to the seven divisions within the *parashah*. Most people can easily recite the biblical verses, which accompany each reading. Each of the seven appointed men approaches the scroll, bows, and proceeds to read. Once the Torah is returned to the *'aron*, we return to the last part of the Karaite prayer book. The acting rabbi recites the *Kaddish* (the memorial prayer) in memory of a long list of deceased Karaites. He ends with a special blessing for those who are ill.

There is a palpable change in mood, shifting from reflection and thoughtfulness to action. We all move toward the door. A few men are rolling up the rugs, while one collects the prayer books and puts them with the *kippot* into the box. Someone folds the chairs, while the older women slowly make their way toward the door. Once outside they search for their shoes, making small talk all the while. It is now time for the big Shabbat meal. On warm, sunny days, the meal is served outdoors near the entrance. Thanks to the efforts of the women, the meal consists mainly of homemade food. Sometimes a particular family prepares the entire meal in memory of a relative who has passed away. The Shabbat meal is always associated with the memory of deceased Karaites and is therefore composed entirely of dairy products, as during the mourning period when Karaites eat only dairy foods. Someone passes around a tray with small plastic cups filled with wine. A beautiful, large homemade challah is placed in the center of the table. Two children sing the blessings over the wine and the bread. The food is traditional Karaite-Egyptian. As Avi, who left Egypt more than twenty years ago as a teenager, points out, "The food that Karaite[s] serve is not a Jewish food"—it's Arabic, like the music they listen to and the films they watch. The main dishes, such as slow-cooked fava beans, brown eggs, vegetables, the typical Karaite matzah crackers, olives, and homemade feta cheese, are served on one side of the table. The sweet desserts—different cookies and cakes like baklava and *masmūsa*—are placed on the other side. An appetizing variety of seasonal fruit trays and large bottles of 7-Up and Coke accompany the dishes. People gather in small groups, chatting and eating happily; the atmosphere is informal and cheery. This is the time to approach new visitors. Daisy tells me about her granddaughter in medical school. Sophia promises a copy of the most recent newsletter to another woman. Lailah mentions that she and her husband will spend next month with her mother in Ashdod, Israel. People gradually leave. By 1:30 the parking lot is empty.

Pure Torah, Pure Blood, and Pure Body: Standards of Karaite Life

The Karaites are a close-knit community; their law, as stated in *Sevel ha-yerushah,* does not allow conversion and does not legally accept the status of those who convert out of the community. Thus, Karaite identity can only be acquired through birth. In light of the increasingly frequent intermarriages with non-Karaite Jews among the younger community members, it is ironic that a leading Bay Area Karaite authority described in an interview the essence of the community as being a *ma'dan 'asil* (pure metal), preserving itself through its autonomy and isolation from the "other." The more commonly used metaphor is the Hebrew *dam tahor* (pure blood). The notion of pure blood, coupled with the claim to pure Torah, is a Karaite religious ideal that has contributed throughout history to the preservation of their conceptual group boundaries while simultaneously reinforcing their Jewishness (Colligan 1980, 146–89). The principle of not intermingling with other peoples in order to protect their own survival is stated repeatedly in the cultural discourse. This historical isolation has instilled in the Karaites a sense of nobility and pride. It is not surprising, therefore, to find some Israeli Karaite leaders arguing for their community's legitimacy and for the personal status of individual Karaites by advocating the use of "blood tests" to "prove" their ethnic purity, as if to say, "Our blood has been clean for thousands of years. . . . No foreign blood entered us. . . . We did not mix with the *goyim* [gentiles]."[6]

Karaite society is patrilocal and, unlike Rabbanite, patrilineal.[7] The identity of the child is determined by the father, meaning that the genealogical integrity of the "blood line" is maintained through the male. This principle further shapes Karaite attitudes toward fertility, conception, and childbirth.[8] As in many other cultures, a male child is considered proof of the father's masculinity and of God's blessing:[9] a male child's birth and subsequent circumcision reconnects him physically with Jewish Karaites, but, more important, this ritual of *brit milah* also binds him to the pre-Karaite lineage, beginning with the covenant between Abraham and God. Reconnecting in this way to the Bible, as in the case of Passover, confirms Karaite historical identity, which anchors its origins neither at the time of the Rabbanite-Karaite split (during the eighth century C.E.), nor at the time of Jeroboam (during the first century before the Common Era), but at the mythic genesis of Judaism itself. Clearly, the Karaites are actively engaging with what Foucault said of the old historians, who "push back further and further the time of antecedents" in order to "have construct recourse of metaphors of life" (1972, 12). This is especially relevant considering that the Karaites' few narratives regarding the origins of their sect were so often and so easily undermined since their very conception. In the Bay Area community, the birth of each son and his circumcision is seen as the metaphoric rebirth of the Karaite community as a whole, securing its future survival.

For the Karaites the notion of reproduction not only stems from the biological need to physically engender Karaism but it is also ideologically tied to the constraints of patriarchy already introduced in the book of Genesis. Such patriarchy works its way in different aspects of culture, from the patrilineal "blood line" to various forms of socialization. In the wider Middle East, patriarchy has developed to "the dominance of males over

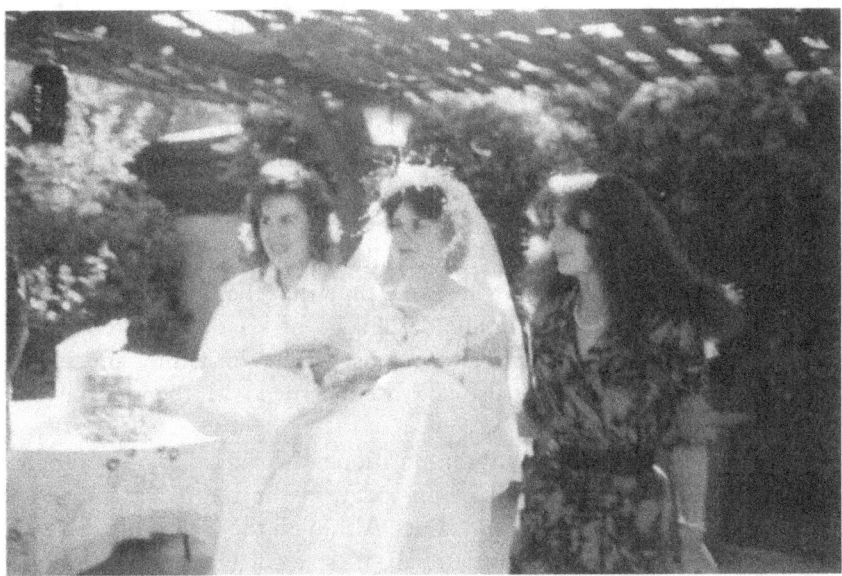

Three women carry the baby boy for a *brit milah* ceremony, 1992. (Photo courtesy of Remy Pessah)

females and elders over juniors (male and female) and the mobilization of kinship structures, morality, and idioms to institutionalize and legitimate these forms of power" (Joseph 1994, 55). In the realm of Judiasm and its relationship to the body, patriarchy as an institution has emphasized over and over again, through different discursive systems, the relationship between history and reproduction. The modern Karaite body is situated precisely in the junction between "the body that produces" and "the body that desires." According to Charles Mopsik: "Insofar as it concerns their collective and individual survival, the relation of human beings to their lineage is one of the most complex and critical questions for all societies and for each individual in society. The place of the body within this perspective must be carefully understood. It is through the individual body that the life of the people—and the level of humanity they have achieved—perpetuates itself" (Mopsik 1989, 49). Accordingly, the ideology of engenderment is conceptualized through the language of the biblical texts and oral writings from late antiquity. It presupposes the notion that "man, a being of language from birth ... is a being of language through his body" (ibid., 50). Whereas Mopsik underscores the primacy of the body and its symbolism in the acquisition of culture—a discussion that surely demands the inclusion of the woman—he also fails to acknowledge, and thus further denies, the role the female body plays in engenderment.

Hayim Halevi's *Toharat ha-Mishpahah be-Yisra'el* (The Purity of the Family in Israel) is a modern guidebook by the Israeli Karaite chief rabbi that chronicles the Karaites' long history as a small community whose integrity can be maintained only from within.[10] The preservative measures, against which the book warns, include birth control, abortion, masturbation, or any spilling of semen in vain—all of which are considered "shedding of blood" (1981, 12).[11] At the same time that these words are articulated in the text, using the familiar language of classic patriarchy in an attempt to reproduce patriarchal relations within the family and in the wider social context, they are also deeply concerned with the very physical survival of the community.

This concern has important ramifications with regard to how Karaites historically construct the body. Even today, in the Bay Area, individual Karaites struggle with these constraints. Although the California community, as a whole, does not conform to Halevi's strict dictates,[12] the emotional repercussions are inescapable, and are most apparent in the relative immediacy with which newly married couples have children and the vestiges of conformity to traditional child-rearing practices. Among European Karaites, this pressure is manifested in a rather more urgent way, as Emanuela Semi describes: "When I was in Vilnius [Lithuania] in 1989, I discovered that the Karaites who wish to preserve a 'pure' Karaite lineage of pedigree take as their first spouse a fellow Karaite from their own community and wait until offspring of the union are born. Once such an unsullied line of descent has been formally established, they feel free to divorce and to choose another spouse who is not a Karaite but who is more to their liking as a marriage partner" (Semi 1991, 101).

Every Bay Area Karaite, for example, inevitably is aware of the fact that childbearing and the rituals and beliefs surrounding it are closely connected, and, in fact, have a strong influence on the way Karaite culture will evolve. Still, almost all young Karaite couples use birth control and limit their family size to an average of two to three children. Indeed, if the significance of circumcision is momentous given this consciousness, even more interesting is the life of the female body around menstruation and breast feeding that carries over and routinizes this momentum in every day life. Moreover, much of the cultural burden of purity and impurity is assigned to the Karaite woman. Reproduction becomes the backdrop against which Karaite identity is informed. Not only are genealogy and social identity prescribed by religion and ideology, but they are also inscribed into a practical, female responsibility over reproduction. Ironically, but not surprisingly, the woman's role in preserving and regulating the community's standards is barely acknowledged.[13]

But while the male discourse serves as a commanding subtext and a guiding motivation, women's culture evolves precisely at the margins of this discourse: when the official text (biblical and legal) does not provide adequate guidance, and where there are ambiguous interpretations, women have been given the space to move beyond male authority and to establish their own code of conduct that is compatible with this authority. Karaite women's commitment to conception, as the pinnacle of the male canon, underscores their attempt to negotiate a position of power through the female material language of motherhood (preferably of a son), and to relocate from the margins inward toward the center. The women's strategies have been drawn from Karaite mother-daughter teachings, from body truisms, and from the folklore of their Rabbanite and Muslim neighbors. They are also motivated by inner aspirations and dreams as much as by a sense of practicality and lack of social choice.

Na'imah

I can still smell her rose water perfume. After we shook hands, said "Shabbat Shalom," and kissed on both cheeks, she would gaze at me with big, serious eyes, saying: "*Ahuhah* [so], what is new?" and look expectedly at my belly to see whether I was pregnant. It was hard for Na'imah, the mother of five sons and three daughters, to imagine why a married woman would not have children. Na'imah looked larger than she actually was. In her mid-seventies she was still tall, and her facial features clearly pronounced. From her eyes emanated deep grief and sadness. She mourned the death of her younger daughter, who had been killed in a car accident. Still, Na'imah's voice was confident, her responses certain. And beyond her words lay profound silence; nodding her head or making a facial gesture, she imparted to me an assumed, shared understanding between us as women, as Middle Easterners, and as Jews. Na'imah, who lived with her son, Joel, and daughter-in-law, Mira, passed away in the spring of 1991 at the age of seventy-six.

When we first met, Na'imah spoke haltingly in English. Once I realized that it was easier for her to express herself in Arabic, we gradually moved to Arabic, using Mira's assistance in translating from Arabic to Hebrew whenever needed. The result was an interesting trilingual conversation shifting seamlessly from one language to the other, using Arabic to convey some concepts, or conversely using English for others. I conducted the interview in all three languages, whichever seemed appropriate.[14]

When I arrived at Mira's large and spacious house, Na'imah was sitting at the kitchen table. It was obvious just by looking at Naʻimah that this interview would be particularly significant. I had been struck from the beginning by the depth of her commitment and sense of duty. Today, she was wearing a colorful dress that she probably wore only on special occasions; she appeared thoughtful and alert and wholly prepared to take it upon herself to represent Karaite women's life in all its vibrant complexity. Only later would I learn of her eagerness to tell me everything she knew—and her curiosity about my exact motives. Several young children were playing in the living room across from us. I sat with Naʻimah; Mira did not sit with us most of the time. Instead, she occasionally answered the phone, made tea, and brought us cookies that she baked. Once in a while, she would join us, translate if necessary, and add her comments. Mira, in her early thirties, was one of thirteen children. She was born in Egypt, grew up in Israel, and moved to California after marrying her husband, Joel. She was a busy housewife and took pride in being the mother of three children.

Naʻimah began her life narrative: "Ahhh, my father, my father . . . and . . . my mom died and I was eleven years old, me, and mama died, mama died. I had a sister and a brother . . . and my father married another woman. Yes. And I married at seventeen." Starting her story with her family encapsulates the Karaite experience within the intimate context of the family, especially since her mother died when Naʻimah was very young. Her husband was a family relative. Naʻimah liked to remember the past. She continued, "We used to live in Ḥarat al-Yahūd [the Jewish quarter in Cairo], in Ḥarat al-Yahūd *kullina* [all of us] *kullina, kullina kullina* were Yahūd [Jews]. I used to live with my mother-in-law; [Naʻimah counted on her fingers as she recalls] my sister-in-law [*silfiti*] and my other sister-in-law, and myself—the three of us and my mother-in-law, we used to live together and prepare for Pessah together."

Naʻimah's use of the collective "we" revealed the vigor of her sentiments regarding the dispersal of the old Karaite community in Ḥarat al-Yahūd, Cairo, and the subsequent disruption and displacement of her extended family, the tight Karaite community and the wider Jewish (Karaite and Rabbanite) neighborhood. But more than Naʻimah's sentiments, the collective "we" also represents the normative sense of inclusion within a communal group. The protecting walls of family fostered and enhanced a sense of selfhood to the point of creating fluid boundaries of self and individuality (Joseph 1994, 55). Naʻimah's reference to Passover further emphasized the tight-knit Karaite community. Her memory, full of women working together to prepare for the Passover, highlighted not only the centrality of the holiday in the Kara'iyot's mind but also the life of the extended women's network in the family working in preparation for the holiday. The Passover celebration poses an important challenge to the females within the domestic sphere, as the women's detailed cleaning and lengthy preparations—shopping, obtaining the kosher ingredients, cooking, decorating the house, baking the matzah—locates the Kara'it and the home at the heart of the communal religious expression.

RUTH: Tell me about yourself in …

NA'IMAH: About myself?

RUTH: In Ḥarat al-Yahūd. Yes.

NA'IMAH: About myself?

RUTH: Yes. You are a child …

NA'IMAH: Me getting pregnant?

RUTH: Or before, growing up …

NA'IMAH: Growing up? Ahhh, all we did was get pregnant and give birth. And first get pregnant. Two years between each baby. Two years *ya'ani* [that is to say] … But we did not really work [outside the home] so we would get pregnant.

In her hurried response about growing up, Na'imah skipped directly to what she considered to be crucial in the Karaite narrative, implying that childhood and growing up, central to Western culture, was not an integral element of the *Kara'it* biography. Instead, Na'imah centered her response on womanhood after marriage, suggesting that childhood and adolescence were subsumed by the constraints that maturation and married life imposed on the individual. Indeed, she viewed her life with a certain consistency, measuring the intervals between births.[15] Na'imah gave birth to eight children over a period of sixteen years, bearing a child once every two years. This two-year period included the nine months of pregnancy, and one-and-a-half years of breastfeeding, common among Karaites.[16] Na'imah expressed the sentiments of such commitment to child-bearing passionately: "Oh, among us we used to get pregnant and give birth only. *Ya'ani* [it means], on holidays and good days, on the Shavu'ot holiday [Pentecost] my mother-in-law used to get irritated: 'Why didn't you get pregnant?' 'What's the reason you are not pregnant?' 'What's the reason …' so that you will give[17] [birth] in the second, next holiday … Ah. *Lāzem tgībī* [You have to bring/give birth]." Until recently, the pressure on a woman to conceive in the Karaite community was tremendous: "*Lāzem tgībī!*" In this context "bring" suggests a gift to the husband, to the mother-in-law and the community, assuming that the female body is an infinite resource of vitality and birth. "It's part of your life to be pregnant, I mean, after you get married you wait sixty days or three months or whatever. . . . And after that you get pregnant. If you don't get pregnant—something is wrong with you."

When in her early forties she experienced a late period, Na'imah was convinced that she was reaching menopause. After four months, however, she found out that she was actually pregnant. While in her mind she had concluded her role in reproduction, her body was still carrying on in that mode. Other women told similar stories. They spoke of how the body—literally and metaphorically—is invariably engaged: an agent, which continuously (re)produces, contests, and impregnates culture.

Not only is a child brought or given into the community (and to the mother), but the mother also is brought from a position of passivity and sexual vulnerability to a source of "authoritative knowledge" promising her a position of honor within the family (Jordan 1993; 1997, 55–79). In general, fertility and infertility are unique cultural constructs that intend to reinforce the ideological concerns of the community. For Marcia Inhorn, for example, infertility among poor urban women in contemporary Egypt is the condition through which gender politics and family life become foregrounded as subjects strongly tied to patriarchal institutions. "Of all of the types of persons that one could be in Egypt, there are very few less desirable social identities than that of the poor infertile woman—or 'Umm Il-Ghāyyib, 'mother of the missing one,' as Egyptian[s] are apt to call her—giving this particular identity all of the classic features of a stigma" (Inhorn 1996, 1). Despite some differences between the Egyptians and the Karaites, Inhorn's description adds another layer to understanding the seriousness of reproduction to the Karaite community: according to Karaite law, an infertile woman faces the risk of being divorced, or of having her husband marry a second wife, a *tsarah*, literally "a co-wife" and "a trouble" (see Dabbah 1985, 274–318).[18] For if the story of the community is told by its physiological reproduction, then not giving birth means that one does not participate in the writing of this narrative. In other words, a woman who has not given birth has not earned admission into the community.

More than other older women, Na'imah was knowledgeable in matters related to the body, a fact that contributed to her position as a maternal authority among the women. Na'imah's attitude of herself was informed by the traditional perspective of orthodox Karaite *halakhah*. This subject position, apparent in her relationship with her body, derived from her respect for tradition as expressed in her relationships with her stepmother and mother-in-law. More than acting as a model, Na'imah insisted on negotiating a new level of religiosity for herself, albeit well within the accepted degree of "traditionality" of a community in transition. Not only did she facilitate my research, she was always available to other Karaite women who had difficulties regarding conception or breastfeeding. She told stories, educated the younger women about tradition, performed rituals, including fertility rituals, and secretly lent fertility objects (Tsoffar 2004). However, it would be a mistake to describe all Karaites in the Bay Area as holding to the same measure of orthodoxy as Na'imah; today, even the authority of Na'imah and other powerful older women (many of whom have been widowed for more than a decade) is somewhat but not entirely diminished among young Karaite women. This continuity has already manifested itself as these women's sons are assuming leadership roles in the Bay Area community, transmitting Karaite tradition to future generations. One of Na'imah's sons, for example, is currently the president of the community board, while the acting rabbi is the son of another visible Karaite woman.

Class is yet another important factor in the shaping of Karaite positions toward infertility and patriarchy. Whereas Na'imah was raised in an urban working-class family, other women in this study represent in Egypt a higher social class status and a higher level of formal education. Other concerns, such as age, degree of assimilation in modernity and Western culture, or exposure to other cultures, all further diversify the voice of the Karaite woman. Moreover, that Karaites are a community of immigrants that was formed in stages, and that has incorporated a considerable number of individuals from Israel (for whom it is a second immigration), makes it obvious that the community is not one cohesive culture. Whereas the women, in general, represent different levels of commitment to Karaite life, the older ones provide the backdrop against which a new American Karaite life is taking shape. Their collective voice claims the discursive authority of tradition, enabling one to imagine, reinvent, and reconstruct Karaite culture today.

A perusal of Karaite literature reveals that representations of Karaite women are essentially limited to motherhood. As individuals, Karaite women, in contrast to men, are mostly absent from the male-authored chronicles of eighteenth- and nineteenth-century Karaite life in Egypt, Turkey, Eastern Europe, and Jerusalem. If they are mentioned, it is mainly in legal documents of this period and only in the context of their personal situation and marital status. It should come as no surprise to realize that the strict patriarchal laws regarding marriage and sexual relations have historically contributed to Karaite women's liminality. In fact, their invisibility, as in other cultures, became a justification for their proper participation in the male order, as determined by the good standing of their husbands. In travelogues featuring sections on Karaites in Europe and Jerusalem, women appear as if frozen in their domestic roles. Those who do not conform—single women, married women who are childless, or widows—are seen as endangering the community's stability, as if they were threatening, demonic creatures who dwell in darkness and poverty.[19]

Eliyahu Dabbah's journal (in Hebrew) of the Israeli Karaite delegation's visit to Egypt in 1980 reports another example of Karaite self-representation of women (Dabbah 1985, 274–318). Chronicling the first visit of Israeli-Egyptian Karaites to Cairo following the 1979 peace treaty between Israel and Egypt, Dabbah delivers a nostalgic testimony of the life that Karaites in Israel left behind. He describes in detail the remnants of the Karaite community in Cairo. Because most of them were women, Dabbah had no choice but to diverge from the typical pattern and make them the protagonists of his account, providing a rather grim depiction of contemporary Karaite women. Throughout the forty-four detailed pages of activities, meetings, and memoirs, Dabbah resorts to much negative and patronizing expressions in characterizing Karaite women, such as a woman who is "clamorous but good hearted" (ibid., 278), another who is "a noble and gentle woman in spite of her obesity" (ibid., 292), and "an old maid who was not lucky enough to have a husband and of course children."[20]

The following excerpt reveals Dabbah's inability to think of and represent women beyond the roles of wife and mother. Jean, one elderly woman he describes, continued to hold on to fifty years of bitterness about her failure to marry and have children:

> At four o'clock we were ready for prayer, sitting in the courtyard. I noticed an elderly woman who was sitting near Kumsa Pessah's room. I asked Luci who she was. She [Luci] then stood on her feet and with her finger she warned us: "This is Jean," meaning a demon. "Indeed her name is Jean,[21] be careful of this woman." . . . She [Jean] asked us suddenly: "Are you going to visit the Hakham Aaron?" We informed her that that was our intention but we didn't have his address. She volunteered to accompany us. On the road, Miss Jean succeeded in telling us about herself. She was a spinster, about seventy. She worked in education and had made progress in this field and had been a supervisor; she then retired and now receives a nice pension. . . . She told us that when she was young she did not have enough money for *nedunyah*, dowry, and even though she had started to work, she did not save [enough] money. She was bitter at the whole community because they did not realize how

difficult her situation was and that's why she did not have the luck to have a husband and children. (Dabbah 1985, 280–81)

Women's behavior, according to Dabbah's report, is typified by quarrels and jealousy, screaming or cursing. In general, Dabbah feels justified in this characterization due to his belief that women who never married and therefore did not bear children could not be happy and would remain miserable in their unfulfilled social reproductive status. In his account, these women lead meaningless lives, "waiting [only] for their death."[22] That these forsaken elderly women constitute the remainder of the Cairo community reflects how their marginality as single women, uninvolved with relationships and families, prevented them from emigrating from Egypt. Their excluded social status led to their literal physical exclusion from the new Israeli community.[23] For Karaites of Dabbah's age group there simply is no social place for women other than motherhood. Note that not giving birth is always assumed to be the woman's fault and indicates a deficiency on her part.

Na'imah's words articulate this experience firmly: "After you get married, you get pregnant. [If] you don't get pregnant—something is wrong with you." Attempting to expand the picture, I asked her how many children her mother-in-law had. She replies: "She had four sons and one daughter. Oh, many! She brought [had] more but they did not live, they died.... Because when my father [in-law] married her she was only nine years old. She was very young. And then when she was pregnant she did not have the power to keep them alive, he [the baby] usually died. He usually died.... Because she was young." And then thoughtfully she recalls: "They say, because she was so young and married, they used to dress her with boots, high like that [motioning with her fingers to illustrate high heels], so she will be tall. Because she was very small."[24]

As I noted earlier, a woman is transformed into a matriarch from a passive, economically dependent, and sexually vulnerable position. She may then fully participate in the communal efforts, not only of reproduction but also of teaching and introducing her knowledge to her daughter and daughter-in-law. Marriage and maternity are the rites of passage that socially condone what was already presumed to be biologically ordained, namely, that fertility and sexuality exist solely for the sake of procreation. The excerpt above (which refers to the turn of the twentieth century) dramatically illustrates not only the Karaite premium on marriage, but more importantly their impetus to produce children, even at the expense of a nine-year-old girl's body.[25]

Marrying a girl or young woman, common in the Middle East, was a way to ensure the availability of a Karaite bride, as well as to be assured of her virginity, which was highly prized. In any case, sex at a young age would not have been considered abusive but was a known cultural phenomenon within the boundaries of marriage. However, Na'imah's story is particularly poignant, as her stepmother was much younger and less educated than her peers at the time of her marriage.

My interviews with elderly Egyptian Karaite women who married during the 1940s, 1950s, and 1960s revealed a broad spectrum of education and preparation for married life and elicited retrospective and reflexive musings about sexuality. In recalling the consummation of their marriages, some women expressed dismay over the paucity of their sexual knowledge at the time. Others were proud of their mothers for the education they provided. In general, it seemed that sex was perceived as potentially dangerous or shameful and was, therefore, alluded to obliquely if at all—as if explicit instructions would trigger discomfort and embarrassment. Their professed ignorance about sex stood in marked contrast to their knowledge about and preparation for menstruation.

The reminiscences of Leah, a woman in her late sixties, are illustrative. A fourteen-year-old in Cairo on the eve of her marriage, Leah told me and the other interviewees that she had no idea what would happen after the marriage ceremony. On her wedding night and thereafter, she kept running back to her mother's house, refusing to stay alone with her young husband. Only after he came to her mother to bring her back with him, promising to approach Leah gently, did she agree to return home and share the bedroom with him. A few younger women, who are more formally educated, mentioned taking feminine hygiene or sex education classes in school. But even the more formally educated women, or those with several older sisters in the household, also professed a lack of specific knowledge about sex and sexuality. Whether or not the women had been the totally naive brides they claim to have been, sex per se remained a taboo subject, especially in the group setting of our interviews. To males was attributed sexual authority and initiative by default.

Saturday Night and the Predicament of Making Love

The Karaite Shabbat frames issues of purity and impurity for individual Karaites as it informs a woman's consciousness of cleanliness, becoming a normalizing force of predicted cycles of time and its narratives. Even more than in Egypt, Shabbat in Northern California is a time of encounter between individual Karaites within the family and the community, between the people and the book. On Saturdays, in the presence of the sacred Torah, the concerns of pure body, pure Torah, and pure blood converge. Indeed, the joy of the monthly meetings, the reading of the prayers, the physical gathering around and touching of the Torah, all provide an opportunity for the sense and experience of a community. To the extent that Saturday provides a time framework that routinizes Karaite practices and provides continuity of tradition, it is also the place where practices is being invented (Hobsbawm 1983). Issues of history and memory, of calendar and future aspirations, are being rearticulated even more forcefully.

The meetings on Saturdays grounded my ethnography. I first met the Karaites as a group, and only after a year did I initiate conversations with individuals. Shabbat provided the opportunity to introduce myself to individuals with ease and to slowly gain their friendship and trust. During the services, I could observe their interaction, the functioning of the community, its hierarchy of power, the impact of generation and age, and the economic distinctions, as well as other important details that presented themselves in that context. It is on Shabbat that issues of women's purity are at the forefront of Karaites' concerns. Yet with its emphasis on purity, the gathering amplifies the female condition: *niddah* both specifies a woman's distance from the book, and also highlights her social inadequacy, prescribing a separate set of rules pertaining to contact with people, handshaking, and touching food and objects. Menstruation acts as a force that sets the limits on woman's intimacy within the world. Although she is less restricted today—for in the past a woman did not cook or even enter the kitchen as a *niddah*—a Karaite *niddah* in California tends to avoid going out and interacting with people, including other women.

The Karaites prohibit making love during Shabbat and holidays, in accord with the biblical injunction of "You shall not perform any work" (Exod. 20:10). For the limited duration of Shabbat, the concern with reproduction is suspended. And in its place, the primary concerns become the pure Torah and the pure body. Yet the fact that the Karaites prohibit sexual relations on Shabbat means that the purity of the body is maintained through abstinence, an ideal that further limits the already restricted time-frame of Karaite procreation. In the attempt to preserve the purity of their "blood," strict Karaite halakhah does not encourage intermarriage, and does not accept conversion. In order for a child to be considered a Karaite, at least, the father must be a Karaite. From the perspective of Karaite survival and concern with "blood lineage," Shabbat overrides the urgency of Karaite reproduction. The concern with the purity of blood is intrinsically connected to the notion of reproduction and to the responsibility of individuals to actively participate in the continuation of Karaite

68   Chapter 2

lineage. Karaite ontological philosophy and their ethno-religious premium on genealogical integrity are tightly connected to tangible issues of cultural endurance and future survival.

I now return to the women of the Saturday morning services in Foster City by describing their understanding of and concerns regarding the prohibition to make love on the Shabbat and the resumption of sexual life on Saturday night.

The conversation I describe took place on a Sunday afternoon, building slowly while we were drinking tea and eating cakes, moving from polite chitchat to passionate debate. The women responded to each other quickly. They not only attempted to reestablish the rules concerning the purity of males, but they were also concerned with their rationale. They move fluidly between English and Arabic. At times when Susana was not satisfied, she continued to explain in Arabic the inconsistency of the argument regarding males' cleanliness at the temple. At one point she posed a contradiction: if the cleanliness of a man, who prays in the temple the next morning, is the reason for the prohibition of having sex on Friday night, then sex should be prohibited at any other time he goes to the temple, and if a man is unclean for the sake of the temple, sex with him cannot be clean. Sophia, the same age as Susana, was less antagonistic and posed different questions. She also answered some of Susana's questions but eventually conceded, accepting tradition even though she did not entirely agree with it. It is interesting to note that different generations of women offer different ideas about sex, sexuality, and cleanliness, and that despite their commitment to pure body and pure Torah, not all of them have followed the law. In general, the younger generation of Californian Karaites, most of whom were born in Egypt, were much more comfortable talking about sex and sexuality than were their Egyptian foremothers.

> **SOPHIA:** So after Shabbat is over, Sol [the husband] sometimes goes and looks.... [*Susana joins Sophia, and both complete the sentence together, laughing.*] Looks at the clock [to make sure the Shabbat has ended].
>
> **SOPHIA** to **SUSANA**: I bet your Josh [Susana's husband] does the same thing. Doesn't he?
>
> **SUSANA:** He used to [*laughing*]. Now we don't have to worry. The kids are not ... [*She laughs.*] No. Yes, it's usually, yes, that's the intimate time.

I ask if young Karaite couples still keep the prohibition of sexual contact during the Shabbat.

SUSANA: It's something we grew up with. I cannot, I cannot change now after twenty-three years. And, my mother [Miriam] never told me that. She never told me that.

MIRIAM: About?

SUSANA: Friday night you shall not do any work. [*She cites the prohibition in Arabic.*]

MIRIAM: No. No.

SUSANA: But all your life you have never told me.

MIRIAM: I've never told you about anything.

SUSANA [*to the other women*]: She never discussed anything with me.

MIRIAM: I never talked to her about that, or about anything. No, with my children? No.

I ask why. She is not sure.

MIRIAM: I don't know [*thinking aloud*]. I was ashamed to talk about ... with my children about that. [*All the women smile.*] Maybe it is a stupid thing, stupid, but I never liked ... my mother, she never talked to me about that.

SOPHIA: You see, that's strange. My mom did.

MIRIAM [*surprised*]: Your mom did?

SOPHIA: Yeah.

SUSANA: My mom *never* ... my husband is the one who did. It was funny because when we first got married he told me, you know, "Shabbat you don't do it," and then the first week we were married then he wanted and I said: "You told me Shabbat you don't do it, how come now?" [*Someone laughs in the background.*] He said: "It's okay; at the beginning you can do it." I said: "No. Either you do or you don't but not in the middle. I don't like confusion in my life." Then he said: "Can't we make an exception?" I said: "I don't make an exception with things like these [*laughing*]. It's my day off."

RUTH: So, he was willing ... ?

SUSANA: Yeah. He was willing. Men are always willing, any time.

RUTH: Are they? [*To Miriam:*] Your husband, was he willing when you were younger?

MIRIAM: No.

RENEE: Friday night?

MIRIAM: No. He always had to go to the temple. Always ... Oh, his father would kill him if he didn't go [*laughing*]. I was living with my father-in-law. [The man would not be allowed to go to the temple on Shabbat morning if he had had sexual relations the night before.]

SUSANA: And won't they ask him, "Why didn't you go? Why aren't you going to the temple this morning?"

MIRIAM: What is he going to tell him?

SUSANA: "I slept ... ?" You cannot do that!

RUTH: So, it is a rule. Yet if he does not go to the temple, can he still ...?

MIRIAM, SUSANA, AND SOPHIA: No, no.

MIRIAM: You never think about that [making love on Friday night].

SUSANA: We don't go to temple now.

RUTH [*to Susana*]: So your husband is becoming more liberal. More ...

SUSANA: Yeah. That was at the beginning when he wanted his way. You know what I mean?

SOPHIA: That's not liberal. That's becoming horny. [*They all laugh.*]

RUTH: Is it very important, you think, for the next generation? Is it one of the ...

MIRIAM [*confident*]: Yeah.

SUSANA [*speaking at the same time with Miriam, her mother*]: I did tell Ben [her son], I did tell Ben. I [also] told Dina [her daughter].

MIRIAM: Yeah. It is very important for the next generation. They are supposed to respect the Shabbat.

SUSANA [*repeating quietly*]: I told Dina.

Miriam: And they [are] supposed to respect . . . to go to the temple, they have to be really clean.

Susana: Oh, Mama, I'll tell you something.

Miriam: *Nu?*

Susana: If you really think about it, there is nothing in between. . . . Everything that happens between husband and wife is sacred and there is nothing wrong with doing anything, it's just, we think about it this way, we grew up this way and we are not going to change it.

Miriam: *Ya-rūḥī* [my life, my love], no.

Susana: Mama? I am not going to argue about this.

Miriam: No, no, no.

Susana: I will not argue, I will not argue.

Renee: But, but, but anyway he can . . .

Susana: Because I argued this thing over and over and over . . .

Renee: But tell me.

Susana: And they don't understand. That's what I think. What happens between the husband . . .

Renee: *El-Rabbanim* [the Rabbanites], they take a bath after?

Susana: *Tant* [aunt], *tant*, yes, *tant*, yes. If you [are] going to say that what happens between your wife is a shame, you and your husband, is something shameful . . .

Miriam: It's not a shame.

Susana: Mama, just let me finish, that's enough, not kosher [pure], it means it's always not kosher and always shameful. It means you cannot go to the temple the whole week.

Miriam: Why?

Susana [*vehemently*]: Why? Because any time you do [make love], you don't go to temple.

[*Sophia tells Susana to get a handle on her apparent anger.*]

Susana: How do these men go to Temple every day? [*Turning to Sophia:*] I know, but think about it.

Sophia: I thought about it. But I cannot talk when you scream that way. So just relax, and then I'll give you my point of view.

SUSANA: No. It . . . it . . . it just . . .

RUTH: It doesn't make sense to you?

RENEE: No, no. He still can go, only take a bath and go, no?

SUSANA: I know. But on Friday night it is *ḥarām*, forbidden.

RENEE: Friday night too?

RUTH: Renee, you didn't know that?

RENEE: Ah, I don't remember anymore.

RUTH: You didn't, wasn't it important enough?

RENEE: I don't think, I really don't remember. I don't remember. I don't remember. I think my husband was not very kosher about it. But I am not sure.

SOPHIA: But it takes twenty-four hours to clean.

SUSANA: Twenty-four hours to clean.

SOPHIA: Yes, twenty-four hours.

RENEE: You have to be . . .

SOPHIA: No, it is not really twenty-four hours, it's after sunset.

SUSANA: Sundown! Sunset!

SOPHIA: After sundown.

MIRIAM: Especially the woman. Especially the woman.

SUSANA: *Tayyib, buss mama* [All right already, mom!].

MIRIAM: The woman can never be clean like the man.

RENEE: Wait, wait, wait, wait. After this story they take a bath.

SUSANA: *Tant*, we all *ya-rūḥī*.

RENEE: *Ha?*

SUSANA: We all do that.

RENEE: *Tov, khalas* [So that's it], he is clean.

RUTH: So he is clean according to you.

SUSANA: To you but not to the Kara'it [Karaites].

RENEE: Why?

SUSANA: That's the way it is. You see? [*She explains in Arabic.*] You have one thing in your mind and . . .

Sophia: *Tant* Renee, it takes until sunset for them to be clean. If they do it [make love] . . .

Renee: Oh, oh, if he takes a bath when it's done and it's midnight, he has to wait until . . .

Sophia: Until sunset when he becomes clean. But what I wanted to explain to you, Susana, when you said it is shameful and it is intimate and everything else, . . . nobody told you that it is shameful, I don't know where did you get, you got this idea.

Susana: No. . . . That . . .

Sophia: Let me finish. I listened to you and now, and now please listen to me. The Torah says that the Shabbat is a day of rest and is a day of remembering, so we never said that having sex is shameful, I don't know, I mean, I am not. . . . I've never considered it shameful and I don't know why you would consider it shameful, or a sin. It's not considered a sin. Having sex is not considered a sin. Except on Shabbat. It is a day of rest and it is a day that you are supposed to remember God.

Susana: And when you do that you don't remember God?

Sophia: The question is not that you don't remember God. According to the Torah it says that you are supposed to do no work and . . .

Miriam [*jokingly*]: And this is a kind of work.

Susana: I'll tell you what, I'll tell you, it's a beautiful tradition, I swear to God, it's a beautiful tradition. Because it's one day that you can go to bed and you have nothing to do and you have no responsibility. It is a relief for the husband and for the wife. You know, you can talk, you can communicate you can . . . without feeling obligated or without feeling any . . .

Ruth: Yes, yes. It's an important point. Sex sometimes can put a constraint on relationships.

Susana: Yes. But, you know, to be able to go to bed and just talk and relax and not think about it. I'm not complaining. What I want to say is that the way we do it or the way we interpreted the Torah, our interpretation of the Torah for that day, I feel, is not correct. In my view. Do you know what I am saying?

[*Miriam is speaking in the background with Renee in Arabic.*]

RUTH: So, you don't like presenting sexual relations in a negative light?

SUSANA: Correct.

RUTH: Because there is also beauty in making love?

SUSANA: Sure, and intimacy between the husband and wife, you know . . . You know . . . I don't know, that's the way I look at it . . . And my husband and I we argued about it and when . . . and we are always on opposite sides. When he tries to make it right I try to make it wrong and when he tries to make it wrong, I try to make it . . . you know what I am saying? So we just, it's something I have never been able to . . .

RUTH: And in spite of that you were ready to make the commitment when you got married and the rule was clear to you.

SUSANA: I had no problem with that. It is a beautiful commitment, like I said, I feel refreshed, I feel happy, I feel good on Saturday morning. You know, it's a different feeling.

3

Talking Menstruation: The Language of Blood

> On Yom Kippur when Benjamin, my ten-year-old son, went to the synagogue and I was not with him, Leah asked him: "Oh, Benjamin, where is your mom?" He said: "She is not here today. It is very personal."
> Sophia

> I grew up in a home in which no one knew that I had my period and when I had my period. But once I got married, I had to tell the whole world [she is laughing] that I have my period. That's what it seems like ... and you tend, at the time, you tend to isolate yourself, you don't want to go to your in-laws because [so] you do not have to explain yourself.
> Susana

Although the verbal root *n.d.h* in Hebrew means, in general, to displace, remove, cast out, expel, banish, or ostracize, the noun *niddah*, as it appears in the Bible, originally referred more narrowly to menstruation. In time, it became metonymically associated with the menstruating woman herself. In the Bible, the term implies both aspects: the uncleanness of the woman and the exclusionary status derived from it.[1] The statement from Leviticus reads:

> And if a woman has an issue, and her issue in her flesh be blood, she shall be in her impurity (*be-niddatah*, in her [condition of] *niddah*) seven days; and whosoever touches her shall be unclean until the evening. And every thing that she lies upon in her impurity (*be-niddatah*) shall be unclean: every thing also that she sits upon shall be unclean. And whosoever touches her bed shall wash his clothes, and bathe himself in water; and be unclean until the evening. And whosoever touches anything that she sits upon shall wash his clothes, and bathe himself in water and be unclean until the evening. And if he be on the

bed, or on anything whereon she sits, when he touches it, he shall be unclean until the evening. And if any man lie with her, and her impurity be upon him, he shall be unclean seven days; and every bed whereon he lies shall be unclean. (Leviticus 15:19–24)

By establishing this analogy between the term referring to the bodily condition of *niddah* and the term identifying the menstruating woman, the Bible gives rise to a new identity, giving the menstruating woman a new name: the *niddah*. In both Karaite and Rabbanite Judaism, *niddah* came to identify a particular female individual in a temporal bodily condition. At the same time, the term underscores the permanency of menstruation in association with the female social body, thus contributing to the conceptualization of woman and womanhood as a cultural phenomenon. Indeed, as a term referring to a condition, *niddah* moves between reducing the woman to the physical phenomena of her body and abbreviating the social praxis, epistemology, and language communicated by this noun. Similar to Bertrand Russell's assertion about proper names, *niddah* is an *abbreviation* of description; it describes "not particulars but *systems* of particulars, *classes of series*" (cited in Kristeva 1986, 234). The gaps in this abbreviated language, I believe, can be found in *Kara'iyot*'s noncanonic and informal language of the menstrual period. *Kara'iyot*, I argue, are the actual readers or "speaking subjects" of a condensed language, experiencing, rather than either assenting to or rejecting, its messages. Ethnographic discourse that narrates women's oral history around *niddah* in the contextual process of narrating vernacular language can articulate best the "signifying process" (ibid., 24–33) embedded in the otherwise immobile language of the text.

Between the ancient language of the religious text, its absolute discursive authority, and the contemporary Kara'iyot's experience of *niddah* in California, there are several semantic gaps and spaces. Even without taking into consideration the historical developments of "reading" and practice, in an immediate sense, one can ask, how are the verses of Leviticus translated into practice? Yet it would be incorrect to assume that the reality of Karaite women moves exclusively between the poles of text and ethnographic experience. In fact, the Karaite halakhah plays a major role in bridging the text, interpreting it, and making it available to women and men. At the same time that Karaite halakhah instructs that all members of the community have to know the "secret," it also provides a woman with a set of rules that exposes her condition.[2] Yet how do contemporary Karaite women speak about menstruation? Do Kara'iyot still refer to menstruation in the language of the biblical text? What aspects of the biblical lexicon and rules are internalized? In what language and terms? In particular, I expand on the conversation at the end of chapter 2 and focus here on how the women's discourse of menstruation sheds light on the relationship between their culturally coded experience and their subjective experience. In other words, I examine the rhetorical clues in Karaite women's discourse that will help us discover the nuances of their self-perception as females who, by virtue of their sex, are divided into two groups: one defined by a cultural norm and the other more specifically by gender.

Although the term *niddah* is grounded in the language of the fathers, in contemporary Karaite culture it is unclear whether the term itself is understood as an external one, imposed by social authority, or as an internal category that ties together deep aspects of the culture, including the text and Karaite native language (of prayer) and memory. It is often the case that the spoken language of the dominant culture will have a great influence on the vocabulary of a minority whose religious language cannot compete with the more pervasive lingua franca. However, Egyptian Karaites, who for the most part spoke Arabic, substituted the term *niddah* for other Arabic terms and expressions, precisely because *niddah* was used in the Torah and by its followers to point out the specific social and legal status of the woman during menstruation, and, in all likelihood, carried specific semantic and cultural meanings that could not be translated. As an objective category, *niddah* neither addresses nor refers to the individual body and its experience; rather it addresses and refers to the social body as well as to its socioreligious representation. Just as this representation was projected upon the woman from within the culture, constantly redefining her spatially and consigning her to the periphery, so too did it impose its vocabulary on female subjectivity, confining her during her menstrual cycle to a liminal status.

In contrast to the official language of Leviticus and the Karaite halakhah, Karaite women's language about menstruation continues to evolve. As evident in the conversation at the close of chapter 2, women talk with one another about their periods informally and in the context of familiar, everyday activities. They also draw upon the familial intimacy of girls in schools, girls' relations with their mothers and female siblings, and other interactions among female relatives in the same household. Names and terms for one's period have become part of the abbreviated, coded language of daily life that women employ to indirectly notify one about their condition when in formal, public settings. The practical details of menstruation—which is mentioned by name only when absolutely necessary—are an additional aspect of the everyday language of menstruation. Mostly unspoken, they are doubly concealed in the secrecy of language and in the coded practices of social exchange, together with the hidden functionality of handling the sanitary napkins, wiping the blood, or washing the body. Similarly, terms that replaced *niddah* do not refer specifically to the menstruating woman but to the period itself, a temporary condition, such as the expressions in Egyptian Arabic, "I got my period" or "The period is upon someone."

Although Karaite women suggested that I study the subject of *niddah*, it would be incorrect to assume that all (or at least many) Karaite women want *niddah* and menstruation to be the medium through which their speech is represented. Indeed, not surprisingly, once I started my fieldwork, the mere mention of the subject made some women uncomfortable. In spite of my increasing academic involvement in the subject of menstruation and my relatively open and uninhibited interaction with Karaite women, especially the younger generations, I found it difficult to speak about menstrual blood, all the more so with people who were not close to me. My mixed Israeli-Iraqi upbringing had taught me that menstrual blood was considered dirty, and that one does not speak about the subject, in part because it is considered tasteless to talk about the subject at length.[3] While not explicitly present as such in Rabbanite Jewish tradition,[4] the general notion I had grown up with was that speaking about things unclean inevitably renders the speaker unclean. In retrospect, I was not prepared for the experience of establishing contact with other women through, and in mutual opposition to, the social prohibition of talking about menstruation. In fact, the Kara'iyot's narratives around *niddah* magnified whatever distorted ideas I had harbored about the female body, forcing me to confront the extent of my own internalized negative cultural projections about menstruation. Once I started listening to Karaite women's experiences, I found that every time a woman opened up to talk about it, something would open up within me as well.

Whether or not the women were willing or reluctant to confide in me, our interviews always provided a constant realization that menstruation was an unusual topic. To directly discuss the body, menstrual blood, dirt, or impurity, and, in general, to place the "shamefulness" of the body at the center of our conversations in nice living rooms and kitchens, was common neither to Karaite nor to Egyptian culture (nor to American culture, for that matter). In Muslim society, for instance, as Fatna Sabbah (1984) persuasively argues, the canons of beauty, male desire, and sexual ideology all presuppose female silence, lack of expression, and obedience.[5] Originating in the legal text, this message is continuously reinforced and restated in all domains of public life. Often the female body is not only physically veiled and covered but also absent from the public space.

At times, our conversations went smoothly. At other times, it was embarrassing for me as well as for the Karaites, filled with moments of hesitation, pauses, questioning looks, anxious laughter, perhaps even mistrust. When I asked Naʿimah how children come into the world, she looked at me with disbelief and replied, "Are you sure you are from the university?" Yet despite the fact that women were not always aware of the importance of the subject, and that sometimes I could feel them wondering where the conversation was going or, even more, how I was going to use this material, they nonetheless trusted me and cooperated in the interviews.

The meeting at Leah's, which I recount below, is a good example of the discomfort that the subject of my study provoked. Admittedly, discomfort could arise from other reasons, such as the language barrier, or my ambiguous status as an "increasingly familiar" stranger. However, since the initial subject of my work at that stage was the Karaite *ʿādah*, an Egyptian term referring to menstruation that is still used by the older generation of Karaite women in California, I identified myself as an academic researcher studying *ʿādah*. The distinction between the *niddah* and the *ʿādah* soon unfolded for me: *niddah* is associated with Jewish scholarship and with following the law of Leviticus. Contrarily, *ʿādah* is a contemporary reference to menstruation. I use *niddah* mainly as a textual reference and *ʿādah* as the term of choice for ethnographic discourse.

By the time of the meeting, I had already been attending the Karaite Shabbat services and other community gatherings for a year or more, and most of the regular participants knew me and were aware of the fact that I was studying Karaite culture. When I first met Leah, I was impressed with how comfortable I felt in her presence. She was in her late sixties, with soft gray-blue hair and a round body, and her loving smile radiated warmth. She frequently employed terms of endearment, such as "Yes, honey" and "What, honey," that reminded me of my aunt. Even after several conversations with her, I was never sure how much she actually understood, and wondered whether the difficulty lay in her English, my Israeli accent, or the subject of menstruation. Only later did I learn that Leah was hard of hearing and used a hearing aid, which might also explain the protectiveness of her husband, Ahron, who was never far from her side. Whenever I approached her, she would immediately turn to Ahron, leaving it to him to figure out what I wanted, to set a time for an interview, and to give me directions to their home. Ahron would also translate into Arabic for Leah; when speaking with me, he adopted a patronizing tone but spoke with a friendly smile.

During the interview, one Sunday afternoon, Ahron sat close to his wife in their living room full of women, and, as the most vocal person present, brought the conversation to a stop by impatiently asking: "What is there to say about the *'ādah*?" Only after I turned to Ahron and said, "You don't get the *'ādah*, do you?" to which he hastily replied, "No, no," did he reluctantly but quickly flee from the room. All the women laughed and resumed their discussion on the *'ādah*. Ahron later returned and, with a sense of horror, told us stories about his encounters with the *'ifrit*, the female demon.

Ahron's behavior alerted me to some of the acceptable topics of conversation—what should be spoken about, what is considered entertaining, interesting, or "really Karaite." He certainly made sure to let me know right away that the subject of *'ādah* was trivial and insignificant. In his view, there was nothing to tell and discuss about the female body, its disorder and (re)ordering. Yet at the same time, he was willing to swear on the Bible that he himself had encountered the supernatural female, the *'ifrit*, and regaled us a detailed personal account of that experience. Ahron's attitude was also illustrative of the void men are allowed to fill in Karaite society. One could argue that the subject of menstruating women does not belong in men's social discourse. Indeed, all conduct related to menstruation aims to mark females as distant, and distinctly different, from males. The female demon, by contrast, appears to assert her existence by violating the male space, and therefore is a fair subject for discussion.

The difficulties of speaking about menstruation are not surprising. Menstruation is not a common subject of Karaite social interaction on beautiful Sunday afternoons, and it was I, the familiar stranger, who framed the meeting at Leah's home around this subject. The context in which my observations were made arose from these difficulties. Thus, my research was shaped by the reservations surrounding speaking about menstruation as much as by the women's willingness to overcome these reservations. The social gathering that provided the narrative opportunity emerged out of Leah's initial refusal to meet me alone, which led her to invite other women for the gathering. The personal effort of talking about the subject was eased by the presence of the other women.

My active role in introducing the subject also provided a narrative opening. Once women started talking about themselves, it became clear that more than the menstrual cycle was at issue. Matters of maternity, sexual education, personal narratives regarding "the first night" (the wedding night), and other topics were discussed and came as a surprise not only to me but even to the other women listeners. Notably, as much as the Karaite personal narrative of *niddah* and *'ādah* is individual, the topic is also not seen as merely concerning the individual but rather the collective social body. Therefore, the term *niddah* has come to represent the whole community and communal condition of purity rather than an individual or a personal one, in spite of its being a private issue. Sophia told me, "It [menstruation] is a very intimate thing. We tried to keep it very private. It is not considered something natural like in the U.S., where people can say it very openly. There, people would look down on you. Especially in a mixed group of men and women. Among women it is okay to discuss it." Earlier I asked Sophia if she would mention the period around men in the family, especially her father and brothers. She immediately dismissed the possibility: "Not men, brothers usually used to tease their sisters. My brother was much older than me, so I did not have this problem. My husband's sister told me that her brothers always used to tease her."

"*Al-'ādah, lāzem bayn al-bint wa-'ummahā*" (menstruation is a matter between a daughter and her mom), warned Na'imah. It is intimate, private, and above all controlled by the notion of *'eb* (shame), which counteracts any sense of the honor that is so highly valued in Middle Eastern society (Delaney 1991; Boddy 1989; Weideger 1976, 3–16). A synonymous usage is *ḥarām*, which means "impure" and "forbidden" in Arabic, and refers to a range of activities that are taboo to Muslims. *Al-'ādah* belongs to matters of the secrecy of the body. Menstruation and its care are private matters. Men are excluded. But the exclusion of men is not because menstruation is a woman's matter, but because it is not a subject one talks about at length. As one Karaite woman stated, "You don't talk about it. There is not so much to talk about it." In a female reversal or reflection of biblical exclusion, the public sphere is excluded.

While men as brothers and fathers are excluded from the day-to-day discourse of the *'ādah*, once a man and woman marry, the subject has an impact on their daily lives in different ways, depending on their level of religious observance. The more orthodox couples not only avoid sexual interaction but also refrain from any physical contact during the seven days of menstruation. In Israel, some Karaite men still maintain the biblical prohibition against touching the food, seat, clothing, or bedding of a menstruating woman. However, to my question as to how a husband and wife communicate about menstruation, Rosa, an Israeli Karaite, gave me a look that implied that she did not believe I did not already know the answer. Full of conviction, she said: "He knows. The husband? He knows" (she stretches out the syllables). "How? *Khalas!* Enough, he knows." And on second thought, realizing that I was still puzzled, she added: "You see, she [stays in] her bed, he goes to his." Rosa was referring here to the fact that most Karaite couples, especially the more observant ones, have two separate beds; when the woman is not menstruating they make love only in her bed in order to guarantee the husband's total purity.

In spite of the fact that the period is not often spoken of, and that there is an obvious effort to conceal the monthly event, the onset of the menstrual cycle is evident. In a practical sense, then, men are not totally excluded from the discourse. The fact that a woman is menstruating is conveyed to them in various accepted ways, both verbal and nonverbal. The prohibition and taboos are highly effective in structuring the reality of menstruation. At the same time, women's attempts to make the bleeding invisible help to veil the phenomenon. In fact, if a woman attracts any attention to the fact that she has her period, she has failed to be a woman with *'aqel* or *'agel* (common sense), a woman of reason who can enter the social realm by understanding and employing the social codes (Abu-Lughod 1986; Boddy 1989, 56–61).

The interview at Leah's home was productive and in many ways successful, since the women talked about a variety of subjects and told stories relating to their womanhood; still I felt that the conversation was not focused enough, that it had often digressed. I also found that the recording I had made was not clear due to the fact that the women often spoke excitedly and at the same time. While I was grateful that Leah had organized the meeting, I still wanted to hear each woman tell her own story. I believed that individual narratives, rather than collective ones, would more completely compose the story of the *niddah*. At the next monthly gathering in the synagogue, I approached Miriam, who, I noted, had a great sense of humor. I hoped that meeting her alone would give her storytelling talent full rein. Miriam seemed extremely excited about this idea when I suggested it.

When I arrived at Miriam's house in South San Francisco, I was surprised to find another group of women sitting in her living room waiting for me. This time the group consisted of Miriam, three women from the previous meeting, including Sophia, accompanied by her son Benjamin, and Susana, Miriam's daughter. Whether consciously or not, Miriam had managed to avoid meeting with me alone by arranging her own communal alternative.

At that stage in my methodology, I was convinced that it made sense to state to the woman I planned to interview that I was interested in talking about the *'ādah*. I hoped that introducing the subject directly at an early stage would give her time to prepare for our meeting. Both the questionnaire I had prepared earlier along with the Human Subject Protocol reinforced this approach in a way that I initially took for granted.[6] I realized retrospectively that stating my intentions at the outset was problematic: my straightforward questions must have provoked discomfort, even anxiety—especially in one-on-one interviews. Their solution of assembling a group of women to discuss the subject of *niddah* probably alleviated their anxiousness. Moreover, it is common for women in Middle Eastern cultures to gather as a group and share both the burdens and joys of life. Our meetings doubtless provided the women with a strategy whereby the social body contained and protected the individual body's secret. At the same time, the social arrangement limited the discussion by confining it to discursive norms acceptable within the women's circle, norms that, nevertheless, were more elastic than those determined by men.

A more peculiar situation occurred one midsummer's day when I arrived by bus for an interview at Rosa's home in Merhavim, a town in the south of Israel. I had been referred to the seventy-year-old Rosa by her daughter Mira, who lives in California. There on a large, sun-drenched balcony sat three people: Rosa, the mother of thirteen children; Lulu, another Karaite woman, in her fifties; and Yosef, a Rabbanite Jewish pharmacist in his fifties, originally from Iraq. They were sitting around a table playing cards.

Yosef, who was loquacious and authoritative, at least at the beginning, kept insisting that there is nothing special to learn or ask about menstruation, and in many ways intimidated the women, who also wanted to speak. In order to cover up her embarrassment and to avoid dealing with me alone, Rosa had surrounded herself with other people, including a pharmacist (perhaps assuming I wanted or needed to know about the biological facts of menstruation). She also set up a parallel activity, card playing, which is absorbing and demands the full attention of its participants. I felt obliged to ask Rosa whether it was all right to continue asking her questions, especially when she was losing the game. She would nod her head and mutter impatiently, "Yes, yes, of course." Rosa's more direct replies to my questions were also unhelpful. To my question, for example, on what women are not allowed to do while menstruating, she stubbornly answered, "Nothing," in a way that ended all further inquiries.

Obviously, women do not ordinarily sit around and talk about the *niddah*. The situation I framed and imposed on them forced them to objectify and reexamine their subjective experiences. True, compared to its secret acknowledgment in the past, the subject of blood recently has become a more socially accepted topic for conversation. Yet, throughout the process of discussing menstruation, a parallel process was going on in which the women dealt with the still somewhat shameful nature of the subject, comparing the Egyptian way, "the way we used to speak" with "the way they speak in the United States." The secrecy of the past highlighted the casual manner in which menstruation is discussed in the American media. As Sophia had carefully noted in our interview in California, "Back in Egypt where I grew up, menstruation is considered a side issue. Children should not know about it. It is not part of life like in the United States." Other women also made sure to mention the fact that in Egypt people referred to menstruation in a manner different from in America.

"Things were intimate. It used to be important to be clean. In the hot weather of Egypt in the summer," said Daisy, an articulate, sophisticated woman in her early seventies, "if it smells it is a disgrace." She pauses, sighs, and then continues. "But now you see it on the TV." Daisy remembered how amazed she was to find herself watching an American television advertisement for tampons. "You couldn't believe they talk about something like that. It [the period] wasn't an interesting topic for us to discuss. It was not a social issue. You had to take care of yourself. That's all." By stating that the period was not a social issue, Daisy meant to say that menstruation was not an appropriate topic of conversation. One does not talk at length about it; one just has to follow the rules privately. Later, Daisy expressed appreciation for the fact that American culture makes menstruation less private, though its publicity is mostly from mass media advertisements for tampons and sanitary napkins.[7] Clearly the image of the *niddah* as an isolated female was fading away as the women repeatedly claimed the responsibility to represent her.

Codes of Secrecy

As mentioned, no Bay Area Karaite woman referred to menstruation with the term *niddah*. This Hebrew word seems to be more commonly—but not exclusively—used among Israeli Karaites. Infrequently, the California Karaites use the term *tame'ah*, derived from the Hebrew *tme'ah*, as a substitute for *niddah*. *Tame'ah* is a more general religious concept that denotes the ritually impure from various sources. The women I interviewed mentioned *tame'ah* interchangeably with *ḥarām* (impure, forbidden). In women's everyday language of practicality, *niddah* and *tame'ah* are further removed. Yet, I believe, the textual language is condensed into the coded references that constitute the subtext, which underlies and feeds the new practical language.

In the Egyptian dialect, as reflected in Karaite culture (at least in my interviews), the term most women used in referring to the period was the Arabic word *'ādah*. In the Egyptian dialect, *'ādah* means habitual or customary. Unlike the term *niddah*, which does not refer to the cyclical state of the physical condition, the Arabic term *'ādah* suggests the ongoing, repetitive aspect of menstruation. Menstruation is perceived as part of the wheel of time, as part of nature. In its contextual usage, according to Sophia's example, the expression would be *'aleeha al-'ādah*, literally, "the period is upon her," as if the condition were imposed on the body from above. The preposition *'aleeha* ("upon her") is important in this specific example, as it encodes female gender by the reference of the pronominal suffix, *ha*, her. Equally important, *'aleeha* also depicts the body as engaged and controlled by time and nature. Sophia introduced another way to refer to the menstrual period in Arabic: "*Gatet li*, [it] came to me. Yes, and everybody knows. *Gatet laha* [it] came to her, means 'she got the period.' And you stop after the word 'laha' [to her]."

Women repeatedly mentioned the term *'ādah* in our discussions and on other occasions in which the subject of menstruation was raised naturally. However, when I asked women in what terms they referred to their periods, several of them replied, "*Gatet li*." Although in Arabic the pronominal suffix is attached to the verb in the past or perfect tense, the third person always requires a specific mention of the subject. It is possible that *gatet li* was originally *al-'ādah gatet li*, literally, "the period came to me," which then was abbreviated to *gatet li*. Therefore, "*gatet li*" is context dependent. While the subject is missing, the woman, referred to by the preposition *li*, is positioned as the object to which the implied subject comes. This process of ellipsis reveals women's tendency to minimize the language of menstruation. While the woman, for practical reasons, needs to communicate (to her sister, husband, her mother-in-law) the fact that she is menstruating, the vocabulary she employs is reduced to the absolute minimum. The result is that the phrase both communicates *and* conceals simultaneously. In this elemental coding, the prepositions and the feminine pronoun suffix gain prominence in the elided message. Thus, the feminine pronominal suffix stands in for the absent menstrual signifier to which it alludes, in effect collapsing the grammatically feminine form and menstruation into a single encoded reference.

Karaite girls and women, like people in many other cultures, learn to speak of the body in euphemistic language (Ernster 1975; Laws 1990, 80–84). A good example is the Arabic expression *'alay al-ḥamra*, literally, "the redness is upon me" or "over me." *Ḥamra* modifies the unmentioned blood and thus, like other adjectival nouns, takes on its feminine form. The speaker is the object controlled by a redness that is seen as a contagious condition of the whole body, rather than as a localized state. The overwhelming effect of the blood on the body, the fact that the body is perceived to be invaded once a month from the outside, the permeability of the boundaries of woman's body, make her dangerous and therefore in need

86   Chapter 3

of being controlled (see also Douglas 1966; Boddy 1989; Delaney 1988, 81; 1991). The result is that the blood is not only controlled and concealed in the social scene but also omitted from social discourse.

Modern language further attempts to hide the body. A more modern usage among younger Karaite women, which Deborah mentioned, is the Arabic expression "I got the x." This expression was mentioned by other women as well. In another conversation, Sophia added:

> **SOPHIA:** The "x" is a question mark. It is something very mysterious. It comes from algebra, x, y, and z.
>
> **RUTH:** So it's from school?
>
> **SOPHIA:** Yes. Yes. In school we always called it x, yeah, and in fact, in Arabic the Egyptians call it "el x."

In school, Sophia says, she always used the expression: "I have the x."

This formulaic idiom is still more impersonal than the terms in Egyptian dialect, for it adds the secretive, Western letter "x," which encodes both a blank space, that is, the possibility of any answer, and simultaneously its opposite, a specific signifier connoting menstruation alone. The x, itself empty of any content, further removes and distances the condition of menstruation from the speaker. The euphemistic use of *'ādah* as x or "it" assumes and reinforces the social familiarity of women and girls in exchanging hidden information.

Another term Mira reported that was common among Karaites in Israel is the expression in Hebrew: *ha-dodah mi-Rusyah* (the aunt from Russia), which refers to the period itself, not to the menstruating woman. Since this term hearkens back to Mira's childhood in Israel, it might have been more common among Israeli school girls and young women in general. When communicating with children, adults use the term *dodah* (auntie), and *dod*, the masculine form, to refer to any adult female, turning the adult stranger into kin. *Dodah*, maternal or paternal aunt, in modern Israeli folklore is a loaded familial referent. This innocent family lore—especially the female *dodah*—is often transformed into a grotesque ironic figure who, although referred to in intimate language, is in fact a stranger.[8] In this case, the *dodah* or aunt is associated with Russia. In a political climate in which communism is reduced to a symbolic color, the red of the Communist Party and the red of blood create an interplay of color signifiers. Redness and communism appear also in another term, *degel 'adom* (red flag), or just *degel* (flag). Although the code word is conceptually and geographically removed from the body and the reality of the speaker, which serves the purpose of secrecy, the phrase links the state of being an adult woman (*dodah*) and the menstrual condition. Yet beyond the secrecy, if anything appears to be concrete, it is the verbal placard of redness, which stands for the condition of the woman.

Two common ways to mask the bodily phenomenon of menstruation include borrowing vocabulary from other languages and implying knowledge. Interestingly, the internal Karaite codes referring to menstruation indicate the multilingual and multicultural environment within which the Karaites exist. Often, a vocabulary of borrowed words consists of evoking semantic fields that tend to contain the uncomfortable feelings about menstruation among the speakers. However, at the same time, borrowing also demonstrates a need to go beyond one's language, or to incorporate into one's own language the foreignness of the phenomenon, the estrangement of women from their bodies.

Niddah is an abbreviation. To start with, the language of Leviticus did not include women's lives or culture of the body. In the matter of laws of menstruation and lactation, the usual tension between the religious biblical text and its contemporary interpretation is ramified and complicated by the dialectics of textuality and the life of the body. The biological experience becomes a coded sociology that manifests itself first and foremost in the most intimate level of experience as it meets both the text and the larger social environment—the family, relations between generations, females and males, or among siblings.

Although Karaite women's language, with all its intertextual obligation, is contextualized, it constitutes a discontinuous text that narrates women's lives as naturally encoded in a feminine language, since it corresponds with female gender in actual life. Paradoxically, the limited language for female experience that does exist gains further importance. In such coded language, the subject is absent or sometimes appears as "it," and is implied only by the social context. The syntax comprises more predicates than nouns, the usage of verbs is extensive, and the prepositions are significant. The female subject does not need to be spelled out, not because she is excluded, but because she is pervasive. As a result, women's language becomes the voice of those who do not speak their body but who act on it or act out its materiality.

While the code of secrecy binds women, it also excludes them from central, socially accepted discourse. From a male perspective, women are not only reduced to the status of *niddah*, but in their very attempts to conceal the blood, they reinforce the perception of menstruation as shameful, thus contributing to, rather than avoiding, the biblical judgment of menstruation as unclean. As a result, women themselves are pushed to the margins, where they hide themselves and their bodies.

Speech can expose as much as bodies do. What happens on the level of the body happens on the level of speech. The dynamics of concealing and revealing are reflected in both individual speech and the submergence of individual speech in collective discourse. Subjective language, we learn, can hide in the body social where individual experience can be submerged. Concealing and revealing appear to be inextricably connected in the discourse of reference to menstruation. Leviticus sets the tone for this paradoxical mode by naming (and thus exposing) the menstruating women and simultaneously determining her exclusion. In women's discourse, the very act of encoding and concealing the onset of menstruation communicates it unmistakably. Concealment by indirection is a remarkably expressive speech act, which performs its message rather than verbalizing it. As ten-year-old Benjamin's innocent assertion at the beginning of this chapter indicates, menstruation is such a personal, private issue that, in fact, every one knows about it; the absence of the woman from social activities speaks of her physical status. Finally, my own attempt to circumvent these strategies of concealment fell into the same paradoxical trap. By confronting my questions with collective rather than individual narratives, the Karaite women managed to signal their individual experiences while submerging them in the discourse of the social body.

4

Mother-Daughter Teaching

> For we think back through our mothers if we are women.
> Virginia Woolf, *A Room of One's Own*

Following de Beauvoir's formulation of the noncoincidence of natural and gendered identity—"one is not born, but rather becomes, a woman"—I wondered to what extent a Karaite would accept an analogous formulation based on ethnic identity: "One is not born, but rather becomes, a Karaite." Moving away from the physical engagement with reproduction, which, as we saw in chapter 3, affirms on a different level that one is, in fact, born a Karaite, this chapter addresses the process of *becoming* (in de Beauvoir's sense)[1] both a Karaite and a woman, or a "Karaite-woman," through mother-daughter teaching. I discuss the way the language of menstruation becomes women's tradition, encompassing the poetics of the flesh, the poetics of everyday corporeality.

The mother's teaching of menstruation to her daughter is the junction where book and body meet.[2] At this junction, the remembered, evoked, and restored texts are transformed and inscribed into a corporeal physical reality. Textual knowledge and authority inform both her body and practices through which gender is constructed in Karaite culture (de Certeau 1984, 166). In the physical sense, this textually informed discourse mobilizes the tradition of reproduction of pure Karaite bodies in its contribution to the preservation of Karaite identity. It tells us how literacy is translated into bodily praxis.

The mother's teaching is best reflected in women's narratives about their experience of the first menstrual period. In these narratives the Karaite mother emerges as a discursive authority, making it clear that female reproduction is inseparable from women's conception of knowledge. Careful, everyday verbal and nonverbal instructions concerning the sites of blood, pads, and washing, as well as physical distancing, timing, and counting, constitute the alphabet of reading the "textual body." Together they compose a unique method governing the blood as it appears on the pads—a blank page of informing textuality. This discourse not only mobilizes the tradition of reproduction of "pure" Karaite bodies, it also further pushes the limits of reading to include the obvious, though less acknowledged, schooling of the mother.

Both Friedrich Kittler's metaphor of "mother's mouth" (Kittler 1990) and Kaja Silverman's "maternal voice" (Silverman 1988) place the mother squarely at a center of the talking body. Departing from Kristeva (according to whom the mother, lacking subjectivity and relegated to the semiotic interior of the chora/womb, is reduced to silence), Silverman approaches textual intersections as both "an anatomy of female subjectivity" and "as a study of the female voice" (1988, x). If voice is "a site of perhaps the most radical of all subjective divisions—the division between meaning and materiality," or between language and biology, says Silverman, the mother's voice, more than "voice-as-being," can be articulated as "voice-as-discursive-agent." As such, it constitutes part of the body that talks (1988, 44).

Less symbolic than Silverman is Kittler's articulation of the mother's mouth in history (Kittler 1990). For Kittler, the mother's mouth in eighteenth-century Germany's premandatory schooling system is a cultural site of the discursive reproduction of pedagogical knowledge. The history of children's domestic education demonstrates how mothers, teaching their children the alphabet and literature, were the consumers of the culture of the time. Kittler persuasively demonstrates that even though the text women taught was masculine and patriarchal, and women as a plurality were excluded from the official discourse, and in spite of the fact that the mother "was a voice but had no right to have one," she emerged as the authoritative producer of discourses aiming at creating and culturally reproducing mothers' knowledge (1990, 66).

Kittler puts the mother's voice at the center of the discussion of mothers' role in individual secular pedagogy, as a home-schooling teacher for boys and girls in the premandatory schooling system. The oralization of the text shifts our gaze from the written page to the mother's mouth as a site for the production and transfer of knowledge. In the Karaite context, I approach the mother's voice as an instructive voice that prescribes, negotiates, and preserves for her daughter the female knowledge that she herself acquired from her mother's words through her practice. Not only are letters transcribed and transformed from visualized images into audible uttered sounds, but the abstract notions of pure and impure are also encoded and materialized in the bodily ritual of actions.

One can assume that in the past, when it was even less common for women to actually read the Bible, the menstrual period and the process of education that surrounds it marked a woman's transition from "illiteracy" to a "literacy" that was introduced to her—not through the actual reading of the text, but rather through the embodied knowledge of this text.[3] In this vocabulary the *fûtah* (Arabic for apron, pinafore, napkin, serviette, or towel, referring to a cotton menstrual pad) is the object introducing this physical discourse, as the woman undergoes a potential change in her status (preparing herself with the proper supplies) even before she starts to bleed. With the placing of the *fûtah* the girl becomes a watch-woman; she, like her mother, is expecting the blood.

In several of the interviews women spoke of relating the onset of their first periods to their mothers. Nadia, in her mid-sixties, reflected:

> When I got it [my first period], I think I told my mother, and I had a bath also and she removed everything, because it was in the morning. I got up in the morning and I found out that I have something and my mother took all the sheets and washed everything although I didn't dirty anything but that has to be done. And I think my sister was sleeping with me and she had a shower too, because she was touching me and sleeping with me, and after that I stayed by myself.

In the case of Na'imah, her stepmother served as her teacher of ritual.

> RUTH: Do you remember your first *'ādah*?
>
> NA'IMAH: Yes. I was with my stepmother. She started telling me, "watch out for the *'ādah*," "pay attention to the *'ādah*." At night, in order not to spot the bed we used to put the *fûtah*.
>
> RUTH: At what age did you get it?
>
> NA'IMAH: Fourteen years old.
>
> RUTH: How long did you sleep with the *fûtah*?
>
> NA'IMAH: One, two months. Once you get it you have to wash.

Having the presence of other maternal figures did not necessarily help the woman to prepare better for the period. Leah's description of the first period was dramatic:

> One year, and . . . I don't know, with my grandma living with us in

the house and I called her: "Nana, Nana, come and see what happened to me. What happened to me." And she said: "Oh, don't worry." I don't know, father was dead and we were six children with my Mom, my Mom worked in the *machina* [factory] to get food, because it was very hard and the lady had six children, yeah, six children, three boys and three girls, and she worked very hard, and my grandma and my aunt helped her. My Mom in the *machina* is working all day. I go to school and I come back every day, me and my sister. And one time I saw the blood: "Mom, Mom, what happened to me?" "Come." She took me to the shower, and okay. I took a bath and she comes back and she gave me hot water and gave me a piece to put it [*fûtah*] and she changed all my dressing and said: "Stay here. Don't go out. Don't go out into the street." "Why?" She said, "Don't go! Stay." I don't know why.

Lailah described her first period as follows:

I learned about the [Karaite] community from *'Ima* [mother]. The first time I got it I was eleven, I was in school and I found it all in the underwear. I went to douche. We have something that we wear, a piece of plastic on both sides and we wear it. *Hufat*, like a baby diaper. It is placed near the restroom behind the door. No one can touch it once you used it, it is *tame'*, impure, defiled. You wash it on the spot, the *fûtah*, a cotton piece, it should be washed and boiled. She, my mother, prepared for me the food and I eat in the corner alone. It is not good but what can one do, *'Ima sheli haytah 'ishah hazaqah*, [my mother was a very strong woman]. Till I got married and came here I used to change everything.

Sophia is the youngest of three daughters and represents the young, nontraditional generation of Egyptian Karaites. She is a good example of today's Karaite cultural hybrid, an interesting blend of Egyptian, French, and Northern Californian manners and style. She was educated in French schools, has a college degree, and is now working in a high-tech company. The wife of the community leader and the mother of two sons, she plays an important social role in the community, especially among the women. She is knowledgeable in Karaite tradition and active in organizing social events, such as an international summer camp for single Karaites. She is an especially striking woman in her mid-forties, open, outgoing, warm. Sophia's mother was especially active in teaching the basic principles of Karaite life to her daughters. Sophia's brief description, like other excerpts throughout my study, demonstrates that her background and mother's teaching make her an informal authority figure on Karaite social and Karaite halakhic issues, especially among the women:

> My mom comes from a religious family. Her father was a so-called rabbi, an extremely religious man. She explained to me that when a girl has her menstruation she is not considered clean during the seven days. Whether she is bleeding during all the seven days is not the point. She is still considered unclean. Being a girl and going to just girls' school, of course I knew what menstruation is. When I had my period, my mother explained to me the principles of the *taharah*, purity laws.

Daisy recalls:

> Oh, of course it [the first period] changed my life, because, I remember, I was very shy. And I didn't know if that [the bleeding] would stay with me my whole life. . . . You understand what it is? . . . I was very ignorant. I remember at school they were starting to teach hygiene and to explain the man's and the woman's body, we were at a private school and I remember I was very curious and they refused to tell me. . . . I was curious, I wanted to know what they were talking about.

In the Karaite community, a woman's memory of her first period is tied to memories of her mother. To my questions regarding their memory of their first *'ādah*, the women responded first by giggling: "What, do you expect us to remember our first period?" Later they would refer to their mothers with words such as "religious," "strong," "difficult," "strict," and "observant," or alternatively "not so strong," "not old fashioned," or "open," describing thus her religious background, personality, and ability to insist on following the rules. As shown in other aspects of the lives of Karaite women, maternity, motherhood, and mother tongue are closely related, as the body, its memory, and future behavior during menstruation are all crystallized through the mother's voice. The fact that subjects related to the body are not channeled through communal institutions or general public education contributes to a dependency on the mother and her authority.[4] At least while apprenticing under their mother's tutelage, girls tended to follow the family's version of tradition, often referred to as the "mother's household." When Mira spoke about crying as a girl, after being removed from the main table at Passover because of her period, Susana jumped in, startled, asking stormily in Arabic, "What, at your mother's too?"

Obviously, referring to the mother is not that surprising, since mothers in Karaite Egypt were important in the general education of their daughters and in preparing them for their future feminine role, and like other women in different cultures, Karaite mothers controlled the process of education about women's bodily maintenance. Nawal el-Saadawi, the Egyptian feminist physician and writer, sums up the dominant place her mother occupied in her childhood: "But it was my mother who controlled my life, my future and my body right down to every strand of my hair" (el-Saadawi 1988, 16). One should also bear in mind the competing social and cultural trends in Egypt at the beginning of the century. In the colonized Egypt of the 1920s mothers were forced to compete against the increasing influences of imported Western and European etiquette, fashion, and manners to ensure that their daughters behaved properly, especially in their body language, and protected their virginity.[5] One can argue that matters concerning the privacy of the body and its impurity tend to be concentrated in the female domain of the household or neighborhood, especially when mandatory schooling failed to address these subjects. Within the Karaite community, the attitude toward religion underwent a tremendous shift reflected in the new efforts among the young urban generation to Egyptianize and Westernize (al-Qudsī 1987). Renee's statement during this conversation, referring to the new secular lifestyle in Karaite households, summarizes this tendency: "Anyway there was no tradition in our house, was there?" Other women on different occasions pointed to a rebellious stage against the rigid Karaite tradition in Cairo. As Sophia's mother-in-law used to tell her: "Oh, don't worry about this or that Karaite thing. It's old fashioned."

In Karaite culture, the mother emerges as the irreplaceable source of knowledge upon whom the daughter depends regarding the bodily ritual of cleanliness. Being the only source of practical education, the mother is thus responsible for the creation of a private text in the process of enculturating the next female generation. The question of a secular lifestyle in a multicultural context is especially important for a minority group such as the Karaites in which the small size of the community, its historical reliance on the dominant culture at large, and its limited access to sources of communal knowledge, further increase the dependency on the mother. Moreover, when the subject is not only a woman's body but also its polluted condition, this knowledge is further relegated to the innermost intimate level of female life, forcing secrecy that by its very nature narrows its availability to others. Nevertheless, and perhaps not surprising, for Kara'iyot, the mother-daughter paradigm is grounded in the context of male dominance and limited women's expression, a context that, to a large extent, determines the content and importance of their speech.

Menarche initiates the Karaite girl child into adult womanhood. The mother introduces a practical set of rules to her daughter, and implicitly and explicitly conveys the meaning and obligations of gender in Karaite culture.[6] Predictably, embedded in the focus on the subject of purity and impurity are the cultural values and norms of sexuality and virginity. As Sophia said, "When I got my period that's when my Mom treated me more as an adult. She explained to me a girl can get pregnant. She wanted to protect me from other evils. Especially in Egypt women always tried to be virgins; it was considered a really bad thing [to lose one's virginity before marriage]."

Na'imah's description of her preparation for and the onset of menarche differed from that of the other Kara'iyot in that her mother had but few words to facilitate her practical preparation for menstruation. In fact, action mediates the language: the *fūtah* in this vocabulary is the object introducing the discourse, anticipating Na'imah's change of status even before her actual bleeding commences. The fact that not all the women mentioned the *fūtah* suggests that it may have belonged to an earlier generation, used by older, more conservative women. While its usage speaks of women's attempts to contain the blood, to avoid spotting the bedding, it might also reflect pragmatic concerns such as the availability of water and the routines of doing laundry. In her discussion of the *fūtah*, Na'imah relates that her father made his second marriage contingent upon his new bride's ability to love and teach his children as if they were her own, perhaps demonstrating that motherhood, as a role, is intrinsically tied to the religious teachings and the family's common efforts to abide by them.

Nadia's and Leah's excerpts depict different situations. In spite of Nadia's education, her family's affluence, and her five sisters, she was neither told about nor verbally prepared for menstruation. In Leah's case, too, the presence of other maternal figures (mother, aunt, grandmother) was of no help to her in preparing for her period. Yet once Leah and Nadia got their first periods and involved their mothers, practical matters were conveyed to the daughters through action: they were given pads, taken to the shower, confined to a certain place, and told to wash the bedding.

Obviously, these conversations with the women present different degrees of menstrual and general bodily education given to girls. Yet in spite of the differences, the mothers' chain of tradition has been preserved and the transmission of knowledge maintained and negotiated through history. Motherhood emerges as a social institution that is intimately maintained within the family unit, even one that is not socially encompassing and hegemonic, with values such as modesty, shyness, femininity, cleanliness, and bodily aesthetics playing an important part in the institution of motherhood. Practical discourse conveys that a lack of verbal teaching can still be perceived as instruction if the girl is introduced to the knowledge of taking care of her body. Specifically, Karaite production of purity is intertwined with more general feminine concerns. To be a Karaite and to be a female are articulated together through the body and through the subject of reproduction.[7]

As a preparation for the *'ādah*, a Karaite girl approaching puberty used to sleep with the *fūtah* rolled between her legs, in case her first period occurred. Na'imah herself used the *fūtah* for two months prior to her first period, at age thirteen, in order to avoid spotting the bedding. How long other girls used their first *fūtah* prior to their actual bleeding is unclear. Na'imah is the only woman who mentions the *fūtah* by that name—most women referred to it as a "cotton towel." For her and other women of her generation, the first *fūtah* was used as a preparatory device to provide warning of impending impurity. My sense from talking with them was that the *fūtah* coached the prepubertal girl in how to read the signs of her maturing body. With every night that passed, the *fūtah* accumulated its coded meaning of potential uncleanliness, psychologically helping a Karaite girl to develop a consciousness of purity, imposing upon her the ideology of blood and stains. As if to mark social initiation into adulthood, when the mother "read" on her daughter's body the advent of menstruation, she incorporated her into the world of womanhood by introducing her to the "cotton towel," along with the projected fear and anxiety of spotting the bedding. The *fūtah*, like a blank page, was usually white; the blood marked it like words on a page. The *fūtah* yesterday and the sanitary napkin today are best understood as the material antecedent of the imagery of the Karaite girl's experience, as their use marked her separation from childhood and her incorporation into womanhood and motherhood (cf. Gross 1980; Paige and Paige 1981).

Another common rite of passage for girls today is the bat mitzvah. Californian Karaites make a point of encouraging young girls—just like boys—to read the Bible from an early age. The preparation for Simchat Torah and the excitement about reading in front of the community become important markers of the new generation of Karaite girls. The bat mitzvah, at age twelve, is the equivalent puberty rite of the bar mitzvah, the male ceremonial reading of the Bible at age thirteen. The bat mitzvah is celebrated mostly among secular, contemporary Israeli Karaites. American Karaites themselves claim that for girls, the study of Hebrew and the reading of the Torah are the counterpart of the bar mitzvah ceremony.

Women take care of objects of menstruation the same way they take care of their bodies. The objects of menstruation are hidden in a designated place. The *fūtah* is kept "near the restroom behind the door." This publicly known—at least among family members—"hidden" place indicates a certain public-private knowledge available to girls. "Public privacy" is a common theme in the encoding and communication of the practice of the *'ādah*, a discourse of actions that parallels the discursive language referring to the period.

The abstract code of secrecy gains its material encoding: textual signifiers are articulated and pronounced through bodily signals. With the first spot, young women start reading their bodies. With the first drop of menstrual blood the body communicates the condition of *niddah*, beginning the time that a woman should guard against being spotted and spotting. The dilemma begins with the fact that the menstrual blood cannot be contained within the body: how can one physically contain that which is boundless? It is now the woman's duty to attend to physical matters, to count the body with the day and hour, and to mark the blood from within with meaning from outside. From this point, until menopause, a woman cannot permit her body to flow freely out to the world. While the care about being spotted starts in a personal, private space, as soon as a woman steps out of her room, it becomes a public matter. The outside world resides in the body, causing self-consciousness and social consciousness to develop.

Some women recalled that after using the *fūtah*, they had to wash it so it could be reused. Both the attitude toward the impure blood and the family's economic situation determined whether a woman had to wash the *fūtah*, or merely soak it (leaving the washing to the maids), or even throw it away. For some women, allowing the maid to wash the *fūtah* would be considered a violation of privacy.

Nadia recalled: "We didn't wash [our clothing] very well but at least we soaked them in water and before . . . we didn't have washer and dryer, we had someone who came every week or two to wash all the linen and everything. We usually were very careful. We used towels. Usually we don't clean the towels which are dirty; we folded them and threw them out." I told her that another woman mentioned that she used to wash the towel. She was amazed: "I never in my life washed a piece. Only our panties. I never did it, not even my sister."

Naomi described her mother, as opposed to the father, as religious: "The material we used during the period was a white toweling material. I would wash it as soon as I changed, soak it in water or bleach. You could not give it to the maid, you had to do it yourself. . . . In the Karaite religion a menstruating woman is unclean." Naomi was animated, and spoke with passion. She was restless, energetic, and responsive. Her answers were alert. Her descriptions implied that although the first period was a private event, it had social echoes. Women who are late in getting their period become the focus of public social concern, suggesting that the experience of menstruation is homogenous and regulated. Naomi's experience of her first period was associated with the development of her body and her body image at the time: "My breasts developed very young [early]. I was shy, so I was walking with my back [hunched] and posture to hide it. I was so skinny it was considered like being sick. Because I got it [the period] late, some relatives used to ask my mother: 'Did she get it?' 'Is something wrong with her?' It upset me that every month you had to wear a belt. It would show a little bit. It caused discomfort to my consciousness."

Many women changed their religious attitudes after getting married. Once they were on their own, the tendency was usually toward being more liberal with the rules. Occasionally, marriage forced some women to adopt a stricter approach, most often because of the mother-in-law's insistence on maintaining the traditional Karaite life. As Naomi noted: "I stopped doing the ritual after I was at home married. I felt clean. When I got my menopause I was lucky. Gradually it came one month, two, a year. I was happy. It was a burden, a necessary burden."

Through the physical cleaning, the concern for the spots, and the engagement with boiling, soaking, scraping, and washing the pads, a woman faced the blood and its meaning. To a certain extent, the bloody *fūtah* was the embodiment of the periodic impurity of women, especially those women who had to wash and reuse it. By doing so, a Karaite woman emerged as the agent of cleanliness. Acts of cleaning constitute her discursive language. The vocabulary of cleaning was detailed in numerous moments of caring for her pads, making sure she did not stain her clothing and bedding, avoiding their public exposure—all of which combine to suggest that despite the religious perception of the menstruating woman (*niddah*) as unclean, her intense engagement with the ritual of cleanliness is a purifying act in itself. Therefore, if the practice of the *ʿādah* can be considered a cleansing act representing the Karaite society at large, the woman emerges not as unclean but as doubly clean. The more she internalizes the stains of culture, the more she scrubs and cleanses herself. It is through the changing of pads, and the close administering to dirt and defilement, that the abstract notion of impurity accumulates its clear imagery, color, and odor for the young woman. Washing the *fūtah* is, in fact, the practice that physically forces the woman to be in touch with her impurity. If impurity is articulated in various ways within the culture, the *fūtah* called for the literal engagement with the stains of culture.

Menarche is the first reading of the social codes that are inscribed on women's bodies, the time when language and physiology merge and converge. Moreover, menarche marks the place where language becomes the action of everyday life, where rules are translated into practice. With the first drop of blood, the *'ādah* materializes its own condition, substantiates the notion of impurity, and presupposes the appearance of the *niddah* and the disappearance of the young girl. Equally powerful, touching objects and being touched by the woman with the *'ādah* bring forth and give concrete essence to the abstract notion of dirt.

Miriam

On a sunny Sunday afternoon at Miriam's house, with Sophia, her son Benjamin, Renee, Miriam's sister-in-law, and Susana, Miriam's daughter, I was reminded of the fact that the mother-daughter relationship originates in and is controlled by the discipline of patriarchal values, suggesting that in the case of a disrupted chain, a new alternative voice might emerge.

RUTH [to Miriam]: You told me last time that you did not keep the rules of the *'ādah* so much. I mean ...

MIRIAM: *Al-'ādah?*

RUTH: That it was not so important to you.

MIRIAM: Yes. Me? Yes.

RUTH: You did not grow up religious?

MIRIAM: No, no, no. My father, he did not let me do it. . . . And since I got married, I . . . just . . . nobody knows about it [the period].

RUTH: Secret!?

MIRIAM: Secret.

RUTH: So you were very private?

MIRIAM: I don't want anybody to know about that. It was my two brothers-in-law in the house, my father-in-law, why [should] they know about that too? [It's] enough. I live with them in the same house. It's too much for me.

SOPHIA: So, how were you doing that, Miriam?

MIRIAM: I keep it in secret.

SOPHIA: So, but wait a minute, they know, naturally, you must have your period once a month.

MIRIAM: I know, they know, but they don't know the time.

RUTH: They did not tell you: "you have to be out"?

SOPHIA: But how can you do it, how can you go into the kitchen? [*Sophia is referring to the fact that menstruating women are prohibited from going into the kitchen to cook or serve themselves food.*]

MIRIAM: I got . . . I don't let them know because I don't want them to separate me from the kitchen. I do nothing.

SUSANA: You never went to the kitchen, anyway.

After a short discussion about not cooking and entering the kitchen we continued:

RUTH: So for you, because you already gave up your privacy living with a large family, you wanted to make sure that they will not tell you what to do about the *'ādah*, that you will do whatever you want.

MIRIAM: Yes. Sure. Don't know, I don't know, I don't let nobody know because I was scared.

SUSANA: She was afraid.

RENEE: Ah.

SUSANA: She was afraid, my mother.

MIRIAM: They going to tell me: "Stay here," and "stay there," "don't touch this," "don't sit here," "don't do that," "don't do this." I said: "What for? I am married to Abraham. Let them give me orders?"

RUTH: So you lived with all your husband's family?

MIRIAM: Yes.

RUTH: And this was much more strict than your family that you grew up with, [and] that's why it was harder to adjust.

MIRIAM: Exactly. Yeah.

RUTH: I see. And you didn't really want them to tell you what to do in your life . . .

MIRIAM: Uh-huh.

SUSANA: Which they did. They did.

SOPHIA: If they could, they would have done it.

SUSANA: My grandfather protected her all the time. My grandfather protected her all the time.

RENEE: They wanted to do something to you?

SUSANA: No, no, no.

RUTH: You just wanted to protect yourself?

MIRIAM: Yeah. Not from the women that were with me in the house. I was ashamed from my brothers-in-law.

Miriam's account revealed a different approach to the *'ādah*, one that was inspired by a lack of menstrual education. Growing up with her father, an engineer whose work took him away from Cairo, Miriam spent her childhood in a nonurban, agricultural village, open to non-Karaite influence. A new protesting voice emerges as she narrates her subversive approach to the practice of the *'ādah*. Miriam's description of that period depicts how the female chain of purity is disrupted once maternal teaching is unavailable to a girl; she becomes isolated from the Karaite community, and the transmission of knowledge is left to her father. When Miriam moved to her husband's extended family, she found her new residential arrangement too challenging and consuming. The voice of Renee, who lost her mother when she was seven years old, is mostly excluded from the conversation, as she was probably even less informed about the subject and more excluded from the discursive ritual itself in her youth. She did not remember well how she approached it. Enveloped by paternal love and protection, Miriam remained excluded from her own female tradition. For whatever unstated reason, Miriam's father obviously did not provide her with the maternalistic education appropriate to Karaite women, and by that omission made her an outsider to her own tradition. On the other hand, the tendency of fathers to be less strict than mothers with their daughters over issues regarding the preservation of traditional rules is interpreted by the two women as an excess of paternal love and protection. Thus, their education was arrested by both fathers' inability to provide or arrange the proper maternal culture, much less with a sense of natural comfort that reduced the anxiety and fears associated with it.

That Miriam's father excluded her from the chain of maternal tradition leads us to ask how this complex feminine discourse plays out within the overall patriarchal tradition and whether they can be reconciled to work together. Men are not entirely outside the discourse. Yet, because the knowledge is so embedded on mothers' tongues and so forcefully engaged with female bodies, mothers' voices and female discourse lack this anxiety, allowing this discourse to be transmitted effectively. By contrast, the father's attempt to teach his daughter about the female body is loaded with contradictory messages. Whereas it seems that there is no normative or natural position for men in this discourse, father-daughter relations are more easily negotiated by and through the mother and other adult females in the house.

Miriam's special circumstances subjectively allowed her to justify not keeping the rules of the *'ādah*. Marriage and patrilocal residency in the extended family household (consisting of several males) further aggravated the absence of other females. Miriam feared that she might be subjected to her male housemates' demands, which she experienced as arbitrary and fearful, and that they could expose her as lacking the proper Karaite education. Miriam's account leaves the situation somewhat ambiguous: one can posit that the men with whom she shared a home as a young woman must have known that she was menstruating yet did not dare (or were unwilling) to make a point about the proper maintenance of the taboos. Like her father, Miriam's husband colluded in maintaining this scheme of silence as well. This case tells us that men's responsibility regarding bodily purification is limited.

Above all, Miriam raises a voice that makes the violation of purity laws seem justified once we realize how privacy is subjectively violated. True, Miriam's malpractice contaminates other women's practice of the *'ādah*; she transgresses family purity, yet her claim that she herself is violated by the family, specifically through the interference of males, and her fear that their demands have no limits, gains a sympathetic ear even among the women listening to her in astonishment.

Indeed, listening to the different women, it became obvious that in spite of multivalent women's voices narrating menstruation, the ABCs of the *'ādah* are, as Na'imah explained it, *lāzim bayn al-bint wa-'ummahā*, "between a mother and her daughter." Since their religious backgrounds were diverse and since their mothers had different approaches to the subject of the *'ādah*, I presented several versions of the practices and different explanations for their consideration. Several factors help to explain women's diversity: objective factors such as age, formal education, residential arrangements and space division, economic status (wealthy Karaites used to hire Muslim housekeepers), and geographic location. Yet in spite of this multivocality, a distinctive thread is woven throughout the Kara'iyot's narration of the *'ādah*, revealing that mother-daughter teaching, however limited in scope, is institutionalized as a guide to the Torah's rules of purity and impurity of the *niddah*. Although not all women actually read the text, their mothers "read" it by the mere fact of following their own mothers who followed the rules. The oral tradition of women represents in the Kara'iyot's context an oral reading not of the text necessarily but rather that of their own mothers.

Whereas Rabbanite Jews compiled the oral tradition and canonized it, the Karaites, because of their political stance that rejected oral tradition, put their efforts into consolidating the written canon, and as a result did not develop an oral code comparable to Rabbanite oral tradition. However, along with the men's discourse concerning teaching and reading the Bible, the Kara'yiot's discourse also has an oral component that is physical and concrete. Unlike the traditional rabbi-pupil paradigm for transmitting knowledge among patriarchal males, the Karaite mother-daughter paradigm is one through which knowledge is transmitted by unofficial borrowing from the practical wisdom of everyday life. Indeed, modernity and modernization further increase the tendency to invent new compromises with the rigid text, facilitating a hybrid solution that, on one hand, makes it possible to cope with modern life and, on the other, maintains the core of what is considered Karaite identity. Purity and impurity are tactics of everyday life in which women are endlessly developing ways to conform to the social body by appropriating the individual body.

The subject of menarche and the menstrual period plays a central role in the Karaite mother-daughter discourse of teaching. In its detailed routine, this discourse reinforces the practical language of everyday engagement with the physical body. While this discourse of the body details the contours and contents of impurity, it actually enlists a unique method of governing the impure individual body in order to maintain the clean social body. But more than the production of the clean social body, the discourse of purity is based on the stained "pages" of the Kara'it, and on her ability to "read" them in order to mobilize the tradition of reproducing "pure" Karaite bodies.

The Karaite-woman reads: if she reads the texts, she also reads her body, the blood. In her culture, maternal reproduction is inseparable from the maternal conception of knowledge. Both are exercised in the female domain around the body, and both are originated, informed, and shaped by the textual, religious lesson. In Karaite culture, the embodied sex-gender system becomes the corporeal locus of cultural meaning, and motherhood emerges as its unpublished, unwritten textbook of womanhood.

5
"Please, No Handshaking": Quantifying the Arbitrary Body

> [T]he story of man's travels through his own texts remains in large measure unknown.
> Michel de Certeau, *The Practice of Everyday Life*

They stand at the entrance near the cluster of women's, men's, and children's dress shoes. Their body posture is telling: they appear almost humble, clasping their hands behind their backs, as if to remind themselves not to extend them instinctively to shake hands with the guests. Craning their necks, they peek into the big hall, trying to catch as much as possible of the scene they are missing. "They" are a small group of women that includes Rebecca, Rosa (the Israeli), and another visitor, all of whom chose to participate in the event in spite of the fact that they would have to remain outside. I join them for a while. When the women realize that they had pushed too far inside the room, they retreat back into the corridor. Today, at her son's bar mitzvah, Rebecca can participate only from this place.

Rebecca's expression is somewhat distant and wistful. Her words reveal more than her face: "I counted again and again to make sure that in Josh's bar mitzvah I would be clean and able to participate. But I made a mistake. Here I am. I cannot shake hands with people. I stand here like . . . like . . . I don't know . . . and cannot be inside. But I am telling you, I counted again and again and was sure that today I would be clean." In part, she is telling me what happened since I, swept up in the general excitement of the celebration, came to greet her, extending my hand to meet hers. She is also retelling the story to herself so that she can figure out where she went wrong. Since Rebecca is the one who chose the date of the bar mitzvah after long calculation, she cannot stop blaming herself. She should have been able to better predict her monthly cycle, she supposes. Several other women in our group look at her with sympathy. Although they also happen to have their period today, they understand that to be the menstruating mother of the bar mitzvah boy is an irreconcilable misfortune.[1]

Rebecca, like all Karaite women, counts. She counts her bleeding into days, believing that the days of bleeding—in fact, that the entire period of bleeding—is easily broken into countable, repetitive units. If wrong, she feels that she should be held accountable; after all, *she* made the mistake in her calculations. But is everything a matter of being simply countable? Or is there something in counting that makes for not just an "accounting" (in terms of responsibility) but that holds the key to decoding an additional Karaite narrative that is articulated in the process of counting? The central issue now is how impurity is counted and how the Karaite narrative of counting reconstitutes boundaries and spaces of purity and impurity. With each act of counting, the Karaite woman narrates her story. This chapter examines the measures of women's impurity. It asks, what are its units? Who counts? And along what scales? I emphasize the specific concerns that emerge from counting impurity in the context of communal worship of the synagogue. The numerical discourse of the Karaite body is expressed in terms of the bodily calendar in female personal life. I thus follow Kara'iyot's commentary on Leviticus (12:1–7), according to which a woman is impure for forty days after the delivery of a son and eighty days after that of a daughter. Ways of rationalizing counting and calendars can explain how text and body function as mutually referential sources. For the Kara'it, counting days is a personal, intimate discourse. It regulates her public appearance and disappearance, providing standards for marked biography and mapped geography.

The root *spr* in Hebrew means both "to narrate" and "to count." The semantic connection of the two meanings is highlighted in the active participle, *sopher*, which can mean both "a scribe," for whom writing religious texts requires careful setting of letters and accurate calculation of space, and "a person who counts numerically." But, more interesting, the acts of *sipper* "to tell" and *saphar* "to count" are juxtaposed; counting is a practice that can generate a narrative, and, any given set of numbers in a sequence of signification results with a contextual story, especially if these numbers correspond with time and history.[2]

It is important to emphasize the centrality of counting and calculation in the Karaite annual calendar and its relationship to the identity it generates. Calendars define time and space, regulates cyclical conduct, and turns arbitrary units and orders into a linear process of signification. Even the simple act of counting people, as Karaites believe, is an action reserved to God. Humans must not be counted, and thus Karaites do not take a census. The centrality of the Karaite calendar in family life is evident in the *ke-*

tubbah (marriage contract) of mixed Egyptian Karaite-Rabbanite couples, dating back to the eleventh and twelfth centuries, and codifies cultural differences between the two groups. There are several *ketubbot* from the *genizah*s in Israel and Egypt, written in Aramaic or Hebrew and published and discussed by later scholars of Karaism. They are an excellent resource for examining the challenge of interfaith marriage at that time. One such *ketubbah* carefully enlists the obligations of the husband (Rabbanite) toward his wife (Karaite) in issues concerning dietary, sexual, and calendary differences:

> He shall not bring into his house, as long as she is his wife, the fat tail, or the two kidneys, or the large lobe of liver, or the flesh of a pregnant animal, or the bread of Gentiles or their wines and their abominations. Further, he shall not light a candle on Shabbat eves and there shall be no fire in his house during the Shabbats. He shall not sleep with her on Shabbats and festivals the way he does on weekdays, and he shall not make her desecrate the [true] festivals of the Lord of Hosts as they fall in accord with lunar observation and the finding of *abib* [ear of barley] in Palestine. For she belongs to the people of the Scripture ['*anshei Mikra*' = Karaites] and adheres to their religious principles. (Ankori 1959, 297)[3]

Counting is a discourse that underscores and further reinforces Karaite philosophy, ethics, and aesthetics into a numerical matrix that materializes numbers with referential obligations. "Referential obligations," according to Scarry, make a claim about the relation between language and material, between index and order, and cultural meaning (1988, vii–xxvii). Practices of counting often developed in vernacular oral traditions of measuring and children's games and rhymes. But scholars have paid considerable attention to the fact that calendars are a "social segregative" (Zerubavel 1981, 70–100) that mark identities and symbolize group cohesiveness through differentiation. It is not surprising, therefore, to find that calendars have played a central role in the negotiation of identity politics between minorities (such as Ethiopian Jews or Samaritans) in Israel, in the past as well as in the present.[4]

All manner of contested issues seem to find their expression through specific timekeeping tactics. Although for the Karaites the Bible has provided the precise temporal index of counting, calendrics and the calculation of the year kept Karaite scholars preoccupied throughout the ages. Whereas the Rabbanite calendar was fixed in the Middle Ages such that it could be calculated in advance, the Karaite calendar was always open to the monthly witnessing of the New Moon for *Rosh Chodesh*, the annual reporting and the intercalation of the leap year and of the ripening of the ears of the barley (*abib*), thus keeping Jerusalem as the ultimate reference point throughout Karaite life in the Diaspora (Ankori 1959, 292–93). But beside the different calendars, the debates between Karaites and Rabbanites are based on the question of how one determines when to start counting and then over when Shabbat and holidays actually fall. If, for example, the date of Yom Kippur is different in the Karaite calendar than in the Rabbanite, it suggests that one method of counting is erroneous (and likewise the theology and philosophy associated with it). Thus, it is around the annual calendar that we find one of the most contested pillars of Jewish religious thought. Briefly, the calculation of the year in the Karaite annual calendar initially began with the "spring principle" in the month of Nisan, which is early spring in Israel. The Karaites determined that the New Year may occur on any day of the week,[5] but the counting of the seven weeks preceding the Festival of Weeks (Shavu'ot) begins on Sunday, the day after the Saturday of Passover (whereas Rabbanites count from the second day of Passover). As a result, the Karaite celebration of Shavu'ot always falls on Sunday (forty-nine days plus the day of the holiday itself).

In Rabbanite-Karaite relations throughout history, calendars became a distinctive feature of collective identity that allude to the halakhic disparity and have marked differently the festivals of each group. Ankori maintains that "the history of any religious sect, whatever the latter's time and brand, is to a great extent a history of its calendar deviations. For such deviations have always been the most outstanding symptoms of the sect's break with its normative environment or with the general body to which its members adhered originally" (Ankori 1959, 293). Accordingly, Karaites' political position of "sectarian counter-institutionalism" is the reason for the different calendars that Rabbanites and Karaites developed, both as a reflection of the rift between the two as well as a contested force that keeps widening the sociopolitical rift between them (Ankori 1959, 293). And thus, "the differences of calendar ... seal the separatist trend and constitute the group's final declaration of self determination and independence." Differences of calendation—similar to the woman counting her days of impurity—are, more precisely, the result of the different reading of the text.

But beyond the calendar's immense symbolic power with regard to the emblematic unity of the people of Israel, calendars have a concrete, tangible impact on the immediate outlining of conduct that they generate. Indeed, the conflict of two distinctly different calendars resulted in religious controversy and accusation, shifting the calendar's synchronic linearity into a diachronic rivalry (Kashani 1978, 76; Halevi 1988b; Mahler 1949).[6]

It is revealing, for example, that Saadia, the Karaites' most vocal opponent, was also the person who fixed the Rabbanite calendar (Kashani 1978). The Egyptian Rabbanite Rabbi Shmuel Vital, in his responsum written in 1657, complains, "And on our holiday they [Karaites] do work publicly in order to humiliate us in front of the world.... We tell them: 'We celebrate the holiday like you by looking at the moon'... and they eat *hamets* [leaven] on the last day [the eighth day] of Passover following our calculation, and they eat on Yom Kippur" (Asaf 1936, 225). Well aware that the calendar had the potential either to unify or to divide Jewish culture, Kashani concludes his monograph *The Karaites: History, Tradition and Customs* with a call to demolish the partitions and unify the tribes of Israel through highlighting commonalities rather than differences: "As a first step, it seems to me, that if our brothers, the Karaites, would agree to follow the Hebrew calendar, we would, undoubtedly, progress towards bridging the extremes. ... We have no interest in the existence of two religious nations on this earth. Only by celebrating the holidays on the same dates will the torn fabric be mended, the generational animosity will dissolve, and the miracle of the fusion of the Karaites and Rabbanites will occur" (Kashani 1978, 77).[7]

Today, the Karaites use the Internet to distribute "New Moon Reports" with the exact time and location at which the new moon was observed and the names of the witnesses, the time of the beginning of the Shabbat, the dates of holidays, and other related concerns. The knowledge, commitment, and meticulous work of Nehemia Gordon, the cofounder of the newsletter *The Karaite Korner*, in Jerusalem, is highly appreciated among the Bay Area Karaites, who rely heavily on his Web site.

A Karaite Bar Mitzvah

Quite some time had passed since I last drove to Foster City for a Karaite Shabbat service. When I arrived I realized that an important event was taking place inside; rather than using the usual small study room, located by the back entrance of the building, the Karaites had made a special arrangement with the Rabbanite Conservative synagogue to use the main sanctuary. The hall was huge and full of people, excited and talkative. Everyone was especially well dressed. The warm, early June wind was a promising sign of another beautiful day on the peninsula.

As I noted at the onset of this chapter, I stayed with the women outside the sanctuary. Soon after, they became engrossed in their conversations, moving smoothly from one subject to the next, and forgot about their restricted entry into the sanctuary. Rosa raves about the comfort of having a separate bed while menstruating, even though it has been many years since she reached menopause. The women smile ambivalently. Not everyone sleeps in a separate bed. The conversation moves to children.

Even from outside, I can sense the excitement in the big hall. Looking in, I can see that it is filled with adults and children, for Karaites have traveled from afar to join the festive occasion, adding to the joyfulness of the gathering. Present are not only the usual family members coming from Chicago, New York, and San Diego but also men and women from other Karaite congregations in France, Israel, and the East Coast who will partake in the approaching singles' summer camp, planned for the end of the month in Lake Tahoe. Today there is even an unexpected surprise for all of us: Linna, a Karaite in her mid-thirties, is here in her first visit from Warsaw, hoping to be introduced to single Karaite men. People in the community are thrilled. As the Karaites compare halakhic details, ways of celebrating holidays and rules of *taharah* (purity), they realize that they have much in common with Linna. She is not a stranger. Several women come to the entrance to tell us excitedly about her.

At a typical Shabbat service there are always a few menstruating women; they keep themselves otherwise occupied, with partial preparations for the meal and a relaxed talk in the synagogue's kitchen. The Bay Area Karaite community is slowly adapting to the needs of modern life, allowing menstruating women to be around the food, even if they cannot enter the prayer room. The other women in the prayer room tend to actively underplay the presence of these women, acknowledging them only at the end of the service. Many women, knowing that they cannot participate in the prayers and must remain outside the prayer room, prefer to stay home if they happen to have their periods. On more important occasions, the festivity of the event, the lights, the special clothing, and the big crowd somehow make the menstruating women blend in. Nevertheless, even as a "natural" part of the celebration, they keep their distance.

It has been a long time since so many Karaites gathered together. There is an expansive, festive atmosphere enhanced by the nice clothing, the celebratory mood, and good weather. People catch up on recent developments in the lives of others whom they have had no chance to see for a while; the couple from Chicago just came back from a trip to Israel, the son of another California family is going to study at Berkeley next year. Many nod their heads, agreeing that time goes by too fast. The young generation is moving on—and a bar mitzvah is exactly about that.

Josh, the bar mitzvah boy, is surrounded by his friends—boys in white shirts and short haircuts. He walks around looking serious, though enthusiastic. Today his ability to read will be tested, and since he is an impressive

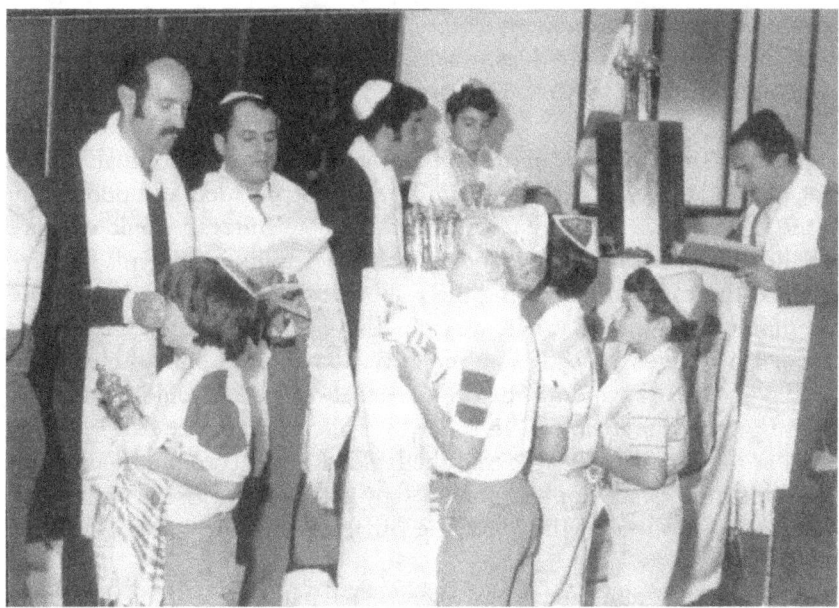

Children celebrating Simchat Torah at a private home, c. 1986. Each one is holding a small, personal Torah. (Photo courtesy of Remy Pessah)

and proficient Hebrew reader, he is less nervous than previous bar mitzvah boys. This ceremony highlights Karaites' efforts to teach children, both girls and boys, to read and sing the Hebrew prayers. The bar/bat mitzvah, borrowed by American Karaites from the Rabbanites, has become the most important individual rite of incorporation, initiating boys and girls into Karaism by having them recite their biblical *parashah*, Torah portion, out loud in front of the community. As in contemporary Rabbanite culture, the child's portion of the reading becomes his or her private text. The congregation's response at the end of Josh's reading provides evidence of his ability to master his text and to read it gracefully. It is obvious that everyone takes pride in his performance. The older woman at my side quietly mumbles a blessing, something against the evil eye. Josh is initiated into the community; he, like the other adults, is now a "reader." He has proven it in front of the entire congregation.

"Teaching reading Hebrew took three to four years," Sophia tells me; her son's memorable bar mitzvah is still fresh in my mind. "Last year, the boys prepared to conduct the whole service. It took a lot of preparation in terms of learning to read not only fluently [the Hebrew text] but also learning the specific Karaite melodies, which meant a lot to Sol, their father. The Torah was shared, as usual, in reading. The boys did not give a speech only because they were so absorbed in learning the Service and the Torah."

Sophia continues her digression on the bar/bat mitzvah ritual, noting that in Egypt, the gathering at Simchat Torah provided an opportunity to the children to read. "We felt that having a bar mitzvah would encourage the kids to learn Hebrew and to read the Torah. So the pros far outweighed the cons [of borrowing the Rabbanite ritual]." Other kids in the community had their bar/bat mitzvah. They learned Hebrew in Sunday schools in different, mostly Conservative, Rabbanite Sunday schools, in the Bay Area. A few months before the event, the rabbi would spend time teaching them the melodies. In order to facilitate the process of learning, Karaites distribute audiotapes that the Israeli Karaite community prepares and ships from Israel. Sophia concluded by noting that girls have bat mitzvahs but do not mount the *bima*, the ritual stage in the synagogue. They read a lot of songs."

The monthly and, later, weekly communal gatherings on Shabbat regulate the social interaction around the reading of the Torah and its distinct Karaite music, facilitating a strong sense of community and family belonging. The pedagogical efforts to weave the Torah with the Karaite narrative present to the children a space to nurture their identity and to make biblical narratives available. Simchat Torah, which occurs on Shmini Atseret, the last day of Sukkot, celebrates the joy of the revelation of the Torah on Mount Sinai. In addition to marking the conclusion of the annual cycle of the Torah reading, the Karaites make special efforts to incorporate the children in the reading of the Torah from an early age. The eve of Simchat Torah is an exciting culmination of the children reading the Torah. The parents and other adults gather excitedly around a wide circle of dancing children who each carry a small, private, ornamented Torah. Each child demonstrates in turn her or his ability to read Hebrew while standing on a stool at the center of the circle; the adults cheer and praise the children. The room is full of clapping, laughing, and words of encouragement and acknowledgment. The young children, especially the boys who have recently celebrated their bar mitzvahs, are the stars of the evening.

The Measure of Blood and Its Schedule

Time frames ritual. It is the central factor that organizes and structures the Karaite female narrative. Although the body defines a spatial matrix of purity and impurity, its temporal aspect—governed by the monthly appearance of the blood—becomes explicit with the rationale of counting. An erroneous calendar is corrupted and corrupting, and could lead to different practices of purity and impurity: the beginning of the Shabbat, the end of the *niddah*'s days of separation, each delineate the pure/impure temporal aspect of the law. The gendered calendar of the woman states that, unlike man, her presence is not always appropriate at religious services. Her periodic menstruation magnifies female cyclicality (as opposed to perceived male stability) and manifests her body within the overall reproductive scheme that disciplines her body (Lander 1988, 102). In the case of women, quantifying the blood and counting its duration is believed to be a strictly textual matter, although in reality, the body is the primary index, and reading involves both the text and the body. In that sense, the oral tradition of women who have been engaged in counting and recounting their bodies is an extension of the textual. Counting days regulates a personal calendar in which annual social events, religious prohibitions, and individual freedom are all marked with meaning.

The Karaite reading of Leviticus makes explicit that a woman's calendar consists of seven days of impurity. The personal narratives of counting reconstitute these temporal boundaries within the personal space of purity and impurity. They aim to preserve the purity of the husband and the community as a whole. Unlike annual cycles and life cycles, the female calendar corresponds intimately with the personal biological life of the female body and the cultural meaning attached to it. Practically, menstrual taboos remove women from the social centers of activity, be it the Torah, the synagogue, the kitchen, the bedroom, the shower, or the main holiday table.

Elaine Scarry's analysis of practices of counting help elucidate Karaite women's fastidious interest in quantification:

> On the one hand, counting makes an extreme claim about its correspondence with the material realm. It asserts a one-to-one correspondence between itself and its subject matter: its vocabulary exists solely to register increases and decreases in the content it calibrates. Its proximity to the physical is also indicated by its inseparability from the body. The act of counting *is* an act, and was called this even before language came to be understood as speech acts. People who count tend to do so with their bodies (tapping a finger; bobbing the head; bouncing the entire body slightly as they number the people around the room); it is as though the existence of matter must be registered in matter itself. On the other hand, numbers and numerical operations are, presumably with good reason, habitually thought of as abstract, as occupying a space

wholly cut off from the world. Even forms of counting that claim to have worldly content sometimes seem instead characterized by the complete lack of it: The "body count" in war is a notoriously insubstantial form of speech. Because numbers fall at both extremes of the spectrum, they provide a useful way of illustrating the more general capacities of language. (Scarry 1988, viii)

On one extreme of the continuum, according to Scarry, one might find a language that is empty; on the other extreme, one might find a language that is loaded with referential obligations. Counting is a form of reference to the materiality of the body, a cognitive, objective precursor that corresponds to its interior. With its ritualistic significance, Karaite counting corresponds to the meaning of impurity as a "language that is loaded with referential obligation" (ibid.). It emphasizes the relevance of purity to sexual life, sleeping habits, the preparation and eating of food, visits to the synagogue, and mourning the dead; it gains further significance as it materializes women's discourse in the conduct of socioreligious life. Perhaps because of its matter-of-factness and repetitiveness, and perhaps because a woman is unconditionally expected to follow it, counting is taken for granted. But in fact, counting attributes agency to the body; it is the scale that provides measurable data. These quantitative data are loaded with referential obligations by virtue of their qualitative value. Careful scrutiny of the body, or the acquired knowledge of reading the immediate body in countable units, is a way in which the abstract, arbitrary notion of *tum'ah*, impurity, is concretely inscribed in Karaite practices.

Notably, counting is the act by which Karaite women measure not their bodies but, more precisely, their blood. In its uncontrolled and uncontained flow out of the body, this blood threatens to blur bodily boundaries, and to demolish society's order (Douglas 1966; Kristeva 1982; Boddy 1989; Delaney 1991). Once society attaches quantitative measurements to the uncontrolled body, it becomes countable. Quantifying the immeasurable bleeding body tames the blood. By introducing the temporal aspect, divided into days and marked by the sunset, the impure body, temporarily banished, is quantified (it is predicated on these units). The materials of the body gain aesthetic, moral, social, and religious meaning because the units are controlled. The body is a timer, an alarm clock that brackets the female condition of impurity. Counting of time becomes the conceptual metaphor that guards women from impurity.

The discourse of counting and social calendars does not operate only in the external realm of Karaite life. As opposed to the objective, arbitrary annual calendars, women's counting and bodily timetables are intimately connected to the issues of family role, sexuality, and reproduction; and perhaps more important, they determine the state of a woman's purity and impurity. According to Leviticus, *tum'at niddah*, the impurity of the menstruating woman, lasts seven days (Leviticus 18).[8] The text's normative time of impurity defines both normative cycles as much as anomalous deviations. The fact that impurity is marked by the first drop of blood and lasts seven days requires a woman to be a careful observer of her own body, for this minimal measure, a drop of blood, further disciplines the personal calendar that divides "time up into bounded units not in order to count and total them but to describe and characterize them, to formulate their differential, social, intellectual, and religious significance" (Geertz 1973, 391). Moreover, according to Leviticus, a woman who bleeds longer than seven days is no longer considered a *niddah* but *a zavah*, a woman with any kind of discharge, and should maintain another seven days of impurity.[9] Thus the Bible constructs impurity according to the duration of bleeding, not by discriminating between different types of blood.[10]

The question remains why the Bible assigns seven days to impurity and not five, six, or eight days since, biologically, the period can last from two to eight or more days.[11] Does the Bible "think" in terms of weeks, as Eviatar Zerubavel (1985) suggests in connection with other occurrences of seven-unit cycles? As a representation of a quantitative unit, the seven-day cycle serves as a mnemonic device; seven is conveniently countable. Its cyclical, repetitive aspect easily converges with the weeks of the annual calendar, which in part is the function of ritual. As Mary Douglas indicates, "Ritual focuses attention by framing; it enlivens the memory and links the present with the relevant past. In all this it aids perception. Or rather it changes perception because it changes the selective principles" (Douglas 1966, 64). Counting in weeks facilitates the counting of the menstrual seven days of impurity, and thinking in weeks encourages the perception of the period as cyclical and promotes structure and orderliness, regularity and periodicity (Zerubavel 1985, 85). Yet the Karaite halakhah attempted to highlight not the repetitive aspect of the week, but rather its progressive aspect, which leads to the purification of the body.

Halevi, following other Karaite sages, explicitly links the seven days of impurity to the linearity of the first week of creation in Genesis 1 (Halevi 1988b). First, he makes a distinction between the historical week, which alludes to the creation story in Genesis, and the metaphoric week, which refers to any seven consecutive days, commencing in the Karaite division from Saturday evening. Second, he differentiates this week from other "cyclical movement(s) astronomically speaking, like the month and the year, which move from one specific point and return to it. And all that because

God created all that exists in six days, and on the seventh day he stopped and rested" (Halevi 1988b, 26). The Karaites' reading of the "week" is in fact analogous to their reading of the Passover, making similar distinctions between "*Pessah Mitsrayim*" and "*Pessah Dorot.*" *Pessah Mitsrayim* is the event that happened in Egypt; it is linear, progressive, and historical, whereas *Pessah Dorot* is the instituted and celebrated Passover throughout generations; it is cyclical and reverts back to the past. Karaite sages were careful in following the instructions that the Bible provides as to how to read and to distinguish between the two, using it as a conceptual paradigm of approaching stability and change, past memory and future aspirations. In that regard, the week as a category of time produces change. Halevi's words follow the spirit of Leviticus, which does not aim necessarily to conceptualize *niddah* as a cyclical event; rather, he focuses on linear progressive time, which suggests a transition from pure to impure, and from menstruation to pregnancy. Counting to seven, as part of the overall attempt to frame impurity, focuses further attention on the boundaries of clean and unclean; it also marks its norm and deviation. Nadia stated very clearly: "After seven days, if the woman is not clean she will wait another seven days. For example, I got [the period] today. If I have blood [at the end of the seven days], I will wait seven days more."

Women expressed their discomfort with the idea of having fourteen-day periods. Most Karaite women attest in their interviews that a menstruation of more than seven days is undesirable since it forces the woman to conform to the rules of menstruation for fourteen days, even if the woman stops bleeding on the eighth day. Adding another seven days to the seven-day period changes the status of the woman from *niddah* to *zavah*, and transforms what is perceived as normal bleeding into abnormal.

At one of our group meetings, Leah, who experienced many periods of such long duration, recounts, "All this week the blood was very very hard, all seven days. I cannot help myself. Every two or three hours I put another one. Every two, three hours ... and after seven days it doesn't stop, more than ... fifteen days." Leah highlights the number fifteen. She speaks with intensity, pausing to see the effect of her story on the other women. The women respond with sympathy. One nods her head, "tsk, tsk, tsk," and another says: "*Ḥarām* [alas]."

Leah continues: "And she [my mother] took me to the doctor and he told her it will go away alone. 'I cannot help her.' Because years ago they could not help. Every month, every month, it comes okay. . . . But two weeks, two weeks. More than a week, two weeks. And it lasted till [I was] sixty-five. Till sixty-five."

Sophia's description indicates that her mother's instructions regarding the time of the period follow Leviticus exactly. Moreover, Karaite halakha elaborates on the quality of Saturday as a day on which purification cannot be performed, thereby introducing the rule of counting eight days. Other women mentioned the counting of eight days even when the menses do not begin on the Shabbat in order to make sure that the counting is correct. As with the Rabbanite approach, women are almost overly careful to follow the rules. Sophia notes:

> When a girl has her menstruation she is not considered clean during the seven days. Whether she is bleeding during all the seven days is not the point. She is still considered unclean. After the seven days she can take a shower and would be considered clean. The shower should be taken in the afternoon and she won't be considered clean to go to the temple until after sunset. There is no *tahara* [purification] on Saturday, so if we have [got] our period on Sunday we [are] supposed to be clean on [the next] Saturday. We have to stay one more day.

That impurity and dirt are issues of time was reflected in Sophia's comment: "Let's say I got stained and I didn't change or even without being stained I didn't change my pad for 3–4 hours. I will smell. So realistically it is really dirty."

Forty/Eighty Days of Confinement: Quantifying Gender

The act of giving birth redefines the Kara'it; the *wālidah* is a woman who has recently delivered a baby, and her body is a new site of impurity. On the one hand, she is considered *tame'ah*, contaminated and contaminating because of her postpartum bleeding. As a result of her impurity, her physical mobility and social interaction are restricted. Still in practice among the Bay Area Karaites to varying degrees are the prohibitions against a *wālidah*'s entering the synagogue, visiting the cemetery, and having sexual intercourse for fear of contaminating the husband, who then might himself enter the synagogue in a state of impurity. The new mother herself is considered vulnerable, since her body is now active in the production of milk and there is considerable concern on her part and the community's in regard to protecting her milk. The evil eye, other lactating women, and especially a menstruating woman's presence can reduce the flow of milk or even stop it altogether (see chapter 7 of this volume).

In spite of the many concessions that modern life has imposed on the Karaite legal code, at least as far as the synagogue is concerned, Karaites make a communal effort to keep the impurity of the *wālidah* away from it. The Bible draws a distinction between the seven days of *niddah*-like separation and thirty-three additional days of impurity (forty) following the birth of a son, and fourteen days and sixty-six additional ones (eighty) following the birth of a daughter.[12] This distinction is simplified by Karaites to forty or eighty days of impurity.[13]

At one of the Shabbat services, Rina and her husband, David, arrived with their newborn son. They were greeted kindly by everyone present. Rina is a Rabbanite Jew who emigrated in the late seventies from Iran and later married David, a Karaite man, in California. On this special visit, her mother, who lived in Los Angeles, accompanied her to the synagogue. Inside the prayer room there was immediately a sense of uneasiness; women started gathering in the back of the room, whispering to each other. When I came out of the room I saw Rachel, a woman in her fifties, speaking with Rina. They were just starting to discuss the *ʿādah* and its rules in the Karaite context when I joined them. Rachel, very cordially and amicably, asked Rina if she knew about the *ʿādah* and what it means. I did not at first realize what the problem was, because *ʿādah* is a generic name for women's bleeding; here, however, it was postpartum bleeding that was the issue. Rachel did not speak much beyond mentioning the term, mostly responded to my questions with one-word replies. It appeared that she was now speaking more to me than to Rina, perhaps thinking that I could help convey to Rina this delicate matter that she herself did not feel comfortable doing. Knowing that I was studying the *ʿādah*, Rachel presumed that I would more easily find the words to address it; this was especially true given that both Rina and I were Rabbanites, and so perhaps would find it less difficult to discuss the subject. Clearly they wanted Rina to stay outside with the menstruating women, but they were afraid of hurting her feelings; indeed, when she understood the situation she *was* hurt and angry but consented to leave the room. She and her husband took the baby, the baby carrier, bag, and toys and went outside.

Obviously, the Karaites were upset that Rina had entered the synagogue before the end of the forty days. "It's *ḥarām*," said Lailah with a worried expression on her face. "I remember the circumcision, it was only four weeks ago," said a younger congregant. "It's really not nice to do that," exclaimed another. After the service, sitting on a chair outside, many people, men and women, approached her to play with her son and to say something to soften the atmosphere. During all this, Rina had a discontented expression on her face. She expressed uneasiness at the fact that this taboo was still observed. She mumbled that she knew the rules, but, as far as she was concerned, four weeks had passed and that was enough. Nevertheless, the rest of the community had calculated the days for themselves, and they knew that Rina did not count the full forty days since her son was born.

To a large extent, this incident reveals the cross-cultural, interethnic differences in reading and misreading internal Karaite codes. Rina, a Rabbanite Jew, was not a frequent participant in the Karaite Shabbat services and considered it a mitzvah (commandment) to bring her son to the synagogue. She felt especially proud that she gave birth to a son, and wanted to bring him to the community and share with the others her new maternal state. To Rina, visiting the community along with her mother, who had come for a visit from Los Angeles, was more important than the fact that she was several days away from being considered ritually clean. The fact that the community met only once a month introduced a sense of urgency and contributed to Rina's less precise calculation. The Karaites, however, took offense at what they regarded as a lack of respect for their observance. It is possible that because Rina is a not a Karaite, the women felt especially compelled to educate her and make their point. Yet once Rina was outside the prayer room, and once the purity of the prayer hall was restored, they considered the issue resolved; they allowed themselves to be more personal and friendly with her.[14]

This episode highlights two distinct attitudes toward tradition. The Karaites are serious about the purity of the Torah and the purity of the body beyond personal discomfort or special circumstances. They count days according to the rules of separation. In contrast, Rina's reaction reveals a different attitude: "So what?" she said to me. "Why do they make such a big deal out of it? I know it's not exactly 40 days," apparently unaware that others would count her forty days even if she did not. Being an outsider whose generation is much less conservative and more assimilated, she represents a flexible approach toward tradition. Yet for Karaites, observing tradition means keeping track of precise numbers and fixed units—and educating outsiders who are new to the community. To read, to count as a Kara'it, means not to add or subtract from what is prescribed, but to be exact.

Whereas most Kara'iyot know about the *wālidah* taboo, they were surprised when I asked why a woman is impure for only forty days after the delivery of a son but for eighty days after the delivery of a daughter. Answers such as "I don't know" or "My mother told me that" or "It is in the religion" or "It's in the Bible" were very common. Clearly these replies were inadequate explanations, but tracing their underlying, nonverbal, perhaps unconscious presuppositions, they may provide a deeper understanding of the reasons that substantiate their systems of signification (Bourdieu 1977).

Leviticus does not provide an explanation for the different durations of impurity after the birth of a son as compared with a daughter: any new mother would require the same sacrificial ritual of purification regardless of the child's sex.[15] Thus, the intrinsic uncleanliness—not only of the woman, but also of the newborn girl—is implied, as if the sexual impurity connected with an adult woman is biologically inscribed at birth. In this way, the sex of the baby determines the biblical assessment of the impurity of the mother, as the assignment of gender, or the social construction of sexual differences, is made at birth.[16] Moreover, impurity is defined not only as a qualitative category but is also granted a quantitative dimension. It may be that being impure longer means being *more* impure.

The asymmetric forty/eight formula evokes some discomfort among the women. Although impurity is attributed to the mother, the assumptions that immediately come to mind is that this difference is determined by the symbolic imbalance of sexual difference rather than by the mother who delivers the child. Mother and child cannot be regarded as separate at this stage, and yet is it possible that only the mother is held personally responsible for the ascribed impurity of the newborn?

Julia Kristeva approaches the mother-child as a primary unit. The symbiotic relationship between the mother and the baby, she maintains, provides a necessary psychological stage for the baby to exert its narcissistic needs and for the woman to nurture her body. Leviticus 12 inscribes, according to Kristeva, "a defiled maternality" for the sake of "confrontation with the boundary between the sexes" (Kristeva 1982, 100). From a feminist perspective, circumcision displaces the mother-child alliance with a God-son alliance, and thus violently interferes with relations between the child and the mother. This replacement, described as separating the mother and son, can also explain the difference between male and female impurity. Although Kristeva does not offer an explicit explanation for the difference between forty and eighty days of impurity, she implies that mother-daughter relationships benefit from the difference of forty/eighty days.[17] The taboo provides more time and space for the mother to bond with her daughter, since she would have to avoid relations with her husband in that period. In contrast, male children have a shorter period of exclusive bonding with their mothers on account of their social and religious role.

Rachel Biale, who explores Rabbanite halakhic positions with respect to women, provides another vantage point: "The reason for the doubling of the impure period after the birth of a girl is unclear. Perhaps it reflects, as has been suggested by some, the disappointment with the birth of a girl, but this would necessitate seeing the state of impurity as partially punitive, which does not seem to fit the intentions of Leviticus. One conjecture is that underlying this legislation is the sense that the birth of a female, who will one day herself menstruate and give birth, is seen as 'doubly bloody' and 'doubly impure'" (Biale 1984, 152). The doubling, according to Biale, assumes that the same substance appears twice, or that the basic units are identical but duplicated and thus can be read as a form of parallelism.[18]

Nadia offers yet another rationale for the longer period of impurity after the birth of the female child as prescribed in Leviticus. She, like several other women, believed that women bleed longer after the delivery of a girl: "I think that the mother of the boy gets clean before when she gets a girl.... Before the forty days she does not have any blood." In other words, the birth of a girl involves more bleeding, which in turn lengthens the period of a mother's impurity. For Nadia, as for most other Karaite women, the prescribed period of impurity after the birth of a girl is based on a perceived biological difference in postpartum bleeding. Her theory of difference shifts the subject (and agent) of impurity from the baby girl to her mother's body, in contrast to Biale's theory of doubling. Nadia reads the levitical formula for impurity through a rhetoric of the body (i.e., longer bleeding), thereby privileging the body as a reference that reinforces biblical instructions.

In opposition to the dichotomies that create different identities and highlight the gender gap, the *Kara'iyot* follow the analogy already made in Leviticus between the *yoledah*'s, or birth mother's, impurity and the rules of the *niddah*. Leviticus 12:2 establishes: "If a woman has conceived seed, and borne a man child, then she shall be unclean seven days; according to the days of the separation (*ki-ymei niddat dvotah*) for her infirmity shall she be unclean." This analogy functions, not within a contrasting paradigm of A versus B, but within the context of evolutionary time in which B follows A. Whereas the analogy in this verse explicitly compares the nature of the impurity of the *yoledah* to that of the *niddah* (or more precisely, the *zavah*, Karaite women take the biblical dictates one step further. They imply not only the same quality of impurity but also draw a similar model of counting. The rules of *niddah* and *zavah* provide the rationale for the forty/eighty-day period of impurity that is tied to the reality of seeing postpartum blood, assuming that if they see blood past the fortieth day, the impure period continues for a second consecutive unit of forty days. Presumably, forty days is a counting unit provided by the biblical text.

Conceptualized counting along new scales is facilitated partially by the frequent appearance of "seven" and "forty" as formulaic symbols, as Eviatar Zerubavel (1981, 1985) and Stanley Brandes (1985, 60–61) have each demonstrated. In the same way that the number three, the pattern of trichotomy, has become a native category in Western and American culture (Dundes 1978, 129–58), seven and forty substantiate units of significance in Jewish and Karaite tradition. Accordingly, the number forty in the context of Karaite culture, and especially in the context of women's frequent pregnancies and childbirths, can be read as an internalized cognitive category, corresponding to the bodily language of bleeding. The women believe in the exact correspondence, or even equivalence, of textual and corporeal reality. They see their bodies as an echo of textual truth, and at the same time perceive the text as an accurate reflection of their experiences. Text and body function as mutually referential sources. Meaning flows from the text to the body, but then also from the body back to the text: the inversion of the referential system becomes dialectic.

This dynamic takes on another dimension. The women's textual reading of the body is also a reflection of the social order. Women's social position is not constructed in opposition to that of men, but rather is situated below or behind that of men. As we saw in chapter 2, in the case of the prayer room in Foster City, there was an unspoken general idea of what constituted the borders of this separation, even though there was no partition between the men and the women and both shared a common space. More generally, having their place behind the men articulates a cultural location that constitutes numerous symbolic ramifications beyond the physical setting, or beyond the distinction of sexual and gendered impurity and its calculation.

The position of literal reality also grants some authority to a Karaite woman's religious experience. Even though she is subject to the *law* of her body, the entire community, men and women alike, is also subject to the *rule* of her body. Karaite women undermine the male/female dichotomy by means of an analogy with the rules of the *niddah* as a model provided by the Bible, and create a more manageable understanding that can serve as an alternative that goes beyond dualism.

Counting of days is a personal, intimate dialogue between a woman and her body. Numbers are not abstract units; they are materialized references. Time, for those who count it, becomes an interpreter of the body, for that body reads and translates its abstract units into materialized being. Whereas men look at the moon to articulate the Karaite calendar, women attach a virtual text to the inside of their bodies. It is a precise, literal discourse that binds a woman and her body to society's limits while at the same time defines her boundaries. With the first appearance of blood, she starts to obey the cultural rhythms *as if they were natural*. From then on, a woman's anatomy will guide her autonomy.

Counting in the context of impure blood converts Karaite cultural, philosophical, moral, and aesthetic ethos into a numerical matrix. Each community has its story, and each community has its own index of counting. Counting is an arbitrary discourse that quantifies the body, a story that chronicles Karaites' specific adherence to the text. Women's narratives are produced on the margins and sometimes, as in Rebecca's case, involve miscalculations and errors in reckoning the numerical figures of the body and its processes.

6

The Site of Impurity

> The anxiety of our era has to do fundamentally with space, no doubt a great deal more than with time. Time probably appears to us only as one of the various distributive operations that are possible for the elements that are spread out in space.
> Michel Foucault, "Of Other Spaces"

The site of impurity articulates the meaning of gender difference and its structure. In order to map out the physical relationship between pure and impure, between the menstruating woman and the rest of the community, it is necessary to trace the contours of the impure body. Since the conceptualization of menstruation as uncontained impurity is repeatedly enforced in the Karaite culture, the question becomes: Where does the female body begin and where does it end? This chapter answers these questions by focusing on the Kara'iyot's descriptions of the experience that is produced by the space of impurity, and the strategies that they have developed over time.

Menstrual blood, the signifier of women's bodily condition, is communicative and discursive in that it travels out of the body through a bodily opening (cf. Boddy 1989; Delaney 1988, 1991). The spectacle of the escaping blood shatters the integrity of the body; the now porous body is characterized by its open-ended boundaries and blurred contours. The configuration of the body and its limits has long been an important aspect in people's imagination in their attempt to construct and give form to anomalous people. Such symbolic bodily representation has further contributed to the construction of gender and ethnicity as either (or both) culturally invisible or over-visible (Gilman 1992a, 1992b; Geller 1992). Feminist studies have addressed specifically the dimensions of the symbolic physical female body, as well as the conception of the woman as capable of losing or transcending her corporeal limits (Bynum 1987; Bordo 1989). Often this power is manifested in the earthly (even grotesque) body and its emphasis on reproduction (e.g., D. Boyarin 1992). In its extreme opposite representation, the female body typifies the infinite, superior power of woman as witch, demon, or other supernatural being.[1] Underlying such a portrayal is the ancient social representation of the woman as "dangerous" and "uncontrollable," a construct that is reconciled through religious and other bodily practices that erect formidable boundaries controlling its movement and fixing the woman within a confined space. While the text directs a woman's daily corporeal conduct, it also redefines her and her body in terms of her obedience and submissiveness.

To a certain degree, social distancing functions as a strategy whose motive is the production and reproduction of the existing hierarchy between men and women.[2] Much of the substantial anthropological scholarship on space has been devoted attention to public-space discourses, such as theater, parades, and demonstrations as a form of resistance and political communication. In the context of the Middle East, studies on *kahwa* and narghile houses (e.g., Chaouachi 2003), bazaars and shopping malls (Abaza 2001), tourist villages (e.g., Slyomovics 1998), and local museums (e.g., Katriel 1997) have added to our understanding of public space as a continual productive process of ideology and identity formation(s). Comparatively less attention has been paid to the politics of private spaces or spaces of silence, although work on sexual, political, and other minorities has stimulated an interest in reading silences and opaque references as a way in which to recover bodies and lives disappeared from or diminished in the historical record, public rituals, and/or collective memory. Spaces of silence, and spaces created through silencing, can also be understood as "a potent form of communication" (Margold 1993, 12). Thus, with respect to *niddah*, it is important both to trace the contours of the silencing space of impurity and to consider it as a site where both ambivalence and active agency are produced in a dialectical process of negotiation.

For Foucault "space is where discourses about power and knowledge are transformed into actual relations of power" (Wright and Rabinow 1982, 14). Always a human construct, spaces can be divided into several types. Most interesting for our discussion is Foucault's notion of the *crisis heterotopia*,[3] in which "there are privileged or sacred or forbidden places, reserved for individuals who are, in relation to society and to the human environment in which they live, in a state of crisis." Drawing on Foucault, I wish to ask what specifically constitutes the perennial Karaite crisis over the space of impurity and its relationship to communal space. I also consider how this space of impurity mirrors and amplifies the imagination of purity. As I see it, religious gender identity and the consciousness of impure spaces are conflated: uncleanliness emerges as a materialized notion at the price of immobilizing the menstruating woman.[4] But mobility and immobility are not limited to physical territories. The graphic representation of women's exclusion from and silencing in the social, familial, and sexual scene is of a void in space. In *Practices of Every Day Life*, de Certeau reads spatial practices as movements within the environment or as perambulatory gestures that can be understood as rhetorical tropes, analogous to figures of speech. It is instructive, therefore, to explore the void of women's geographical silence and see what kind of story it tells us.

"After That I Stayed by Myself"

The dry heat of June can really "melt the brain," I thought to myself in Hebrew as I rolled down every window in the car. I was on my way to visit Nadia at her home in Livermore, an hour's drive east from San Francisco. It was the late 1980s and Nadia had just moved from her apartment in the heart of downtown San Francisco to a small house here following her son's divorce,[5] because she wanted to be closer to him. While in San Francisco, Nadia kept a relatively busy schedule of shopping and interacting with other female friends, relying on public transportation, since she did not drive. Now in Livermore, she had become totally dependent on her son or daughter for transportation. As a result, Nadia did not attend Shabbat services or other community events unless she rode with them.

I was looking forward to meeting Nadia at her home. In larger social gatherings, this petite woman tended to "fold" herself, almost disappear, and I was hoping that she would be less inhibited at home where she could express herself more freely. Nadia was among the more formally educated Kara'iyot of her generation. She had wanted to attend medical school but ended up studying philosophy; married in her junior year, she never graduated.[6] In spite of her early interest in medicine, Nadia often expressed frustration with her limited knowledge of the female body.

Shy in public, Nadia exuded forthrightness and courage in private. Though hesitant, she was nevertheless committed to speak about her life. She was the fourth of seven children, of whom the first six are females, suggesting that she grew up in a female-centered household. Throughout most of the conversation Nadia, like Na'imah, uses the pronoun *we*, which could refer to both the girls and women in her home and to Karaite women as a whole. "We" depicts a sense of solidarity and connectedness, and perhaps even a nondiscrete communal construction of female subjectivity.

Nadia's experience of menarche, provided below, reveals some efforts to organize and structure the space of the menstruating woman in the household:

> When I got it, I told my mother, and I had a bath also and she removed everything, because it was in the morning; I got up in the morning and I found out that I have something and my mother took all the sheets and washed everything although I didn't dirty anything but that has to be done. And I think my sister was sleeping with me and she had a shower too. . . . Because she was touching me and sleeping with me. And after that I stayed by myself.

I asked her where. She replied: "Where? In my room."

> RUTH: In a separate . . . ?
> NADIA: Yeah.
> RUTH: Did you have a separate room for each kid like . . .
> NADIA: No. Two sisters sleep in one bed.
> RUTH: So, when you had the period you slept on one bed alone?
> NADIA: Yeah.
> RUTH: So that was a special bed for it, that all the girls used?
> NADIA: Yeah. Everybody had to use it.

What did Nadia mean when she said, "I stayed by myself"? Her expression camouflages the distinction between being alone and being by oneself. Perhaps the fact that Nadia's words were conveyed in a melancholic tone made me pay attention to the literal meaning of her expression, and to the distinction between the speaking "I" and the "self." I understood her to mean "I stayed by my self." Menstrual rules of separation remove women not only from their family, their sisters, or the comfort of their bed, but from their own body. The linguistic split between the self and the body goes back to de Beauvoir's assertion: "Woman, like man, is her body, but her body is something other than herself" (de Beauvoir 1974, 33), whereby the woman is reduced to her body, and to the imposed cultural separation between a woman's body and self. It points to the historical objectification of the female body and to its accumulated layers of separation from people as much as from objects.

Nadia's description of her menarche responds to several of the prohibitions by which a Karaite menstruating woman is confined. Showering and washing the bedding and clothing reflect the desire to limit the contaminated area into which the woman moves at the onset of the period. The objects she touches are considered unclean precisely because impurity is considered contagious and controlling (see also Good 1980, Delaney 1988).[7] Thereafter, she should remain within a designated territory of impurity, complete with its own small dining table, dishes, and bedding. The bedding arrangement is significant. When close in age and of the same sex, young siblings usually shared a bed, but when one was menstruating, she was separated from her sister. Thus, Nadia's sister, who typically shared the bed with her, had to shower even though Nadia had not soiled the bedding. Touching Nadia had also rendered her impure. Throughout married life and until menopause, this act of separation is reconfirmed. So even if today a couple is more permissive and a woman shares her bed with her husband, during her period—as well as on Friday nights and on holidays when sexual intercourse is prohibited—the husband usually moves to his own bed. The woman then sleeps alone in her bed.

I asked Nadia to continue the list of prohibitions that she had to follow while menstruating.

Ruth: And you did not cook, you did not . . .

Nadia: No, no, no. All [that] we do is wash our dishes. . . . And we have to put them in another special place, you can put them in and take them out when we want to, when we are ready to eat.

Ruth: These dishes were special for the one who was menstruating?

Nadia: Yeah. Yeah.

Ruth: It was not for every one in the house?

Nadia: No, no, no. It is a kind [that is] not like the other [one].

Ruth: How?

Nadia: Less fancy. Maybe older. The good set is for everybody and then there are some maybe from previous sets . . .

Ruth: Uh-huh. Older pieces?

Nadia: Yeah.

Ruth: The same for tablecloth?

Nadia: Yeah, yeah.

Ruth: And was it at a different table that you sat?

Nadia: Yeah. At a small table. We had a small table especially for

... the one who has the period.

RUTH: Would someone serve you when you sat near the table?

NADIA: Yes. My mother or any other people who serve us. We got our plates and sat at this table.

Alone by Herself

When I asked Naʿimah to outline the rules of the *ʿādah*, she giggled, though with some bitterness. Mira was making lunch, occasionally participating in the conversation, praising, and commenting on her mother-in-law's words. Mira's respect for Naʿimah and for what she had to say accentuated Naʿimah's authority. A girl who gets her *ʿādah*, she said slowly, "for seven days she should not enter the kitchen."

MIRA: She does not enter the kitchen at all. She cannot touch anything. She cannot touch the kitchen ... the food in the kitchen.

NAʿIMAH: For seven days we bring her [the] food. And if she wants to get into the kitchen? No. No.

MIRA: She is *tameʾa* [impure].

NAʿIMAH: For [the whole] seven days she is not allowed to do anything. She can eat and drink. ... She sits near the table *waḥda waḥdahā* [alone by herself].

Like Nadia, Naʿimah also emphasized the specific location of *niddah*. The Arabic articulation of the adverbial expression *waḥda waḥdahā*, literally, "one with her oneness" or "alone with her aloneness," duplicates and deepens the sense of the separation and loneliness of the girl or woman.

RUTH: Where does she sit?

NAʿIMAH: In the corner.

MIRA: Not in the kitchen, not even in the dining hall. She has to sit in a different corner.

RUTH: What does she wear?

NAʿIMAH: Regular clothing. But whatever she uses for seven days she has to wash.

I reviewed the prohibitions she just mentioned: "So, you will not prepare the food and not enter the kitchen, right? It is *Ḥarām*?" Naʿimah jumped:

Ḥarām 'awi, a severe ḥarām. . . . Not only entering the kitchen. And you [in female gender] should not cook,⁸ and not bake, and not enter the kīnīs [the synagogue], and not hold the Torah. When I got married, I had a bed and he had a bed. So he can go to the kīnīs. His suit, which he wears to go to the kīnīs, was not hung in the closet, in case she has a period and touches it. So they used to hang it to the side so she would not touch it. . . . Everything was to the side [in the closet]. The books of the Torah, the talit [prayer shawl], . . . if she had the period she would not touch it. On Friday after he would take a shower I would not touch him. Otherwise he would be *tame'*, impure.

Na'imah mentioned the usual prohibitions against entering the synagogue or holding the Torah, but her first thought emphasized the prohibition against entering the kitchen and cooking. More than other places, the kitchen is a female space; the reality of the woman in the kitchen and her role as nurturer informs her perspective on impurity. In Egypt through the fifties and sixties, most women did not work outside the house; in a typical extended family several females resided in one household. Female networks consisted of the mother, mother-in-law, sisters, sisters-in-law, aunts, and housemaids at all different ages, which made them available to take the menstruating woman's place in the kitchen and the house. In California, however, a new reality forced changes and modifications in family life that have affected the networking of Karaite women.⁹ The sociogeographical changes in California have changed the way Karaites relate to menstrual prohibitions and the menstruating body. Often the only adult female in a household, a Karaite woman cannot rely on other women to cook and take care of the house, nor can she rely on her husband, who in most cases does not cook.

Unlike Na'imah, whose generation of women was confined mostly to the kitchen, Lailah represented the emerging modern Israeli Kara'it, whose proficiency in reading Hebrew aloud gained her a better place in the prayer room. At prayer, aside from her highly distinctive powerful voice, Lailah also marked her place with one square meter of white bed sheet that she would spread on the rug along the southern wall right behind the men. During the prayer she would sit and stand there, as it provided her with an added measure of purity. Most of the other women sat on chairs at the back of the room.

The fact that we were both Hebrew speakers no doubt was a source of comfort for Lailah.¹⁰ She was born in Cairo in 1941 in Ḥarat al-Yahūd, the Jewish quarter, and immigrated to Israel (via Paris) in 1971, where she settled with her family in Ashdod. Only after her mother died was Lailah (at age thirty-seven) willing to accept a marriage proposal. Nissim, from California, a humble man in his early forties, traveled to Israel for their arranged marriage. Their relatively late age at marriage may explain why they have no children. Lailah's place within the community, therefore, must be considered in light of this fact. From Cairo she knew several members of the Bay Area community, and she even studied in grade school with some of the more educated men (a point that she mentions with pride). Yet unlike the men, Lailah did not have the opportunity to further advance her education. Today, she works in a garment factory in South San Francisco with several other Karaite women, and often complains, in disbelief, about their non-Jewish boss who forces them to work on Shabbat. "There are only a few years left before I retire," she says impatiently, "then me and my husband, Nissim, will go home." Then she asks rhetorically, "Anyway, what is there for me here?"

For Lailah, home is Israel. But being away from the synagogue while menstruating is the most painful restriction for her. She said, "If I have it [the period], I do not go anywhere. I don't like people to know that I have it. I didn't go to the synagogue today. . . . I have it." She looked directly at me: "And I started going to the synagogue when I was seven years old." Paradoxically, in order to be a fully observant Karaite she has to remove herself from the religious center during her period. Because society does not designate a specific place for the menstruating woman within the boundaries of the religious space, she is temporarily driven from it. It is true that since Lailah moved to California she is less observant, yet she still rarely misses services. While there, she participates actively and reads with devotion. Outside the prayer room, however, Lailah is modest and reserved. She almost appears timid and exudes a certain sadness and embarrassment. She often concluded our conversations with a resigned expression: "*Mah la-'asot? Kakhah zeh ha-chayim*" (What can one do? That's life). As mentioned, changes in the structure of the family and the shift of women from domesticity to the workforce have contributed significantly to the expansion of the space of the menstruating woman. Lailah, who has immigrated twice in her life and experienced the transition from Israeli Jewish culture to a modern California lifestyle, felt this shift even more dramatically than Karaites who had settled there earlier. She summarized her experience in a listless tone: "It is hard to be religious here."

A few women still sleep separately from their husbands during the seven days of their period, but most of them cook and enter the kitchen. Yet there are two times of the year that the women strongly reassert their commitment to the rules of separation and purification: Passover and Yom

Kippur. In California especially, both Yom Kippur and Passover strengthen camaraderie among Karaites and redefine their community's sense of individual belonging and family ties. As a result, these holidays are times when issues of purity and impurity are particularly salient and carry added significance. They combine collective history and personal memory into a meaningful contemporary framework. And it is the special juncture of both cycles—the monthly-personal menstrual period of the woman, and the annual-religious period of the community—that reconnects the Kara'it to the ritual she may overlook during the rest of the year.

Niddah, Yom Kippur, and Passover

Yom Kippur is the culmination of the ten days following the New Year in which one reassumes his or her relationship with God. Purity of mind, body, objects, and space articulate sacredness; specifically, the purity of the body assumes its highest significance on Yom Kippur. The act of fasting focuses attention on the totality of cleansing, emptying, and ridding the body of its internal impurities, making it a symbolic site of ultimate spiritual holiness. Menstruation on Yom Kippur, therefore, takes on a special significance; the menstruating woman cannot participate in the prayers at the synagogue. Indeed, most women, and especially teenage girls, dread the idea of having their period on Yom Kippur, fearing both the attention that it will attract and the exclusion that it entails. When Sophia told me about her experience as a menstruating girl, I could not resist asking, "Did you pray, when you were a kid, 'I hope I won't have my period at Passover and Yom Kippur?'" She responded with a smile. "Oh, Yes. Oh yes. Especially on Passover and Yom Kippur when everybody else goes to the temple, [and] we cannot go to the temple.... I did not take it negatively, but I was always happy not to have my period."

Nowadays, Sophia sums up her approach to menstruation in one sentence: "The only positive thing about menstruation is that it is no pregnancy." She attempts to find creative alternatives, striving to create her own personal experience of purging and renewal, despite being removed from the collective ceremonies. Regarding the festive meal that precedes the fast on Yom Kippur, Sophia recalled: "I told my sister: 'Look, I got my period and I don't know what to do. I understand that you invited us.' And she said: 'I know how you feel. I will not feel hurt if you do not come. But if you come, I will make room for you in such a way that you will not feel awkward. You will be sitting with us at the table but away from everybody, even though I know that if mom were with us she would not allow it.'" Sophia concluded: "I did join them. I went and I stayed away from everybody."

Free of their mother's authority, the two sisters negotiated an alternative that both acknowledged the fact that Sophia was menstruating and impure, yet at the same time recognized her feeling of exclusion. The question is what kind of attitude will the *niddah* develop for the fact that she is not included in the visits to the synagogue, recitation of the prayers, touching of the Torah, or celebrating the holidays? Before examining the issue with regard to Passover, I first discuss the specific significance of this holiday to the people of this community.

Exodus and Exile

In April 1988 the Pessah family invited me to celebrate the Karaite *Pessah* (Passover).[11] There are approximately one hundred members of this family descended from a grandfather who was born during Passover—Pessah or Pesach, in Hebrew—hence, the surname. Sophia, who married into the family, commented amusingly on this parallel: "For many years, our son Benjamin was sure that [on Passover] we are telling the story of our family." For Benjamin, who at the time was only ten years old, the event represented an intimate narrative about the transformation of his immediate family. Joe Pessah, the acting rabbi, said it most explicitly: "So we had our own exodus for the second time.... We did it again. Same story" (he is shaking his head from one side to the other). In their accounts, Karaites tell of their forced departure from Egypt, first at the onset of Israel's Sinai campaign in 1956 and then in 1967, during the Six Day War. Nasser's act of jailing Karaite—and allegedly Zionist—males between the ages of sixteen and sixty-five evokes the ancient image of Pharaoh and his decree that every newborn Israelite male would be thrown into the Nile. The end result, however, was the same: the mass exodus of the Karaites and other Jews from Egypt. The story of the Pessah family has been fully allegorized.

I came to the Karaite Passover celebration with much anticipation. Not only would it be a place where we—Rabbanites and Karaites—could meet but it was also a communal crescendo on the annual calendar, connecting past and present, memory, story, and food into an accumulated, continuous narrative of freedom and renewal throughout generations. More specifically, I was haunted by the Karaite claim that "there is no elaboration among Karaites," as Joe Pessah proclaimed. In light of their double Exodus, I wondered if "oral tradition" still alluded only to *Torah shebe-'al peh*, the rejected Rabbanite tradition of oral elaboration that includes the Talmud, the Mishnah, midrashic collections, and other literary and halakhic texts. The celebration of Passover seemed like an ideal occa-

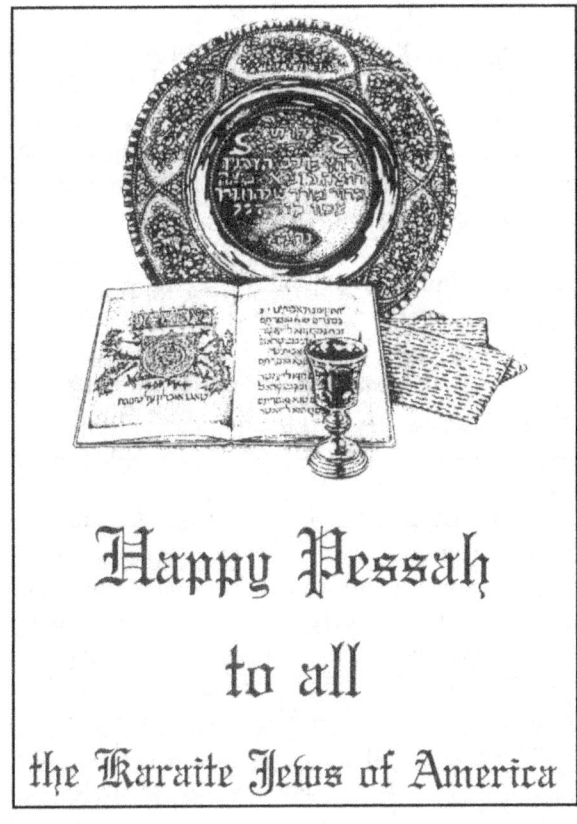

Passover greeting. (*KJA Bulletin* 1994)

sion for me to challenge the Karaite claim of extensive reliance on biblical textuality and to explore alternative modes of oral culture formation.

The ritual meal on the first night of the Rabbanite Passover, known as the Seder, is storytelling at its best: it is productive and generative and persists in large part due to the text's oral repetition. But the event of the departure from Egypt has been told and retold throughout generations, and its narration has become a multilayered experience of many times and places. The Seder combines both the method of celebration and specific instructions for its order, along with the story. The Haggadah (from the Hebrew root *ngd*, "to tell," "to recite," or "to narrate") tells the story of the departure out of Egypt, from slavery to freedom. The written story has evolved from a long Jewish tradition of celebration and elaboration on the holiday; in addition to the biblical verses that compile the story of the exodus, it includes post-biblical commentaries by rabbis, medieval songs, and more recent and timely material. The text, with its different additions, changes from land to land, culture to culture, family to family. My parent's Haggadah is bilingual; the Hebrew was accompanied with Judeo-Arabic translations and instructions, all in Hebrew transliteration. Especially today, the typical Israeli Haggadah is colorfully illustrated and often includes photographs. It tells both the story of the Exodus from Egypt and the history of its storytelling. As such the story is expandable, inspiring various narratives of freedom.

The Karaite Haggadah is a compilation of biblical excerpts—primarily from the book of Exodus, which together compose the Karaite narrative of Passover. "In the Karaite tradition, the Haggadah is composed of verses from the Scripture, so Pessah could be exactly observed for seven days, as written" (Pessah 1983, 1). To build on this sentiment of exactitude, the Haggadah itself is small and unadorned. The recitation is performed by all who are present at the Seder.

The Seder is an important part of the holiday, and the Karaites celebrate only one Seder meal during Passover.[12] The food and the drinks also indicate symbolically their concern with preserving their culture. The matzah, or unleavened bread, appears in the Torah as early as Genesis 19, portrayed as the ultimate fast food—easy and quick to prepare. Egyptian-Karaite matzah is a home-baked mix of flour and water that is formed into flat square biscuits. There is no yeast in it, and it should be baked within three minutes to avoid any leavening whatsoever. Leavened foods are prohibited on Passover, including bread or beer. Furthermore, Karaites also forbid cheese and wine during the holiday. Thus, preventing the fermentation of food during the seven days of Passover is crucial.[13] To substitute for wine, Karaites drink a homemade liquid made from raisins that have been soaked in water the day before the Seder.[14] Because it is fermented, regular wine is a transformed and transforming substance: an "alibi of dreams and myth" as it converts and reverses identities (Barthes 1972, 58). The Karaites' unfermented "drink" resists transformation. The raisin wine and the matzah, much like the Karaite Haggadah, remain unchanged; they are metaphors of the wholesomeness of culture that is brought into a pure body and soul.

As a literal model for storytelling, the Karaite Passover story restores redemption and survival. But going back to its mode of narration, what does it mean to read "exactly"? Can tradition remain unadorned? Not only does Karaite textual orientation toward reading have its own distinctive practice, but it also redefines the nature of oral tradition and the attitude toward it. Like their Passover raisin wine, Karaite history is kept unfermented, or unaged, yet preserved. Within the austere body of the Haggadah, the only relevant account composes history, as if history is equal to story.

The Karaite Passover, I came to learn, with its emphasis on the departure from the old and the encounter with the new, plays a major role in stabilizing the Karaites' sense of identity.[15] By preserving the solid principles of that identity, their historical awareness of Passover continuously renews Karaite selfhood, providing a bridge to their past. But, at the same time, the Exodus is also the moment in which travel begins. Unlike its biblical model, however, the Karaite exodus did not end up in the promised land of Israel, but in California.

"We Are the True Exodus"

"We are the true Jewish people, the true exodus," asserted Dr. Victor, who fled Egypt at seventeen on a boat sailing from Alexandria to Marseilles and finally ended up in Northern California. The Seder had ended. The meal, prepared by the women, was extraordinary; a blend of flavors, tastes, and smells that could only be found on a Karaite Passover table. The *maror*, the bitter herbs, for example, was made of different kinds of lettuce, chopped mint, dill, and small cucumbers, all in pickled lemon. The lemon had been carefully cut so that its peel formed a single spiral; it was set aside the night before to marinate with lemon juice and chopped hot chili pepper. We were still sitting around the tables, engaged in small conversation. A faint smell of barbequed Pessah lamb prepared by the men permeated the big hall, carried on the early evening wind of April.[16] Kids were running around and the echoes of people's laughter ricocheted off the walls, creating a noisy din. "We were lucky," mused Dr. Victor:

> We left Egypt in 1966, a few months before the Six Day War, and the situation was still not that bad. Most everybody had planned to leave for years. All the families in Egypt . . . and especially after 1967, the Six Day War, many left in a hurry, and all the Karaite people knew that their days were numbered in Egypt.
>
> We started to get a suitcase, buying clothes, and preparing for the family to leave for four, five years. We were under the impression that we were going to go to Europe, and life is so expensive there that we needed to take money with us so we could have enough food. The time frame was very different. In Egypt it took years for my mother to liquidate our resources, and even when we left, she had to sell some of the property for very little money to the Jewish community.

Eventually, they lost everything.

At twenty-three Simone was already married and had a son, Daniel, who was five months old. She turned amicably to her sister, Mimi (who left Egypt when she was thirteen):

> It was almost twenty or nineteen years ago, in 1969. The war started in 1967. I waited a year and then I decided to leave. All the men were in concentration camps. They took all the men, teenagers from nineteen years old and up. My dad, my brother, my husband, my uncles, my cousins, and many friends, many friends, all of them, there were no men outside. I told my mom, "We have to leave, I ran out of money." My mom said, "No, we are not going to leave the men in the concentration camps." I said, "We are leaving." So I could not work. My husband was a teacher and the contract ended and I could not get more money. I told my mother, "We are leaving," she said, "no," "yes," "no." So I showed her my passport. She said, "I am not going to let you go by yourself." I said, "Really?" She paused, and then said: "They are not going to let you go by yourself."

Ahron, Simone's father, approached us with a sympathetic smile on his face. "My dad," she introduced him. "He was in the concentration camp for three years." "And three weeks," he corrected her. He continued:

> As a rule, those with Egyptian nationality were taken for three years, and those with foreign nationality for two. They took all men. All Jewish men, Karaites and Rabbanites . . . in three hours they collected everybody. They had a list. Including old people. They brought people from the hospital, operated patients, amputated, injured, because they used the Jewish hospital as a hospital for Egyptian soldiers. They treated us badly. All seventy-two persons were sleeping in one small room, on the floor. We got blankets, and a plate to eat. We used the plate as a pillow. Seventy-two persons in one room. You know the box of sardines? This is how we lived. Unshaved, with no sanitary conditions, with long beards.

Ahron concludes that in the long run, being imprisoned was an act of protection of Jewish men from the angry, mourning Arabs. As he said, "If we were out . . . their heart was boiling. They would become enraged. So they would probably attack us. It was good for us." Ahron's story was a story shared by all the men, along with the radical Muslim brothers, the Communists, the Rabbanites, and the Karaites.

The Site of Impurity   139

The Exodus reclaims Egypt as the former homeland of contemporary Karaites. At the same time, it is the place associated with the trials and tribulations of their recent displacement. Egypt appears in written texts as well as in verbal communication, as an ambivalent site of nostalgia, reflected in Karaites' attempt to historically define their attachment to Egyptian culture: were they more "Arab" or more "Egyptian"? To what extent do variants such as modernism and secular lifestyles in the metropolitan areas of Cairo and Alexandria figure in Karaites' new attempts to negotiate their categories of identity? As a minority within a minority, the narrative of their exodus is the story of the transformation of the twentieth-century Karaites. It tells a continuous story of their cultural exile.

In fact, Exodus is the modus operandi of Karaite history. Within the wider context of Karaite experience, migration and physical mobility were not uncommon. Darʻi's biographic map gives us an idea about the span of Karaites' itinerary around the Mediterranean basin as early as the twelfth century. He was born in Alexandria, Egypt, to a Spanish family, and traveled frequently between Syria and Palestine. Ultimately, he settled in the small Moroccan town of Darʻi (Nemoy 1952, 133).

The itinerary of Naomi, a Karaite woman in her early sixties, reflected a contemporary journey crossing five continents. As she tells it, with intensity and passion:

> I emigrated from Melbourne, Australia, to California in 1974 with my husband and daughter. I was born in Cairo in 1937 to a father who was originally from Turkey and a mother who was born in Abu-'Ir and raised in Tanta [both towns in northern Egypt]. As Turkish nationals we could not remain in Egypt after the expulsion of the Turkish king [in 1952], especially as Jews, and because we did not want to immigrate to Israel, we settled in Turkey in August 1954. So, when it was clear that we [Naomi's husband and child] were leaving Turkey [after four years in Istanbul and two in Ankara], my mother and brother immigrated to Israel, and we, after fifteen years in Australia, moved to California.

Karaites' travel record emphasizes the need of Karaites to preserve their unique culture and genealogy as they move from one location to another, and to rapidly adjust to the new external demands of a different language, economy, national allegiance, and ethnic affiliation. As such, the case of the Karaites in the Bay Area convincingly ratifies James Clifford's call to approach ethnography as a "travel encounter," in that travel constitutes "practices of crossing and interaction that troubled the localism of many common assumptions about culture" (Clifford 1997, 3). In fact, the Karaite narrative suggests that traveling complicates the localism of indeterminate extremes of exile and exodus in Karaite history. As such, it conflicts with the mythological Egypt of the ancient Bible, being the ultimate historical peril of exile of the forefathers.

And yet, despite the significant differences between Egypt of antiquity and Egypt of the twentieth century, the similarities between the two are striking. It is, perhaps, impossible to tell exactly how one Passover folded into the other, nurturing at time of crisis a sense of belonging, engendering communal Karaite ties and an imagined peoplehood among the next generation. Their symbolic significance, however, appears magnified in light of an improvised Karaite celebration of Passover in the prison. The unique hybrid junction of old origins, genealogy, and name system, with the traumatic displacement from one place to another, might have become a stabilizing force in history and an act that reaffirms the intimate relationship between God and Israel (Yerushalmi 1989, 11).

Passover, the spring festival, focuses on the symbolic act of filling and impregnating the body by means of food, experiences, story, and memory. The sacred center moves from the synagogue to the home. The extended family enacts the Seder ceremony on the first evening of the seven-day holiday. These gatherings can include over one hundred people. An alternative ritual is available through the observance of *Pessah sheni,* or *Pessah Katan* (Second [Little] Passover),[17] celebrated a month later by those who were unable for any reason to participate in the actual holiday. Several women related having used this option. Susana chose not to use this alternative and to remain, instead, a part of the family.

Susana

A few weeks before Passover, Susana told me that she would have to sit at a corner table during the Seder because she expected her period to fall "exactly" on Passover. Though this was disappointing for her, it was clearly an opportunity for me to actually observe what I had only heard about so many times: a *niddah* at the Seder. Susana, who was born in Egypt and came as a teenager to the United States, was an attractive, youthful woman in her forties. Her two children had left home for college, and she was able to devote more time to her career as a bank manager. She did not come to the services often. Yet when she did come, her cheerful aura was always a welcome presence; her manner of speaking was powerful and empathic, even when she spoke about casual, trivial matters.

When the evening of Seder arrived, everyone was dressed in holiday clothing. The spirit was festive, light, and celebratory. In the middle of the room was a huge table, covered with a crisp white tablecloth and set with fancy holiday dishes and vases filled with colorful flowers. The large living room had been transformed into a dining area. People embraced with greetings of "*hag sameah*" (happy holiday). This year the celebration was relatively small: Naʿimah, her three sons, their wives, and children.

The transformed living room was a large space with three doorways: one leading to the front door, a second to the kitchen, and a third connecting to the dining room. Naʿimah, wearing a bright holiday dress, was sitting close to the head of the main table. Next to her was David, her second son, and his two teenage sons. As the host, he led the ritual meal. Joel, Naʿimah's youngest son, and Saul, his own four-year-old son, were seated to David's left. Susana was sitting at a corner table set especially for her in the normal dining room. Susana's husband, Josh, and her son, Ben, were facing her, on David's right. Since the seating arrangements at the table were relatively flexible, I wondered to what extent their choices were deliberate, perhaps to ensure some contact with Susana during the evening. As it happened, the men and women sat across from each other, including Susana, who sat behind the women. The women formed a virtual wall of separation between Susana and the table. I sat facing Joel at the opposite end of the table from Naʿimah. Susana was sitting directly behind me, close enough to touch.

David was impatient to begin the ceremony. The grandchildren were excited, full of anticipation; they were talkative. On the count of three we began reading out loud the Karaite Haggadah in one unified voice. Once we began there was no interference in the flow of the collective recitation. There were a few songs that express gratitude to God that were added to the biblical text and that had a repetitive, chantlike melody. We all repeated the blessing of the wine and the matzah. Occasionally, I glanced over my shoulder to see how Susana was doing. The psychological distance was palpable; it was clear that she resented her current situation, as she sat with a sullen expression on her face. Despite the obvious efforts to include her, she nevertheless was excluded and could not enter the "space" of the Seder. She had been banished to the outside, relegated to looking in. Her expression revealed her sense of alienation.

Once the Seder was over, I approached Susana, aware that I was catching her in an awkward moment. Perhaps because of her ordinarily good nature she was able to pull herself together quickly and smiled. Her body language revealed that she was now more comfortable, maybe because the ordeal was over, and once again she felt included; indeed, my presence with the small tape recorder made her the focus of attention.[18] She seemed full of energy and wanted to talk.

"How does it feel to have your period and celebrate the Karaite holiday?" I asked, and she repeated the question. She stopped as she searched for the right words. "You feel silly, stupid, by staying by yourself isolated from your family [she laughs nervously, embarrassed]. But it's ... you have to respect traditions, and then when you grow up with it, you adjust to it." And then qualifying, she added:

> It's not as bad as someone who is ... it's not as hard for me as it would be for you, coming from a totally different environment or traditions, to adjust to this tradition. ... The reason why it's easier for me is because I am used to it; when I have my period I cannot go to the temple. It's one of those things. I have my period—no love making. Shabbat and *'īd* [holiday]—no love making. You know, you adjust to stuff like this. Things that you grow up with, you kind of say this is it, you know, just like something else you probably do that I would see it ... "Hah, you do this?" The only thing that feels bad, when you have such a small family, having a son and a husband and you cannot even share that day with them [Passover], that's the only bad thing. ... That's the only bad thing, but [there's] nothing you can do about it.

She seemed pensive for a while and then suddenly added:

> It's very awkward when you are sitting by yourself. It really is. It's just ... you feel like a dog, honestly, you do feel like a dog. But what can you do? You're just doing it for respect for an older person, and you know, you have to realize that that's how she [her mother-in-law, Naʿimah] lived all her life, and she is seventy-seven or seventy-eight and I am not going to come now and change your [her] life just because of one holiday. Silly! And I feel it's good with the little children to do that too, they respect ... they know tradition.

The way Susana spoke about sitting apart was as important as what she said; her voice rose, she asked rhetorical questions, she hesitated, she thought aloud. She examined her position from within and from without, as if for a moment she had traded places and identified with me, the outsider ethnographer. She then returned to her position as an educated insider living in a relatively secular home. Did it make sense to her? For Susana, her mother-in-law was the maternal point of reference that informed her understanding of the site of uncleanliness. For her, Naʿimah's voice and authority represented the entire Karaite tradition. This point is important, for it designated the site of impurity alongside the traditional female voice and the memory of its history. Sitting in this space, alienating and distancing as it might feel, she was still close and in contact with the memory of her maternal ancestors. In fact, the story of Karaite sisters and mothers sitting afar has been told and retold to her, creating a nexus that communicates that she, the *niddah,* is not separated but rather a part of a long tradition of Karaite women. This consciousness nurtures the solitude of the Kara'it and soothes the harshness of her displacement. It is especially relevant to the experience of the young American Kara'it, who is unlikely to be in this countersite during the rest of the year.

Susana's ambivalence about being separated from the main table reflects the attitude of women of the younger generation. Nadia, for example, who belongs to the older generation, assured me that being separated is not so bad. "We get used to it. I saw my mother, [and] my sisters doing that." In fact, when I asked, "Did people talk to you as if you were included or as if you were not?" she responded decisively: "No, no, no. We are not like dogs." The evocation of the dog in both Susana's and Nadia's statements is interesting: in Egyptian folk culture the status of the dog is associated with the street, and serves as an expression of abandonment, hopelessness, and forsakenness.[19] This claim, in which one aims to dissociate oneself from the dog, still presupposes a certain degraded status even while denying it.

I continued to explore Susana's experiences.

Ruth: Do you feel any connection? Could you exchange some glances with your family? Did you feel, sitting here, that . . .

Susana: No, you see, my husband is not that kind of a person. My husband concentrates on what he is doing. He doesn't, he doesn't understand because he grew up with it. He grew [up] in a home that with his sisters, when his mother had her period she wasn't at the table, with his sisters . . . so to him it's something normal. . . . There is no difference. You know what I am saying?

Ruth: Uh-huh.

Susana: He cannot relate to my feelings. You know.

Ruth: Even though his mother or his sister might not feel good. But he doesn't know about it.

Susana: He doesn't understand that. He doesn't understand that.

I asked her about her children's responses, especially her daughter's.

Susana: They know. They do know. My children know.

Ruth: How early did you start explaining it [to them]?

Susana: Keren knew it maybe . . . when she was six years old, seven years old; when her mom has her period she cannot sit at the table. And then that's one of the things I would worry about. As soon as she got her period, you know, she was always praying that she would never get her period at Passover because it would be awkward. Thank goodness it never happened. She always was able to sit at the table.

Upon meeting her future husband, Susana had to embrace a new identity. Susana's mother, Miriam, was a non-observant Karaite. She did not provide her daughters with Karaite education regarding menstruation and did not follow all of the rituals herself. But Na'imah, her mother-in-law, was more observant. The following description of Susana's first encounter with Karaite orthodoxy reveals the clash between the two traditions and the ensuing shift in her approach to her identity.

Susana: When I went to my husband [to meet his family for the first time]? Yeah. [Imagine] a fifteen-year-old girl . . . a young man comes and asks her, when he is introducing her to his family, telling her, you know, if you have your period. . . . I felt like slapping the man because it's none of his damn business if I do or I don't, but when he explained to me their tradition, and their way, that his mother is religious, I understood, and then I didn't feel as bad as when he asked me in the beginning. And then when his mother explained to me that I won't be able to sit at the dinner table with them, he chose to come and sit with me with my . . . with me at my dinner table, although it is demeaning to a man to sit with a woman who has got her period and eat because, you know, it's like *tame'ah* [polluted], I don't know what you call it in Hebrew . . . Ḥarām, it's not clean food anymore. As long as he sits with me at my table, so . . . he chose to do that.

Ruth: You did not grow up with the ʿādah . . .

Susana: No, nothing, I grew up in a home in which no one knew that I had my period and when I had my period. But once I got married I had to tell the whole world [*she is laughing*] that I have my period. That's what it seems like.

Ruth: Is it embarrassing?

Susana: It sure is.

Ruth: You feel the tension between having it as a private thing and having it declared.

Susana: Certainly. Certainly. And you tend, at the time, you tend to isolate yourself, you don't want to go to your in-laws [so] you do not have to explain yourself. Although now my mother in-law is a lot easier, during the regular days she does not mind, it is only on the holidays that she cares.

Shadows of Impurity: Space and Counter Space

Whereas the taboo against touching during menstruation appears cross-culturally, the delineation of the menstruating woman's contaminated space is different. The "counter places" are fed and materialized in each society by its architectural imagination of "purity" and "impurity." While speaking about the matzah and its sacredness, Sophia asserted that a menstruating woman should avoid proximity with the matzah, but the borders of this proximity move beyond the parameters of the physical body, as she elaborated:

> **Sophia:** During the period, my mother explained to me, we are not supposed to stay with the rest of the family at the table, but at that time she was no longer so religious, conservative, or orthodox, so I continued to stay with them during the holiday. So for Passover, touching the matzah was considered sacred. If I am not clean and I touched the matzah, God forbid, nobody can eat from that matzah. Even the shadow of the woman is considered unclean. If the shadow falls on the matzah—that will be considered *tame'*, impure. So she [my mother] was trying always to get the matzah [that was planned for the whole family] three weeks before Passover and if I have it [the period] she'll put it in a place [where] there is no traffic in the house so nobody will touch it.
>
> **Ruth:** How do you protect your shadow?
>
> **Sophia:** You stay away from the traffic.

Shifting the center of sacredness from the synagogue to the home increases the demand for extra stringency within the domestic sphere. The inevitable presence of the menstruating woman becomes further regulated. The matzah, in this environment, gains a heightened sense of holiness as the focal point of the ritual reenactment of the Exodus. As the "bread of affliction," it is an embodiment of nonfermentation, and as such a paradigm of freedom from time, place, and attachment. So is Karaite Passover wine an unfermented blend of raisins soaked in water. It is interesting to consider menstruation as a converse process of fermentation that expands the body's material limits via its contaminating shadow.[20] It is the time in which impurity bursts out of the physical body, threatening to invade and contaminate the domestic sphere. To claim that a woman's shadow is contaminated is to add to the language of distancing yet another marker of impurity, yet another degree of separation.

Women elaborate on this discourse beyond the prohibitions on Passover and Yom Kippur. In addition to the prohibition against cooking or entering the kitchen, several women among the younger generation, who do not necessarily obey this rule, still maintain that a menstruating woman should not bake. "*Mis te'gini,* do not bake!" In addition, Na'imah instructs me while listing the things a woman with the *'ādah* should avoid. The Arabic verb refers more precisely to the act of kneading dough. Bread is a main staple for Karaites, "the staff of life," and the prohibition on kneading dough represents cooking at its primary level. As in other cultures, making bread is a creative act, like sexual intercourse, and a religious ritual that highlights the "notion of creativity and generativity" (Delaney 1988, 90).[21] The rising of the dough makes bread and the act of baking it highly symbolic of reproductive activities. Whereas bread and the rising of the yeast are metaphors for creation and procreation, menstruation is seen as a competing fermentative impediment to the creation of both bread and children. In the context of Passover, menstruation is especially threatening, as the fermented body and the unleavened (unfermented) dough are at odds with each other.

Not surprisingly, Susana directly warns against baking, even when matzah is concerned and rising dough is not an issue. Due to its much appreciated taste and the relative ease of its preparation, the Egyptian-Karaite matzah spiced with salt and cilantro is eaten all year long.

> **Susana:** A woman when she has her period and she bakes the matzah, it doesn't come up good. The matzah will never come out good. Would you believe that?
>
> **Ruth:** I believe it, I believe it.
>
> **Deborah:** I've never tried.
>
> **Susana:** When I have my period and I have to do the dough of the matzah, my husband does it.
>
> **Ruth:** But the dough does not have to rise.

Susana: It doesn't rise or anything but in the body you have things, you know, the oil of your body is different. The dough does not work as well. And it will never stick together. And that is true. And it is known in Egypt when a woman has her period she should never bake bread. [*She knocks on the table along with the syllables for emphasis.*]

Ruth: Your mother told you that?

Susana: It's known, yeah. Don't make dough because it's not ... you can try to bake. And the baking, even if the dough is good, something will happen with the oven. It doesn't come out right.

Ruth: Women bring something of their own [body] into the dough?

Susana: You do, you do. You do, when you knead the dough you bring something from your body. They tell you no matter how much you wash your hands, and you clean it and then when you have your period ...

Mira: I have a friend. She is Jewish Sephardi, Sephardi. And she says when she combs her hair or brushes her teeth or combs her hair ...

Susana: You can't, you know, my mother always told me don't have your hair cut while you have your period, you never cut your hair because you have to go back, in a week and have to cut it again. Because they can never straighten it, it is different, your whole body goes through changes.

Experiencing the body as essentially different and unpredictable during menstruation, the women expand the corpus of limitations associated with the menstruating woman. Attempting to explain related phenomena during the time of menstruation, they are predisposed to perceive them as anomalies and attribute them to the "malfunctioning" of the menstruating body (cf. Buckley and Gottlieb 1988, 21). Like other folk beliefs, the validity of these convictions is confirmed through personal experience and reinforced by the stories of other women.

Is it that the Kara'it needs to compensate for her inability to take a central role during the days preceding the holiday? Indeed, if she tries to bake the matzah, it is certain to fail; thus she justifies her removal from the ritual site. As the highlight of Jewish domestic festivity, demanding that a woman fulfill her responsibilities scrupulously (cleaning and koshering is the most important part of the preparations), Passover itself exaggerates the unclean posture of the menstruating woman. But ironically, it is her distancing that generates a personal narrative. Almost all Kara'iyot had stories about this "unfortunate" time, memories of being removed from the communal Passover table, associated with tears, sadness, and anxiety. Her desire to remain part of the community conflicts with her compliance with tradition.

Between clearing the table, taking out the dessert of assorted cookies, and washing the fruit, Mira and Deborah joined in my conversation with Susana. We spoke in loud voices and giggled with excitement. At the main table, the men were conversing about personal finances and the economy, while the children played joyfully in the living room. The women, all in their early forties, spoke fluent English, though at times they shifted to Arabic in search of familiar expressions. Talking together about the experience of menstruating during the holiday allowed the women to compare notes. This occasion came with surprises: they were amazed to discover that not all Karaites observe the exact same rules.

> RUTH: Isn't it a relief, that you don't have to do anything for Passover?
>
> MIRA: It's not a relief, you feel guilty.
>
> SUSANA: I don't feel good. I did not make grape leaves [stuffed leaves with rice, called *dolma*].
>
> MIRA: But usually you feel good that you cook and your house is full of...
>
> SUSANA: I had to cook food, the whole week [in spite of the fact she had her period], because I am giving everything to Ben [her son in college] tonight.
>
> RUTH: I am trying to see the positive stuff about the...
>
> SUSANA: *Tame'ah* [*all laughing*]. What's positive?
>
> MIRA: I told her it's an awful feeling. One time I had it over at my mom's, and I cried... I hated to sit down in the...
>
> SUSANA [*in Arabic*]: At your mother's too?
>
> MIRA: Only in *Pessah*. All the rest of the year she does not care. In *Pessah* she is very picky.
>
> SUSANA: At my father's [*in Arabic*]—never. Never.
>
> RUTH: And you cried—what did she do when you cried?
>
> MIRA: Nothing. And she just explained to me: "Nothing we can

do, you just have to sit down." Because I did not believe in that. In my opinion we are clean.

During another interview, Sophia recalled:

> I remember one day a friend of mine came and her parents were not so religious and she came during Passover time and she had her period [*she pauses dramatically*]. My mom won't even let her pass a certain counter. She left and she started crying. She understood, but not to that point. She just could not take it. And afterward she reminded me: "Sophia, do you remember that day I went out of your home and I was crying?"

The holidays that frequent the annual calendar are not the only occasions that highlight the uncleanliness of the menstruating woman. Life-cycle events such as the *brit* (male circumcision on the eighth day after birth) and the bar mitzvah require that the female participant be ritually clean. These celebrations appoint a particular location for those who are considered unclean and are forbidden from entering the ritual space. At the *brit*, a menstruating woman cannot deliver the baby to the *mohel*, the circumciser. Instead, three women, typically close relatives, carry the baby into the room on a white pillow, arms outstretched in a dancelike ritual. And as discussed in chapter 4, at the bar mitzvah, while a boy is celebrating his entrance into communal adulthood, his mother, if menstruating, is not allowed to touch him and will greet him from just outside the prayer room. Yet, regarding the degree to which the woman internalized the notion of being unclean during menstruation, I received an interesting variety of answers, at times contradictory:

> I know I am clean. But that [*she points to her crotch*] makes you feel dirty, makes you feel unclean. [*A pause.*] Yeah, yeah, you just feel unclean. You just feel unsanitary. [*Laughs uncomfortably.*] But you know, she [Naʿimah] realizes now, there is hot water, that you can take a hot shower twice a day. (Susana)
>
> *Al-ʿāda ḥarām* [the period is impure]. (Naʿimah)
>
> Actually, it isn't really dirty but that's what it is. . . . We feel dirty. . . . Well, we feel dirty because something is wrong and we know that we can't touch this and touch that, so . . . why? Because we are dirty. (Nadia)
>
> Just the idea of having something coming out of me is not very

pleasant. I have pain and blood and spots. (Lailah)

SOPHIA: Well, it's sure not clean. . . . [Sophia here refers to "the smell," which signifies for her the unclean nature of menstruation.] So, realistically, it is really dirty.

RUTH: What about the symbolic aspect of the body as clean and dirty?

SOPHIA: Yes. There is some truth to it. When Sol was in college one guy said: "*Yebayyen 'aleeha al-'ādah*" [literally, "her *'ādah* is noticeable" or "she looks like a woman who has the period"]. She is ugly, pale.

According to Susana, menstrual blood is not inherently dirty. She is convinced that she is clean. Whether supported by biological truth or by legalistic status of *niddah*, it is the woman's impure location that designates this condition. Unlike theories that tend to view pollution as an involuntary psycho-physical response of the body, regardless of the symbolic context, the attribution of impurity as a culturally constructed source relieves the physical body from its responsibility of being impure. At the same time, it confines the impurity to the woman's body. Physical sites of impurity, therefore, not only represent bodily status; they are embedded so deeply in the Karaite cultural system that they themselves stain the body. They are polluted and thus polluting.

The impure site stands in striking opposition to all presumably pure spaces, thus attributing to these social sites the notion of ideal places. Inspired and "nurtured by the hidden presence of the sacred" (Foucault 1986, 23), women learn to distance themselves from both people and objects. Thus, being both pure and impure can be perceived in terms of cycles of proximity to different physical centers. Viewing Passover as an intensified example of the increased significance of the domestic sphere, we can see how the already marginalized space of the *niddah* becomes even more restricted. Being prohibited from participating closely in a family ritual in her own home raises the question of whether a woman *can ever* feel at home. Home at other times assumes a protective function during menstruation. Women reported that while menstruating they refrained from visiting other female friends and in general preferred to stay at home. For example, during Yom Kippur, Sophia, because she was menstruating, was unable to go to the prayers.[22] She says: "I stayed home with my period." At home, she would not touch the prayer books and would formulate her own prayers. Calling another menstruating friend to meet, as I suggested to her, would have been possible but she did not do it because she did not want to drive.[23]

Physical placement and spatial relations define and delimit women's consciousness—a consciousness that emanates from her experience of everyday life. The construction of the woman as unclean during her menstrual period is a cumulative process that crystallizes over time. The politics of space defines a woman's access to that which is valued by the community; distancing what is considered the impure from the pure also requires a woman's total exclusion from, and inaccessibility to the validity that informs, the pure space. In other words, women are removed not only from the "main table" but also from all other metaphoric "pure tables": the Torah, the synagogue, the kitchen, the shower, the living room, the environment of pregnant and lactating women, the marital bed, and the cemetery. In addition to interfering with the woman's desire to participate, the removal of the woman to the margins of culture further reinforces existing binary paradigms of social relationships. While clean and unclean are an obvious binary pair, the articulation of the menstruating woman as "Other" reproduces other dichotomies in which her position is perceived negatively. The impairment of women's religious, social, sexual, and physical interaction is, therefore, inevitable according to this system.

To my question of what they *can* do while menstruating, women answered simply: "Nothing." Linguistically, the emptiness of the impure space is furnished with this banal, colorless response, which is common in the discourses of women and minors. As the opposite of ideal space, where everything is possible, "nothing" suggests that the women associate impure space with a lack of productivity and noneventfulness. In contrast, the sacred, social space is imbued with validity and liveliness. Inhibited by the social meaning of their impure bodies, women self-consciously limit their mobility and social interactions. One could say that whereas menstruation as a discourse of impurity is visible and a subject of great consideration, in aiming to conceal the monthly phenomenon, the woman herself effectively disappears.

In light of the social and religious changes that the Karaite community is undergoing, impurity emerges as not a settled category but a negotiable one. The impure space of females, formerly constrained by the public body, has gradually become a zone of cultural debate in which a woman engages herself in order to set new social standards to guide her private body.

Blood and Water: The Shower of Purification

As we saw in chapter 3, gendered language is contextual; being "clean" and "unclean" does not describe the actual cleanliness of the body, but symbolically refers to moving in and out of the periods. When a woman refers to herself as "clean," she means that she is not having her period, and conversely, that she is "unclean" while menstruating. According to biblical law of the Temple period, a woman was required to bring the sacrifice of two doves to the priest at the Temple on the day of her purification (Leviticus 15:29–31). After the Temple period, Karaite halakhah maintained that a woman must still perform the ritual of purification after sunset at the conclusion of the seventh day of her bleeding. Her ability to do so depended on whether her period stopped on the seventh day at noon. In lieu of the sacrificial offerings, a woman could either fast for one day, give charity, or light a candle in the synagogue (Halevi 1988b, 129). Today, although unmarried women follow the seven-day impurity regimen dictated by Karaite law, most married Karaite women currently wait eight days (adding an extra day to the biblical seven) and then take a concluding shower.[24] This additional day is especially significant in that it demonstrates how women have assumed control over this particular section of halakhah. The principle that impurity is contaminated and transmittable underscores the rules of this enactment of purification. All that the woman touched during her period, everything that came into contact with her body, had to be washed (Leviticus 15:19). That includes her bedding, the clothes she wore during the seven days, the chair on which she sat, and her eating utensils.

Karaite women associated menstruation with an unclean, dirty body. Nadia, when considering what other objects, places, or parts of her body she would consider "dirty," said, "The genital parts are dirty. What comes out of the body is dirty," and, in general, "the bathroom"—although the bathroom at her small house was immaculate.

For the Karaite women, the showering area emerges as the enveloping site of impurity. Nadia's perceptions of both body and home yielded a spatial "map" of cleanliness. Domestic space, thus, can be divided according to a symbolic hierarchy of cleanliness; like the body, any room that is "touched" by menstrual blood is rendered unclean. In this highly evaluative scheme, the bedroom—although associated with sexuality and sexual parts—is considered cleaner than the bathroom, which is space where impurity is washed away. Undoubtedly, the fact that in my experience Karaite bathrooms are always sparkling clean is the result of an internalized awareness that aims to scour away any trace of impurity. The logic is familiar: if the bathroom is considered the most unclean place in the house, then it gets special cleaning attention and, as a result, becomes, like the female body, "doubly clean."[25]

While the Karaite women I interviewed almost unanimously claimed that bathing is prohibited during menstruation, the prevailing attitudes toward washing and showering vary. When, on which days, and how much water is permitted are issues that women did not necessarily agree upon, although they all agreed that a woman should neither bathe during her period nor, as Sophia added, swim in the sea or a swimming pool.[26] Moreover, showering and washing during the period is also restricted, which is often emphasized among other prohibitions that a mother teaches to her daughters. When I asked Lailah, for example, "What would your mother tell you not to do [while menstruating]?" she thoughtfully replied, "Not to take a shower on the first day and not to run [to take it easy physically]." Laila especially avoided washing on the first day of her period. On another occasion, when I asked Sophia why showering is forbidden, she replied, "Because during the period, or at least in the first three days, there is a constant bleeding [and] the shower would get impure. And if the husband has to take a shower and go to the temple, he would get impure as well."

By way of *tum'ah mishtalshelet*, transmitted impurity, the ritual of body purification contaminates the space of the shower.[27] The prohibition on showering originated with and is indirectly related to a concern to protect male purity. Female bodily ritual guarantees male bodily purity (Buckley and Gottlieb 1988, 3–53). The fact that, as Nadia claims, the bathroom is the most unclean place in the home indicates that the site in which purification takes place is marked as impure.

Laila, Susana, and other Kara'iyot mentioned that a woman with the *'ādah* washes both during and after her period, but the reasons and significance of these acts differ in each case. Studies of health beliefs and practices confirm that these beliefs and fears prove to be similar to those commonly held among some Arab communities, including Egypt, with regard to the impact of water and showering on fertility, virginity, and, in general, increasing menstrual pain and cramping (Kridli 2002). But more important, in the Karaite community, water encompasses a dichotomy of pure and impure—for at times the very site of the shower is either potentially contaminating or potentially purifying. Even though Karaite halakhah specifically states that "a *niddah* does not contaminate water" because of the very fact that water is instrumental in her purification, women still perceive the direct contact of their body with water as polluting the water. The problematic dialectic embedded in the washing and purifying of the impure body is manifested in all physical contact that a woman has with water. As a result, the first sight of blood introduces a special water discipline for a woman so that her bodily contact with water is limited and washing is restricted to specific days of her period.

Susana was emphatic, elaborating on the potential harm to the female reproductive system should a woman overlook this rule, although she clearly distinguished between Egypt and the United States:

> In Egypt when you have your period, you know, you don't take showers. You don't take showers because they tell you it's not good for you for your reproduction... reproductive system. You can turn out to be impotent. I don't know what they call it, for women not to be able to conceive.... [More secretively:] That's one of the things they tell you, you have to be very careful about. You don't douche. ...You are not supposed to douche. You know, like here you douche, you clean, but in Egypt you cannot do that. You cannot do that. ...I remember when I had my period in Egypt I would just wash myself.

Though fully convinced that showering or douching, or both, is harmful for reproduction, Susana cannot explain the reason. Symbolically, water was believed to interfere with the flow of the blood—itself a process of cleansing—vital to the woman's reproductive wellness.[28] Susana's explanation concerns the vulnerability of the female body and was focused on protecting the female reproductive system, rather than the threat of her polluting condition (see Buckley and Gottlieb 1988, 10).

"The reason for the controversy regarding the shower during menstruation," Sophia suggested, "is the fact that this rule is not written in the Torah." Sophia described an occasion when she consulted with the wife of the Israeli Karaite chief rabbi (during the wife's last visit to California, in 1990), who asserted that a woman must take a shower on the first and fourth days of the cycle. In contrast, Nadia insisted that women should not shower at all during their period, but perhaps could wash themselves on the third, fourth, or fifth day. Thus, we see that Karaite women were forced to develop rules independent of any biblical reference that they based on their own understanding of the cultural mechanism of cleanliness and on their mothers' methods of maintaining and attaining purity; as a result, they suggested several ways of using water during the menstrual cycle. These different rules can be accounted for in part by previous historical circumstances with regard to water's availability, premodern plumbing, and personal comfort.

Modern plumbing modified Kara'iyot's attitudes toward water and washing as hot water became more widely available. A Karaite man now in his early sixties recalled his mother being restricted to one room for seven days, but today women have greater mobility. These factors contribute to the fact that today most Karaite women seem to regard washing during menstruation as a relatively trivial issue. Daisy, who was surprised that I raised the question, said: "It is individual, not a rule, not important." Then she explained: "You see, her hands [of the woman washing] were not yet purified. If she takes the water by herself, she is unclean and contaminates the water. The modern showerhead lets women take a shower without touching the water and thus she can purify herself. But this [prohibition] is an old, old, old, habit. It belongs to my mother's generation and is one that she herself fought against."

Bathing, showering, and washing provide a vocabulary that denotes different actions, and each woman is careful to construct her own washing standards. This vocabulary is precise: "bathing" refers to an immersion in water, while "douching" (both French and Arabic), as Daisy explained, is "water coming from above. The water is touching the body but the body itself does not touch the water."[29] As long as the body is passively washed by the water, the water is not polluted by menstrual contact. "Washing" entails the use of a restricted amount of water and a wet cloth. Running water is the Karaites' metaphor of "dissolving" impurities and restoring life; thus, it is not surprising that the principle of changing water is consistent throughout Karaite culture.[30] As mentioned, not only do Karaites prohibit immersion in any source of standing water during menstruation, they also insist on the private *rahatsah*, washing, by means of running water as the concluding shower of the *'ādah*.

The Cairo Genizah reveals that Karaite and Rabbanite practices of *niddah* were especially contested in mixed marriages with the question of which law the couple will follow. We learn about this from Maimonides' responsa, written in Judeo-Arabic, in 1167 c.e. Maimonides, along with nine other rabbis and judges, protested against the "heretical custom" of Karaite *niddah* that had become common among Egyptian women. According to this responsa, women not only avoided immersion in the *mikvah* and counted only seven days of impurity, they also "have followed the heretical custom of relying on washing in 'drawn water. . . .' Even worse," Maimonides continues, "most of the women rely on complete heresy, a matter not spoken by God, and it is this: the *niddah* takes a woman who is not a *niddah* to sprinkle [*yetzikah*] her with water that she supposes is pure."[31] (Cohen 1999, 91–96). This situation was so threatening to Rabbinic authority that Maimonides mandated that a woman who deviate from rabbinic law with regard to *niddah* must be divorced.[32]

Yetzikah, or pouring in Kara'iyot's language, is a term that we can trace to Anan, who established that "a *niddah* must clean herself in a vessel only" (Nemoy 1952). Once bleeding has stopped, water acts as an active purifying agent; the measured and contained water acts against the immense symbolic power of the uncontained, unquantified blood; not only purity is constructed, but the female (her body and her power) is articulated according to cultural measures. Impurity is washed away.[33]

This quality of purification becomes evident in the concluding shower that facilitates the woman's reentry into her community. Sophia explained, "After the seven days she [the menstruating woman] can take a shower and would be considered clean. The shower should be taken [in the] afternoon and she won't be considered clean, to go to the temple, until after sunset. There is no *tahara* [purification] on Saturday, so if we still have our period on Sunday we are supposed to be clean on [the next] Saturday. We have to stay one more day."

Sophia explained about the symbolism of seven: "I am always relating seven to the days of the week." "Cupping" the running water, the body "drinks" purity seven times, corresponding to each day of impurity. In this cleansing act, two women meet; the maternal authority conducts the ceremony and validates the younger woman's new status. Performed in the privacy of a woman's home, in her own bathroom, this ritual, like Passover and the special prayers on high holidays, locates the domestic sphere as the central place of communal and personal connectedness. While standing naked under the shower, the *niddah* has seven cups of water poured over her by another woman (often the mother, the mother-in-law, or a sister), who also instructs her to recite the *Shma'*. The *Shma'*, perhaps the most significant prayer in Judaism for both Rabbanites and Karaites, is concise; it is a speech act that affirms and avows the sacred oath between an individual and God. The inclusive nature of the prayer in the plural voice attests to one's full presence and commitment to uniting the supreme covenant with one God of one people. "*Shma' Isra'el, 'Adonai 'Elohenu 'Adonai 'ehad*" (Hear, O Israel; the Lord our God, the Lord is one) is recited out loud, in Hebrew, emphasizing God's accessibility to the voice of the individual.

As a verbal transition, the prayer usually accompanies rites of passage. It is interesting to note that whereas in Rabbanite Judaism, one is prohibited from reciting the *Shma'* without wearing clothes, in Karaite tradition, the nakedness of the woman is an important aspect in the sacred moment of purification, constructed by the sprinkled or poured seven cups of water, the prayer, and the presence of the second woman. Emerging from *niddah* to purity and marking her sexual availability requires that she reveals herself fully—in body and in spirit—under the water, reiterating the biblical affirmation, "I will sprinkle pure waters upon you and you shall be pure of all your impurities" (Ezek. 36:25).

The presence of the second woman is necessary because, as Daisy explained to me, if the *niddah* were to touch the vessel herself, it would become contaminated. In the past, she would have had to lift it up in order to pour it over herself, inevitably contaminating it even before purifying herself. The presence of a second woman, therefore, has a practical, physi-

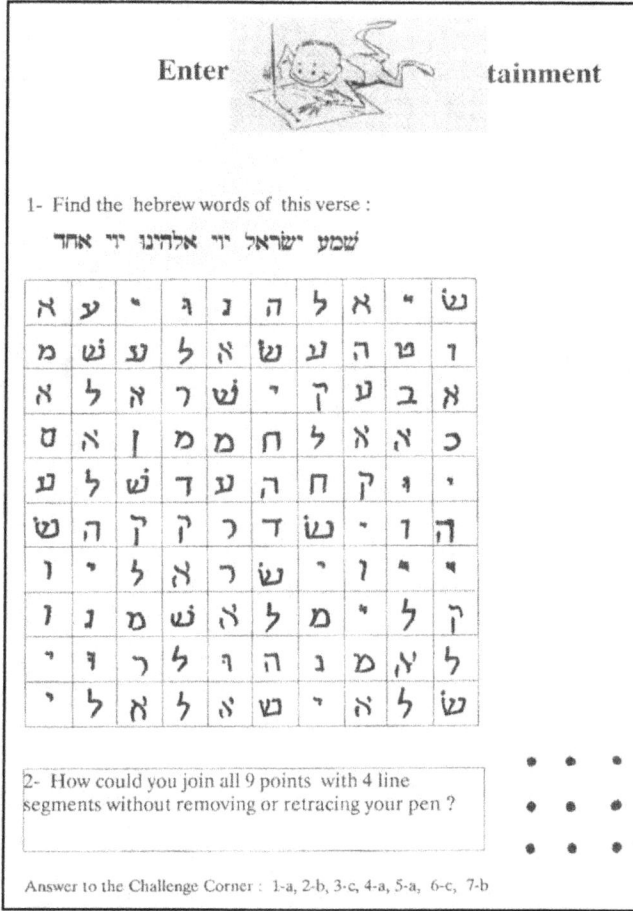

A Hebrew acrostic for children based on the first verse of the *Shma'* prayer. (*KJA Bulletin* 1994)

cal function. It keeps the water external to her body. Nowadays, however, modern plumbing makes it possible for a woman not to have to touch the water, which has led more women to purify themselves without the help of the other woman. Moreover, the more prudish modern nuclear family may frown on the presence of another female to perform this ceremony. Still, the women continue to recite the *Shma'*. Running water is the essential substance in this act of purification. Washing on the last day of the period taps the flow of water, blood, and body. Running water embodies the notion of renewal, especially coming down over the top of the head.[34] Its flowing animates movement in time, enabling a new identity to emerge. The inscription of the blood on the body is now dissolved, washed away.

7

Resolution from Within:
The Encounter between *Niddah* and *Yoledah*

> And yet that woman-thing speaks. But not "like," not "the *same*," not "identical with itself" nor to any x, etc. . . . It speaks "fluids," even in the paralytic undersides of this economy.
> Luce Irigaray, "The 'Mechanics' of Fluids"

The Experience of Childbirth

The Karaites have traditionally regarded themselves as the intellectuals of their time. Folklore, as stated in Karaite halakhah and as regarded throughout Karaite history, is an unfavored category, since it stands for all that is irrational or nonconcrete. Even in their formative period, the Karaites juxtaposed folklore with the privileged category of truth and history: distant from that which is referential, folklore was associated with the mystical, a perspective that the Karaites disavow. In contrast to the articulation of Karaites' self-perception as *dam 'asil* (the pure, unmixable, blood), folklore and oral tradition were created through multiple renditions of the "real." If *pshat*, "naked reading," is the Karaite model of approaching the text, then folklore dresses up the textual body, covers it up, hiding the real meaning. Consequently, Karaites considered beliefs in demons, magic, and power of amulets and mystical ritual to be witchcraft, prohibited by the Torah (Birnbaum 1971, v; Mahler 1949, 10). This might explain the relative absence of folktales and legends (among the other genres) in Karaite culture, and the Karaites' discomfort in claiming the validity of several beliefs.

Historically, the preoccupation with truth not only governed and inhibited the Karaite creative processes in producing fiction, but also left its mark on the community's discursive patterns. Often during our conversations women stated that a particular prohibition, belief, or idea originated in the Bible. Sometimes the reference was actually in the Bible; at other times not. The point whether the Karaites' memory *of* the Bible corresponds exactly with what is written *in* the Bible is interesting, primarily because it reveals that the referential mechanism from the body to the Bible is as productive as the one from the text to the body. This correspondence, or lack thereof, tells us about women's need to legitimate their daily culture (beliefs, thoughts, and actions) with an authoritative stamp of the perceived Bible. It is not surprising that the Kara'iyot compensated for the limited textual concerns with womanhood by expanding beyond the Bible's concrete pages, as contained in the book itself. At the same time, the appropriated Bible that they internalized speaks for its immense role and control in their consciousness.

Being the sole reference for God's truth and its law, the Bible has become a "discursive authority" or "total discourse" that governs the mechanism of producing knowledge. Often, the conceptual notion of reading negotiates with oral materials by redefining and connecting them to the realm of the textual. But more than a conflict between oral and textual, the main issue becomes how to reconcile text and body. From the women's perspective it is a question of how one complements established knowledge without contesting and undermining its authority. Reading as a woman, in this sense, means that she must rely on her body. This establishes an interactive didactic between the referential system of the Bible, building on its validity, and the body, enhancing its symbolic aptness as a scientific, real reference for reconciliation between the two. Contesting the claim that Karaites have no folklore, therefore, this study shows that a specific internal oral tradition, largely concerning body praxis, has developed among Karaites, particularly among women. For women, this oral tradition is in fact an extension of the written law, working to resolve the tension between text, body, and everyday life. In the Karaite reading, meaning is always evaluated in terms of both its truthful value and its textual origin.

In chapter 3 I showed how the coded language women use among themselves to communicate the subject of *niddah* is similar to their "ethnographic," oral language of describing their practices in our meetings, underscoring the secrecy around the female body, coupled with their internalized shame and discomfort regarding the subject ("It is all the dirt of the body"). Whereas the social collective Karaite body is at the discussion of Karaite purity, the private body is hidden and its language is limited. In fact, the secrecy surrounding the female body implies a certain level of "working" of the mechanism of cleanliness in the culture. Speaking and indulging in the subject of cleanliness and purity is considered tasteless and lacking in good sense. Silence, in contrast, is taken as a matter of fact until there is an absolute need to address abnormalities or deviations: in the realm of narrativity, crisis provokes the narrative process. The discussion in this chapter makes clear that when secrecy and discomfort frame the space for counter narratives, they are not only presented in more dramatic tones and ask for immediate solutions; they are also further abbreviated, reducing language and symbols to the level of the ritual itself. But abbreviation—or ritual—does not stop at the level of language and practices; it reclassifies the integral body into discrete, fluid-based components, such as blood, breast milk, and urine.

Childbirth, Milk, and the Evil Eye

"If this is the Karaites," explained Eli, then "this is the Rabbanites." He moved his hand from one side of the table to the other, mapping a scheme of historical relationships and using our coffee cups as props to illustrate the great distinction between the two cultures. Eli, a fifty-five-year-old Karaite scholar and writer, was intense, with a good memory for details that he usually communicated with a nostalgic sense of loss and pain of the "good old days back home." When he described the adjustment of a few Karaite families in Rochester, New York, twenty years ago, he made sure to mention that for many years, he taught his daughters to hide the fact that they were Karaites. "What for?" Eli asked, with an incredulous expression on his face. "It is enough we are Jews from Egypt!" As Jews from Egypt, they were already subject to ethnic discrimination within the Jewish Ashkenazi community, he explained, and to reveal his daughters' Karaite identity would expose them to humiliation that he was not willing to face.

Once Eli began talking about his childhood in Cairo, his fingers became a counting index for his family history. In his attempt to figure out his sister's age, he calculated according to his mother's breast-feeding period for each child. He counted the interval between each of the children, as he bent one finger for each sibling. His mother's body, a veritable familial timetable, recorded his family biography. The interval between pregnancies is a year and a half, including the nine months of pregnancy and the nine months of breast feeding. Five siblings amount to a total of seven years and a half. This is Eli's perception of the bodily experience of childbirth and breast feeding.

Until the early twentieth century, Karaite women spent most of their reproductive years either pregnant or breast feeding, a fact that dramatically cut down the frequency of their menstrual periods. As Harrell (1981), who focuses on the symbolic transitional state of women in the Third World, warns, assuming otherwise "would be a misperception for modern Western societies, where menstrual cycles repeat themselves ad infinitum and lactation is an unusual occurrence." In Egypt, most Karaites lived in an extended family household where mother, mother-in-law, aunts, sisters, and sisters-in-law were present and available around the *wālidah* bed.[1] The breakdown of the intimate walls surrounding the Karaites had already taken place in Egypt through the shift from home to hospital delivery, in the 1930s in Cairo. This had an impact on the Karaite indigenous system of childbirth, redefining it along new medical and public interests. The communal solidarity and networking of women, the woman's individual experience, her relationship with her body, and the economy of her milk (cf. Jordan 1993, 146) all underwent a major change and adjustment.[2] Such a move against Karaite values and codes of honor undermined not only the traditional overtones of Karaites' practices; they hurt the subtle, more intimate, fabric of their sentiments.[3] Julia is in her fifties. She is a quiet and gentle woman. Her magnifying glasses strengthen the impression given by her eyes of a warm and sincere person. She still recalls her mother's strong reaction to the male doctor's presence. She said, "My mother insisted on giving birth at home because in the hospital there are male doctors and that means shame." She shook her head in disbelief. But more important, she added, is the fact that "a woman's milk will stop once two breast-feeding women are in the same room." Not only shameful, she disclosed, the production of milk is vulnerable to the presence of other women who just gave birth, the *walidāt* (plural of *wālidah*). As a result, all of Julia's brothers and sisters were born at home.[4]

Julia's mother justified her insistence that Julia deliver at home by pointing to the danger that her milk would stop if she were around other breast-feeding women. This belief recalls other folk beliefs associated with the danger of the evil eye: although the lactating woman is vulnerable throughout the period of her breast feeding, it is mostly during the first days after delivery that she must be careful of exposure to outsiders, since anyone can cause her milk to stop—anyone can inflict the evil eye, even herself.[5] But in the context of public breast feeding, other lactating women are more dangerous because the flow of milk is not always regular and a woman who cannot produce milk can easily inflict the evil eye on a woman who has abundant milk. Milk, so valuable and vital (Kara'iyot believe that each breast produces a different flavor, one sweet and one sour), is a resource of "limited good" and cannot flow in two women's bodies simultaneously (Foster 1972).[6] This belief had tangible consequences on women's social interaction by motivating them to limit their exposure to other breast-feeding women.[7] Still, the articulation of milk as a limited good is not surprising, as even its whiteness was associated with the sacredness of giving birth.

To a certain extent, childbirth and lactation reveal Karaites' ambivalence toward women, since even as these states speak of women's ultimate performative (biological) destiny, that of bearing children, they are perceived as liminal due to the fact that the woman is still bleeding. *Tum'at ledah* (postpartum impurity), as we saw earlier, is said in Leviticus to last forty days after the birth of a son and eighty days after the birth of a daughter. Indeed, another factor relevant to the Karaite woman's discomfort regarding hospital birth was the notion of being unclean after her delivery. The woman's impurity due to postpartum bleeding shapes her perceptions and further divides the *wālidah*'s body into two separate areas: the upper/clean and the lower/dirty. This corresponds with the woman's newborn identity as she enters the social institution of motherhood, with her lower body now neutralized and her upper body becoming the center of life. Obviously, the postpartum shift from genitalia to breast is part of the natural movement from birthing to feeding. For Karaite women, the impurity of the *yoledah* and the taboo on sexual intercourse create a more pronounced discontinuity between her lower and her upper body, between her own blood and her own milk. The moment highlights the interplay between these two body zones as they are related to the production of blood and milk, and to the two personas, the breast-feeding mother, the *wālidah*, and the menstruating woman, the *niddah*.[8]

In this section I discuss how the *wālidah/yoledah* (breast-feeding mother) resolves the crisis when she is approached by the *'ādah/niddah* (menstruating woman)—a woman who is considered more polluted and dangerous. I examine two narratives that describe such an encounter and reveal the valorization of mother's milk within a discourse of female bodily fluids (i.e., blood, breast milk, and urine), followed by a discussion of the trauma of the open, fragmented body and the resolutions that the women provided.

Mother's Milk and the *Yoledah / Wālidah*

When a Karaite woman has a baby, the act of birth transforms her as well, giving her a new identity—the *wālidah*. *Wālidah* in the Egyptian dialect of Arabic designates a woman who has recently delivered a baby. The Egyptian term, used by the Karaites today, refers to a woman's condition, including her impurity, following delivery.[9] *Wālidah*, or *yoledah/yoledet* in Hebrew, is the nominal active female participle, which morphologically and semantically conveys the sense of the woman as an active agent in the act of giving birth. At the same time, the fact that the child (*walad* or *yeled*) and the mother (*wālidah* or *yoledah*) are semantically related informs her status; giving birth blurs the distinction between the woman who gives birth and she who is herself being born into motherhood.

Motherhood in the Karaite context is an all-encompassing role that defines a woman's totality. Tied so tightly to fertility and community survival, motherhood plays a key role in the reproductive process. But more than that, it is the main institution that generates Karaite identity. As a nubile woman, she is responsible for protecting both the fertility of her body and her capacity to conceive. Once a child is born, it is the flow of breast milk that becomes her main concern. Breast feeding is an intimate discursive event that establishes the framework for the mother/child bond. It also serves to initiate both mother and child into the community.

Both the *niddah* and the *yoledah* have, on the level of praxis, a special social status due to their marked physical condition. This status subjects them to a wide array of prohibitions and restrictions (cf. Buckley and Gottlieb 1988). The body of the *wālidah* becomes both a site and a vulnerable receptor of impurity. Her forty/eighty days of postpartum confinement restricts her physical mobility and social interaction. Still practiced among the Bay Area Karaites to varying degrees are the prohibitions against a *wālidah* (like the *'ādah*) entering the synagogue, visiting the cemetery, or having sexual intercourse (for fear of contaminating the husband, who then might enter the synagogue in a state of impurity).[10] A new mother is considered vulnerable because her body is actively engaged in the production of milk, and both she and the community concern themselves with protecting this milk.

The point of encounter between the menstruating woman and the lactating woman is in fact a zone of "confrontation" between two "liminal personae" (Victor Turner's term, 1979, 235). Symbolically the two women compete not over an abstract position of power but rather over matters of immediate physical significance: fertility and the production of milk. The liminality of the body—or time of interstructural transition—calls for the construction of two mutually exclusive categories, which can be further defined and polarized: the *niddah* (the menstruating woman) and the *wālidah* (the lactating woman).

The conception of the *wālidah*'s vulnerability as fundamentally rooted in her production of milk is both biologically and socially contingent. As the symptom of the mother's good health in the present, the milk mainly reflects the Karaites' desire for the well being of the baby in the future. The occasional occurrence of infertility among women, or women having insufficient milk of their own, contributes to the tenaciousness and uncertainty surrounding the flow of the milk, a fact that on the one hand further marginalizes anomalous women (in Douglas's [1966] terminology), and on the other further articulates the milk as a substance of limited good. The evil eye, other lactating women, and, most of all, the presence of a menstruating woman trigger dangers that could impede or even prevent the flow of milk. Thus, when a *wālidah* and a menstruating woman meet or interact, an elaborate defensive strategy is required.

Sophia was half-smiling when she started with a disclaimer: "This is a superstitious thing." Only then did she continue. "If a woman just gave birth and I got my period, I am not allowed to go, walk to her, first. She is supposed to walk first toward me." When I asked what would happen, she replied: "She may not have enough milk for the baby." Seeing my puzzled expression, she added, "But if she approaches me, it is okay." Only later when I met Naʿimah did I realize that Sophia's description has special importance.

Here Sophia presented herself as a thoroughly modern woman, since she probably would not want to be perceived as a superstitious person, in spite of the fact that she does have a tremendous respect for tradition. Nevertheless, her position also reveals a somewhat ambivalent worldview. By initially classifying the belief as a superstition, Sophia expresses a degree of critical distance from its truth value. She is aware of the fact that this belief, not originating in any text, probably belongs to the folklore of women, part of their life experience. Her claim that this practice is based on a superstition is a rhetorical device that allows her to express the belief while freeing her from being considered superstitious herself. Other women also claimed that the prohibition against a menstruating woman visiting a *wālidah* is rooted in belief rather than textual truth. One of them even mentioned that this belief used to be quite common among many women, including Muslims and Christians. In universalizing it and disclaiming its specific religious source, she effectively legitimized and secularized the prohibition.

The danger to which Sophia refers is relatively minor: the mother might not have enough milk. The internal logic is familiar from the Bible: if the *niddah* is a site of impurity, then contact with her transfers her state of impurity to another and renders the person as impure. All this is nullified if the *wālidah* approaches first. Women's folklore takes the textual threat of menstruation further, as if by metonymic extension, in that the menstruating woman is not only polluting through direct physical contact—her mere physical presence is impurifying. The preoccupation with protecting cultural purity is so significant that the notion of the impure expands beyond the physical body and the shadow to include the body's presence. The impurity resulting from the encounter between the *wālidah* and the *'ādah* does not pollute the *wālidah*'s milk, or for that matter, sour it; rather, it interrupts the flow of milk.

Sophia also offers a resolution as a way of reducing the potential conflict: as long as the *wālidah* is the one who approaches the menstruating woman and is told of the other woman's "presence" (i.e., condition), her milk is safe. Physical approach, in this case, as part of a symbolic power interaction, becomes a preemptive strategy. Being informed thus enables the *wālidah* to make cognitive calculated choices and counterbalances the physical threat of menstrual pollution. In other words, she who approaches, she who is mobile, maintains the dominant position. Thus, the spatial entanglement of the two has its mental correspondence; the movement of the body is permeated by the actions of the mind. Being mentally and physically active allows the lactating woman to keep her boundaries intact and prevent them from being invaded by the polluted menstruating woman.

In spite of the fact that the physical aspect of this interaction is highly explicit, the meeting between the two women is both symbolic and literal, in the Hebrew sense of *milluli*, which includes the practiced verbal utterance. The encounter introduces a line of order according to which the *wālidah*'s cognitive awareness restrains the chaotic potential of the other body by instituting a social "management" over emotions and disorder. The body is implicitly conceived as a Durkheimian *homo duplex*, a closed container of emotions and antisocial desire controlled from above by a social order that is the result of internalized cultural and political constructs (Durkheim 1961 [1915], 29; Scheper-Hughes and Lock 1989, 10–11; Turner 1984, 37). The spatial tension created by two bodies coming into proximity—the bleeding body with the lactating body—is similarly hierarchical and asymmetrical: what the *wālidah* is to the menstruating woman is not what the menstruating woman is to the *wālidah*. A hierarchy of impurity is constructed. If we follow the contours of the violated physical body, we see that the *wālidah*'s body is considered open, above and below. The integrity of the body is flawed, leaving it vulnerable to the threat of penetration.

A transgressed system, once it is represented within the rubric of the radical dramatization of the vulnerable body, with a bleeding vagina and dripping nipples, testifies to its inability to remain in control. Underlying this construction of the deviant, transgressed body is the unconscious prototypical conception of the body as a self-regulating system, closed and defined. Similarly, in his discourse of the grotesque body, Bakhtin suggests that "[t]he stress is laid on those parts of the body that are open to the outside world, that is, the parts through which the world enters the body or emerges from it, or through which the body itself goes out to meet the world" (Bakhtin 1968, 26). Moreover, the lack of representation of the female body as a space of differentiation is precisely a result of the fact that she is an "open container" or a volume without contours, and thus more threatening (Irigaray 1991).

Studies of Middle Eastern cultures, such as Boddy's study of North Sudan (1989) and Delaney's of a Turkish village (1988, 1991), emphasize as well the conception of the female body as an enclosure whose integrity is violated during menstruation and childbirth. This is all the more apparent when language bears witness to such physical articulations. In Hebrew, the word *guf* (variously translated as "body," "self," "substance," "person," "element," or "matter") is related to *le-hagif*, the infinitive form of the *hif'il* pattern, which means to "shutter," "to close off."[11] The drama of the open body is enacted through the flow of its fluids and the way these fluids, in moving from one body to another, physically communicate health and control, or danger and lack of control.[12] Mary Douglas defines the marginal in reference to the external/internal paradigm (1966). She regards marginality as the inevitable inherited disposition of any given system, especially the body: "All margins are dangerous.... Any structure of ideas is vulnerable at its margins. We should expect the orifices of the body to symbolize its especially vulnerable points. Matter issuing from them is marginal of the most obvious kind. Spittle, blood, milk, urine, feces or tears by simply issuing forth have traversed the boundary of the body" (Douglas 1966, 121).[13]

The problem of the invocation of body boundaries is forcefully expressed in the following conversation with Na'imah. We were still talking at Mira's about the prohibitions of the *niddah* in Karaite culture. As usual, Na'imah formulated the prohibition in the second person, making sure that I myself would know to follow the rules. I repeated after her: "So it is *ḥarām* [impure, prohibited] for me [while menstruating] to be with a *wālidah*?"

She approved: "Yes, you should not enter her place. "It's not good for a woman who has the *'ādah* to go to the *wālidah*."

"So the *'ādah* with the milk is . . ." I was thinking in terms of *ḥarām*. She completed the thought: "Not good, not good . . . because of the milk." I asked her if she knew any stories about other women whose milk stopped. She replied stormily,

> *Wahh, 'ana,* oh, myself [pause]. Myself. It happened to me [when I was young and living in Egypt]. I was still a three-day *wālidah* and one who had the *'ādah* entered. At once the milk stopped.

There was no milk [pause]. Then we found out who it was and we told her, I told her: "Come, did you come and I am *wālidah* and you carry the *'ādah*?" She said: "Yes, what will happen?" I told her: "The milk will stop." I told her, "Come," she came, she peed in the bathroom, and then I peed after her.

I was surprised. "In the same toilet? Without flushing the water, right?"

"No," she answered. "*Fi el-'ardh*, on the ground, on the ground. In the *hammam*, in the shower, on the floor.[14] Then we had supper and that's all. I had milk all the time. Do you see? If you do this the milk will come back." Na'imah had an eager expression on her face, making sure I understood the immense significance of the matter.

Na'imah described a similar ritual in Cairo that was performed by a woman who, attempting to conceive, recalled that while breast feeding she had been visited by a menstruating woman. After four years of living away from the neighborhood, unable to conceive, Na'imah's neighbor, a mother of one child, recalled Na'imah's visit in her house ("She [the neighbor] was a *wālidah* and I [Na'imah] was still a *bint tame'a* [an impure young girl/woman]"). The neighbor tracked down Na'imah and asked her to do the urination ritual described above. One month later, Na'imah claimed, the neighbor became pregnant.

Na'imah's narrative, in comparison to Sophia's, introduces an element of urgency. On the one hand the narrative of the milk, which stopped, is told in the first person as personal history. Yet because of the speaker's involvement, it contains all the conventional elements of a good story: repetition, the use of the number three, a dialogue, and a concluding address to the listener, in the second person. With its short sentences and extensive use of verbs, the poetics of this narrative adds detail and concreteness to the emotional intensity of the speaker. There is a deep connection as well between the verbal text (the dialogue, the speech act of invitation: "come," "put," etc.) and the semiotic-symbolic acts in this narrative.

Na'imah's narrative also underscores the conception of the body as a closed unit. The underlying anatomical assumption of her narrative is that if the production of milk stops, or if a woman fails to conceive, there is an external reason for such malfunctions. Once the reason is found and the appropriate ritual is properly performed, the obstacle is removed. In other words, by virtue of the fact that she has had a child and is lactating, the *wālidah*'s body is no longer a closed defined entity, and as such is vulnerable.

Beyond supplementing prescribed methods of correcting the transgressed body (or bodies), this simple, lucid story posits a structure in which the resolution of distinct binary oppositions leads to an elegant plot. Whereas the function of the prohibition is to restrict the mobility of the two women and to create well-defined boundaries, the narrative begins with the violation of the prohibition. Thus, both narration and fertility begin with the opening of the body and the transgression of its borders.

Both folklore and ritual, especially rites of passage, have the tendency to abbreviate messages, to codify language by omitting irrelevant information in favor of magnifying basic principles or codes, at times to the extent of becoming what Zora Neale Hurston identified as "folklore": "The boiled down juice of human living" (Hurston 1976, 41–42).[15] Hurston may have intended her remarks as a valorization of folklore, but my own reading of this Karaite reductionist discourse of the body brings to light the ambivalent nature of folklore. Women pay for this particular reduction with their marginalization and the silencing of their own narratives.[16] In the case of the *wālidah* and the *'ādah*, social and biological benefits are achieved at the cost of female solidarity. There is a direct causal relationship: the more devoted mother a woman is—and the more protective she is—the more she tends to avoid the company of other women.

In the following paragraphs I suggest that one read the narrative in the context of the discourse of reduction, attempting to interpret the story of the reduced body in a literal way. I follow the course of this representation first from the body to menstruation and lactation, and then from its physical condition to its fluids. At first I remain with the events and context in order to demonstrate how the text is embodied in the very presence of the body—reduced, divided, and open as it is—in the ritual. I then explore the discourse of the coded language, in the absence not only of the subject but also even of the body, traces of which appear only in bodily fluids.

The female body is the locus of the social forces of purity and impurity in Karaite body politics. From a mere female, associated with what is considered a normal condition, she becomes an *'ādah*, and from pregnant wife she becomes a *wālidah*. The lower part of a menstruating female's body (womb/genitals) is the dominant part which identifies the *'ādah*, as opposed to the *wālidah* who is controlled and identified by the condition of the upper part of the body (breast).

It is as if the body of the menstruating woman were represented in a caricature by exaggerated genitalia coupled with a restricted mobility of the legs, reflecting the prohibitions on intercourse, visitation, and unrestricted participation in social religious events. Perhaps one can even speak of a surrealistic mutilated body in which the lower half becomes the radical synecdoche of the menstruating woman as a whole. What accompanies this caricature is the cultural significance attached to the lower body: blood, dirt, smell, and the anxiety associated with these substances.

The lactating woman, while not fully divorced from her genitals (for her postpartum bleeding continues to define her as impure), inhabits the opposite extreme of this cultural spectrum: the upper part of her body reflects a symbolic exaggeration of the enlarged breasts and nipples of the nursing mother. The cultural signification of this state is health, abundance, and nourishment. Whereas the upper body is productive, the lower body is restricted. As two discrete beings, the menstruating woman and the lactating woman not only are reduced to their bodily conditions, but their bodies themselves are divided and fragmented by the social, religious, moral, and aesthetic significance their society attaches to menstruation and lactation. Thus, the very sociolinguistic documentation of and reference to bodily phenomena undermines the integrity of the female body as a whole entity.

The tension created by juxtaposing these two oppositions, the upper and the lower, culminates in the dominance of the lower body: the flow of milk is interrupted. The interaction proposed by Sophia, in which the *wālidah* approaches the menstruating woman, can be construed as the upper body regaining its dominance: it is now mobile, and while it "sits" on the lower body it (b)locks its ability to move and stop the milk flow. Naʿimah's account, which ends with the subversive conspiracy between the *wālidah* and the menstruating woman, further suggests that menstruation and lactation are two dynamically opposed poles that push in different directions in the same body. Once the upper body (*wālidah*) is controlled by the presence of the lower (menstruating) body, it becomes paralyzed. Moral categories that view the upper body as pure and the lower body as impure are further internalized by the claim that when juxtaposed, the necessary dominance of the grotesque lower body over the equally grotesque upper body results in the interruption of the flow of milk. While the menstruating woman is perceived as an active, aggressive agent, the lactating woman is perceived as a passive, victimized body.

The language of these narratives further reduces the woman with the *ʿādah* to blood and the *wālidah* to milk. But it is the ritual of reconciliation, in which urine mediates between blood and milk, that retroactively maps the body onto its fluids. The body, in other words, is represented through its three bodily fluids. The liquid paradigm is further clarified by the polar symbolism of each fluid, which then itself becomes a distinct category: milk and blood are extreme categories in direct opposition while urine is the neutral, mediating substance (within the boundaries of female bodily interaction).[17] The three bodily fluids are engaged in a material discourse, and once loaded with social meaning, the urine is able to resolve, "wash away," the contradictory residues of blood from milk.

Despite Naʿimah's stated belief that the power of menstrual blood to stop a mother's milk extends to other cultures, and in fact to all women ("Not only the Jews were afraid of the *ʿādah*, [so was] every one, the Muslims and the Christians. Our family was very careful"), this interaction and the attribution of a specific characterization to each bodily fluid might very well be unique to Karaite culture. It may be worthwhile, nonetheless, to situate Karaite practices among European models of the cultural economy of bodily fluids.

Thomas Laqueur, in his work on the politics of reproductive biology (1990, 25–43), finds both the fungibility of fluids and corporeal flux to be important characteristics in the construction of the one-sex body whose higher form is male: "Like reproductive organs, reproductive fluids turn out to be versions of each other; they are the biological articulation, in the language of a one-sex body, of the politics of two genders and ultimately of engendering" (1990, 39). In this relaxed economy of bodily fluids, not only could menstrual blood, mother's milk, and semen be "interconvertible"; the borders between "other residues and food, between the organs of reproduction and other organs, between the heat of passion and the heat of life [are] indistinct and ... porous" (1990, 42). By comparison, one could claim that the Karaite construction of the body is modeled on the gendered body and is based on gender differences and sexual specificities. Oppositions are enhanced in accord with the sex-gender paradigm informing the hierarchy of female impurity at different reproductive stages.

In a rather broad discussion of Western culture, Roland Barthes, following Bachelard's binary opposition of wine and milk, elaborates on their semiotics and identifies wine as the fire element as opposed to milk, which is antiwine and antifire. Regarding milk he writes, "Its purity, associated with the innocence of the child, is a token of strength, of a strength which is not revulsive, not congestive, but calm, white, lucid, the equal of reality" (Barthes 1972, 60). Barthes's notion of milk as "equal to reality" is problematic. If we think of reality in its simplicity, Barthes's articulation can perhaps justify a universal representation of milk as an unambiguous substance. Yet if we problematize the notion of the "real," applying Irigaray's critique, we could argue that Barthes's idea is still within a framework modulated by "the ruling symbolics" of writing "solids."

Fluids, according to Luce Irigaray, constitute a discourse that marks sexual differences. They are female languages or objects that have been excluded from the dominant discourse for which solid (rational, logic, real, metaphoric) constitutes the only mode of symbolization. This mode "continues to resist adequate symbolization and/or signifies the powerlessness of logic to incorporate in its writing all the characteristic features of nature" (Irigaray 1985, 106–11). Irigaray insists on developing a basic taxonomy of the attributes of fluids that correspond to their physical reality, prefiguring the discourse that should have been written. Milk, according to this description is, like other fluids, not equal to itself. It is both "potent and impotent owing to its resistance to the countable." Always "unending" and changing, it refuses "static identification." More than that, "it mixes with bodies of a like state, sometimes dilute[s] itself in them in an almost homogeneous manner, which makes the distinction between the one and the other problematical" (Irigaray 1985: 111).

Based on Mieke Bal's articulation of the (s)word (Bal 1988, 1–32), one can further argue that milk in the culture, like the (s)word, adheres to an ambiguous space between thing and event. As a "thing," milk is the fluid of the female body. In its exclusive performative act (Searle 1969, 18) between the female body and the child, milk reaffirms its meaning as the predicate of the postdelivery mother-baby bond. As an "event," milk states and restates the conceptual framework exclusive to the creation of this bond. Mother's milk, through its specific role in the Karaite culture, is articulated through and by its discursive constitution. I will return to the subject of milk in the next chapter.

It follows, then, that the economy of urine is different from that of either blood or milk. In the hierarchy of bodily fluids, urine is the least threatening: generally asexual, it is neither gender-marked nor associated with the reproductive system. It is also relatively colorless, associated with the absolute neutrality of water.[18] In Karaite culture, urine, like all other bodily emissions, is impure. One of the reasons Karaites take off their shoes before entering the prayer room is their fear that impure, defiling substances such as urine have come into contact with the shoes. The impure urine is used as the medium of exchange between the two women in the *wālidah*'s purification ritual, generating a new communicative capacity for the body.[19]

Na'imah's resolution also relies on the body as a self-regulatory system. The urine of the lactating woman flows over the urine of the menstruating woman in order to reconcile the tension between two poles. If urinating is a symbolic act that grounds the presence and reality of the body, then what we have at the end of the ritual is a conjunction of the two bodies over the ground with the breast milk covering the surface of the blood. The conflict between the two women fades in this territorial and geographical resolution of contested identities. The intense red (blood) and white (milk) colors, which represent the exaggerated "postures" of the women, are mediated by the more neutral yellow (urine) in an entirely physiological enactment, which restores the flow of milk.

It is crucially important to realize, however, the discrepancy between the biology of the body and its cultural construction: in most cases, as Karaite women are well aware, after the postpartum bleeding a breast-feeding woman does not ovulate or menstruate for at least six months. It is no surprise, then, to find that in our meetings, many women spoke at length about the importance of breast feeding. Lactation tends to suppress menstruation and thus the possibility of conception, and perhaps in this way empowers women to exercise some agency over birth control.[20] Karaites also believe that the menstruation of one woman can potentially suppress another woman's production of milk.[21] The insistence that blood subdues milk (and fertility) reorganizes the orientation of the biological dynamic and conceptually reverses the channels through which fluids flow.

As long as a woman breast-feeds, the culturally constructed superiority of the upper body over the lower body is incontestable, and as long as her body produces milk, two systems of oppositions are acting together, constantly shifting the defined contours of the inside and the outside, the upper and the lower body. Following Bakhtin (1968), we can conclude that through the inversion of the biological order—the lower body overpowering the upper rather than the reverse—the classic achieves primacy over the grotesque, and the body enters into the correct social-religious order. Entry into the social-religious order comes only at the price of dividing the female body: while its upper part submits itself to the text and becomes its embodiment, the lower part designates the totality of the whole community.

Within Karaite culture, a synecdochic bind between the fluids and the female body is but one in a chain of tropological modes that formalizes this poetics (White 1973, xii). As the locus and consciousness of the community, it defines and constitutes the social categories and presupposes that departure and separation is the norm. Kara'iyot thus make mediation with the world possible through other sources of power even if they happen to be polluting. It is remarkable, though, that at the same time they come up with a resolution through which they can protect the cohesiveness of the community. More than that, they resolve the "superstition" through a shared ritual. If Karaite women can urinate together, they can also bridge over the symbolic differences of *niddah* and *yoledah*. The organistic strategy commits itself to a praxis that keeps intact the social body and preserves it.

The koshering quality of women's rituals of the body may "kosher" other areas in Karaite life, such as feeding and dietary habits. As mentioned, Karaites (in accord with *Sevel ha-yerushah*) follow their own dietary laws. Unlike Rabbanite Jews, they read the Bible literally and understand the milk-meat taboo, "Thou shalt not cook a kid in its mother's milk," simply as an injunction against cooking an offspring in its own mother's milk. Whereas for the Rabbanite Jews, the two categories of dairy and meat became an organizing principle of time and space and of keeping and being kosher, for Karaite Jews mixing meat and milk poses no difficulty.

Yet the fact that I was directed to study purity and impurity in the Karaite community by the women of the community themselves is of utmost significance. It indicates that the personal accounts, which separate the woman with the *'ādah* and the *wālidah*, might be their way of claiming that Karaites keep kosher—despite the contrary view entertained by Rabbanites. Categories of milk-blood, accordingly, are but another variation on the theme of cleanliness as it relates to milk and meat. Again, it is Karaite women who tell us that Karaites, just like the Rabbanites, signify impurity and quantify it. Significantly, it is the female body that provides these categories and women's perceptions of the body's biological functions that set the definition of being a *kosher* Karaite Jew. The shift moves from the familiar Rabbanite axis of food consumption to the intimate realm of the woman's body, from the digestive process to the reproductive one. The discourse of orthodox Karaite women articulates the double message that their bodies bear the paradigms of their society *and* form the medium through which categories are experienced.

The ethnography of the body experience is a shift away from absence toward presence, from invisibility to visibility. It is a call to establish an inner reference of subjectivity, a new presence that can describe a community and its history through the disciplined mobility inscribed on the female body. As a category of knowledge, the body is the site within and around which practice and experience evolve. Their bodies claim Karaite women as kosher (against the historical Rabbanite invalidation of Karaite genealogy), and as the legitimate guarantors of Karaite Judaism. In that respect, the Kara'iyot's voice cleans, legitimizes, and redefines the whole community in terms of its religious and halakhic propriety. And bodily fluids, like other travelers, are storytellers that narrate for them—and for us—the politics and poetics of everyday life.

8

Beyond Binarism:
Mother's Milk and Karaite Dietary Law

> The only sound approach is to forget hygiene, aesthetics, morals and instinctive revulsion ... and start with the texts.
> Mary Douglas, *Purity and Danger*

Rahuni's cow has just given birth. Her Karaite owner is entirely dependent on her animals to make a living and perceives the calf's birth as a miracle. Despite fear of her neighbors' evil-eye, she makes an offer to her Rabbanite neighbor, Malkah: "Take one of your vessels and go milk the cow, because in the first seven days the milk and the vessels that touch it are *trefah* [not kosher] to us Karaites, but to you Rabbanites, it is permitted." When Malkah comes back with the full steaming bucket of hot milk, she laughs to herself wickedly: "Such a righteous one: meat and milk she mixes, but the *niddah* of a female cow she insists on observing" (Fahn 1928, 207–9, my translation). This tale, which Fahn includes in his collection of European Karaite folk tales, gives us some sense of daily cross-religious interactions between a Karaite woman and her Rabbanite neighbor. Told by a Rabbanite, the story supports the Rabbanite hierarchy of pollution, in which a cow's postpartum purity is less significant than avoiding the mixture of meat and milk. In addition, the term *niddah* is used by Malkah, the Rabbanite neighbor, to refer to something other than a menstruating woman. In the rural jargon of turn-of-the-century Eastern European Jews, *niddah* evolved to mean the term used to describe the marked status of any female animal, not only during menstruation but also after giving birth.

In the preceding chapters, we have seen how the Karaite ethnography of the body and the internal communal discourses provide what can be called an authentic description of contemporary Karaites without needing to rely on external sources or comparative methods. If the initial question was what kind of ethnography is generated by the study of a community that continually reimagines itself under the ultimate authority of the Bible, then it will be instructive to follow the ethnographic Karaite mode of reading from the field back to the text. This allows us to shift the question: What kind of understanding of the biblical text can this ethnography spark? If Karaites read the text through their bodies, and if the text is the maternal body through which Dar'i's fire of Karaite peoplehood persists (see introduction), then to understand their reading of the dietary law, one must remain at the specific site of the maternal body, and specifically within the wider conception of maternity, motherhood, and lactation. In making this transition, it becomes clear that the Karaite ideological construction of motherhood provides the key to understanding the Karaite reading of the biblical prohibition, "Do not cook [seethe] a kid [goat] in its mother's milk" (found in Exodus 23:19 and 34:26 and Deuteronomy 14:21). Thus, reading against the grain of categorization and separation shows how this dietary law, located within the mother/child relationship, acts as another coded formula of metonymic relations that positions and situates the female body. To a certain extent, this relationship consists of a critique of patriarchal control over the female body, as much as a valorized site of Karaite culture.

The juxtaposition of dietary restrictions and the maternal discourse emerging from my ethnography brings to the center of the discussion recent works on sex and gender that attempt to articulate symbolic and semiotic spaces as they relate to the maternal body (Kristeva 1986; Butler 1993). Traditionally, Jewish scholars have not associated the dietary law of prohibiting the cooking of a goat in its mother's milk with the actual mother's milk, but have approached it in terms of a general category. In fact, given the apparent centrality of this prohibition in the form of *kashrut* (Rabbanite dietary laws) within everyday Rabbanite life, it is somewhat surprising that commentators and scholars throughout history have given it so little attention. Even the Talmud, having its solution "so removed from the plain meaning of the text" (Milgrom 1990, 144), does not elaborate on the meaning of the verse, instead pointing to the corollary association of the three appearances of this prohibition in the Bible as three distinct prohibitions: "*Cooking* meat and milk together, *eating* such a mixture, and *deriving a benefit* from such a mixture" (BT Hullin 115b). Even among Karaites, the prohibition has attracted little scholarly attention and generated limited discussion, suggesting that the verse was taken to apply only to the particular case of a mother and her kid, as seen in the concluding paragraph of Karaite scholar Hachakham Shmu'el Hakohen's work, *Concerning Slaughtering:* "An *additional* prohibition exists concerning the subject of slaughtering and it is the *warning* of 'do not cook a kid in its mother's milk.'"[1] Indeed, some Karaite writers even ignored the subject entirely.[2] However, the Karaite reading of this prohibition often makes direct reference to the "mistaken" Rabbanite reading, indicating the tension surrounding the problematic issue of Karaite identity—its integrity and differentiation—as expressed through this biblical verse.

It is impossible to understand the Karaite position on this verse without considering their dialogical relationship to Rabbanite legal discourse. Here, intertextuality amounts to an attempt to "correct" prevailing perceptions of legitimate reading in the Bakhtinian sense of dialogism, where accumulated interpretations of texts are debated across different periods and time and in which, in addition to the appropriation of language and ideas, the subject actually reads (Bakhtin 1981). In part, by positioning itself in contradistinction to Rabbanite Judaism, Karaites opened themselves to the vast history of Rabbanite reading and practice, competing with it, correcting it, and replying to abstractions or ambiguities. Bearing this in mind, while treating the issue of the meat and milk diet in Karaite history and legal commentaries, I also refer to the relevant Rabbanite position and compare the two when appropriate, but I do not intend to sharpen the Karaite/Rabbanite dichotomy. My interest in their differences informs my discussion of the role these differences play in the ideological construction of the Karaites.

From the Bible to Women's Bodies

Diet and eating habits play an important role in the social politics of all cultures, and as far as the Rabbanites and Karaites are concerned, no subject has been as vehemently disputed as the observance of the dietary laws. As a Karaite "sign of separation" (Ankori 1959, ii), their interpretative stances not only generated differences in practice but were also infused with wider symbolic significance, central to the representation of Karaites and Rabbanites by each other. Already during the tenth century, at the time of the Geonim, an annual ritual was performed on the Mount of Olives on Hoshana Rabba by the Rabbanites in Jerusalem "proclaiming a *herem* against the Karaites who were eating *basar be-chalav*, meat with milk" (Mann 1972, 62). Here, *herem* denotes an excommunication of Karaites for their dietary practices. In Ibn Ezra's commentary on the meat-milk prohibition, Karaites are reduced to *chasrei ha-da'at* (ignoramuses) for their apparent misreading of this prohibition (Ibn Ezra 1977, 160). Karaites made similar charges against Rabbanites as misunderstanding the verse in question. Rabbi Hachakham Hatroki elaborates:

> And our Rabbanite brothers, following the laws of their sages, add to the prohibition [of meat] chicken with butter and milk, and take an extra stringency, and are so careful to guard the mixing of meat utensils and dairy utensils that they put [store] meat utensils and dairy utensils separately. They use special utensils for each and they are as careful with them as with the laws of purity and impurity. And this is an addition to that which is written in the Torah. And on the subject of impurity and purity—they make light of it. (Hatroki 1960, 24)

The ongoing debate surrounding the verse "Do not cook a kid" is especially evident today when much of the identity of Rabbanite Judaism is articulated by one's position as halakhic *shomer kashrut* (guarding *kashrut*), entailing strict dietary separation between dairy and meat products. Briefly, the motivation for Rabbanites' strictness was the desire to avoid any possibility of mixing between the two categories of foods. As one prescription within Rabbanite symbolic language, it is not enough for an animal to be ritually permissible, even when slaughtered, salted, and cooked halakhically; kosher meat itself can threaten the kosher paradigm if brought in proximity with dairy foods. Consequently, *kashrut* became a systematic metaphoric model in which eating demands a consciousness of marked distinctions, with attention to aspects of both space and time. For example, specific intervals of time—usually between five and six hours—are imposed between eating meat and eating dairy. *Pareve* is defined as a neutral category that is neither dairy nor meat, and that can be mixed with either. In this hierarchy of metabolic processes, time intersects with space; *kashrut* also requires a strict physical separation of cooking and eating utensils. This conduct is all-important in the production of the "conscious mouth," which becomes the site of control over hunger and desire.

The Karaite legal system, however, explicitly permits the mixing of *basar be-chalav*, meat with milk, unless the kid is the biological offspring of the mother. In order to prevent such a violation, Karaites reframed the verse with the biblical prohibitions against slaughtering or cooking either a pregnant animal or an animal that has given birth within the past seven days.[3] In addition to the strict rules of slaughter, Karaites are careful in their preparation of meat. In contrast to English, the Hebrew equivalent *basar* does not distinguish between "flesh" and "meat."[4]

The transition from inedible to edible is made through the detailed koshering process, which primarily involves extracting the blood, for "the blood is the *nefesh*, the soul." Draining all traces of blood from the meat includes the removal of its sources: veins, arteries, and organs. Salting and rinsing ensures that any minute remnants of blood will be absorbed and washed away. Karaites also avoid the *helev* (fat) and extract *gid ha-nasheh* (the sinew of the thigh). Although chicken and fish are not included in the prohibition against mixing an offspring with its mother's milk (as they are not mammals), the extraction of their blood before cooking is still of the utmost importance. In observing a young Karaite woman koshering a chicken, her Rabbanite friend commented: "What are you doing to the chicken? You are killing it." Indeed, in her zealous preparation of the meat, it seemed as though the Karaite was killing the bird all over again! In California, kosher meat is purchased from local Rabbanite butchers. Modern methods of food production have nearly eliminated the possibility of bringing together milk and meat products originating from an animal and its offspring.

Jean Soler and Mary Douglas's structural analyses set the tone for the inclusion of the dietary laws in the discussion of purity and impurity, especially relying on their contextual appearance within chapters 11 to 18 of the Levitical codes of pollution (Douglas 1966; Soler 1974, 24–30). Douglas states, in a claim that has been uncritically accepted: "For the only way in which pollution ideas make sense is in reference to the total structure of thought whose key-stone-boundaries, margins and internal lines are held in relation by rituals of separation" (Douglas 1966, 41). Arguing (after Lévi-Strauss) that the body symbolizes and represents the collective worldview, Douglas points to the question of sexual difference and the danger associated explicitly with female bodily fluids (see also Grosz 1994, 192–95). Kristeva develops this further into a critique of monotheistic Judaism, whose "strategy of identity" is to impose legal and semantic systems that are represented by the Temple and the Law. Through the reproduction of metonymic relations, Judaism articulates its meaning through a series of separations: bodily, oral, and material. In order to be separated, "one must wage a struggle during the entire length of his [*sic*] personal history." Separation, then, means "to become a speaking subject and/or subject to Law" (Kristeva 1982, 94). Like Douglas, Soler, and other scholars who have attempted to interpret the prohibition "do not cook a kid in its mother's milk," Kristeva reads the verse fully aware of the practice it inspired in Rabbanite Judaism, rather than concentrating exclusively on the text. Granting the dietary law its prominent role within the taboo system, she emphasizes that "the dietary domain will then continue to be the privileged object of divine taboos, but it will be modified, amplified, and even seem to become identified with the most moral, if not the most abstract, statements of the Law" (Kristeva 1982, 97).

This might explain why (and how) Karaite Judaism chose the meat-milk separation (or lack thereof) to be a site of difference. Through the differentiations that have developed in the two strains of interpretation, it is evident that dietary taboos (like calendar systems or purity systems) occupy a place in the identity politics of marginal cultures, and are another aspect of social life that goes back to the origin of differentiation. Dietary prohibitions are a means of cutting a people off from others. As Jean Soler puts it, "The cut is that the origin of differentiation and differencing is the prerequisite of signification" (1979, 25). From the perspective of the history of the two groups, it meant that the different readings of the dietary law were translated into daily interaction in which "no observant Rabbanite Jew could accept an invitation to dine with a Karaite" (Goitein 1954, 118). The paradigm of separation and the prohibition against mixture is inherently attractive for a lucid structure within Karaite culture, which strives for a dichotomous matrix. Structural analysis occupies these oppositions, a fact that suggests some redundancy or excess in this specific representation.[5] Positioning categories as oppositional highlights their potential violation. It is important, therefore, to consider the way Karaites overcame these polarities, ultimately permitting their mixture.

In light of the strict approach that Anan took in consolidating the Karaite legal code, refusing to mitigate rabbinical biblical stringency, the meat/milk taboo could be read as a permissive prohibition. Indeed, Mann and Harkavi find that this is the only biblical taboo that Anan "tolerated" in contrast to his other rulings (perceived as stricter than those of the Rabbanites) that revolved around abstaining from women,[6] food and wine, and fixing more fast days on the Karaite calendar. Mann and Harkavi concluded that this tolerance does not, in fact, conflict with Anan's overall doctrine.[7] It "had little value as an allowance because, after all, Anan prohibited the daily consumption of meat to those living outside of Israel" (Mahler 1949, 124–73, 142, 143).

The Karaite interpretive rules are extremely relevant to the subject of slaughter, especially with respect to how they interpret Leviticus. Certain principles were applied throughout the reading of Leviticus to guide methods of interpretation. As I mentioned in the introduction, *hekesh*, or analogy, unlike history, is "nonchronological," theorizes Bal (1987, 68–88).

Operating on the notion of sameness, analogous principles compare the unfamiliar with the familiar, expanding the space of the signifier and opening the range of referentiality. At the same time, this referentiality reframes a subject within different contextual associations. *Hekesh* is the dialectical mechanism that the Karaites use to deduce—and to make parallel—meanings. Karaites commonly employ analogy, resisting other interpretive methods (Ankori 1959, 217).[8]

The Karaites were meticulous about providing specific analogous references to understanding the verse "do not cook a kid in its mother's milk," coding the process of its interpretation with their own internal language of abbreviated formulae. The following three principles of interpretation appear repeatedly in Karaite literature:

1. *Lo tikach ha-'em 'al ha-banim* (Thou shalt not take the mother with the young [Deut. 22:6]).[9] "Take" in this context also refers to killing and eating them. In his book *Eshkol ha-Kofer*, Yehudah ben Eliyahu Hadassi (Byzantium, twelfth century) suggests that mixing a kid in its mother milk is analogous to any situation that involves taking a mother and its offspring. He provides a detailed ecological explanation, saying that by taking the mother and the offspring together, one "annihilates, uproots [*me'ashel*], and wipes out the root and the flower from God's world" (Hadassi 1836, 240). The principle adheres to the beneficial rule, which condemns destroying multiple generations of animals at the same time.

2. *'Oto ve-'et bno* (And whether it be a bull or a lamb you shall not slaughter *it and its young* on the same day [Lev. 22:28]). The second *hekesh* replaces the maternal pair ("*ha-'em 'al ha-banim,*" mother and her offspring) with a paternal pair (*'Oto ve-'et bno*, it [masculine] and its young). This analogy amplifies the concern for preserving nature, moving beyond the mother/son link to include the father/son.

3. *'Iqar va-ferach* (the root and the flower). The inseparable pair appears in other Karaite sources as "the root and its branch," or the principle and its end result. The specific use of the conjunctive *vav* in Hebrew intensifies the tight association of the two. Karaite commentaries substitute *'iqar* for the parent (father or mother) and *perach* (or *ferach* when preceded by a vowel) for the offspring.

In attempting to establish semantic distinction between an animal and its offspring, the Karaites have used all three principles interchangeably. The following are some examples of the treatment of this dietary taboo by primary Karaites sources. Eliyahu Bashyazi's *Aderet Eliyahu* (published posthumously in 1490) is a standard manual of belief and practice, equal to the Rabbanite's *Shulchan Arukh* (Ankori 1966, 26; Nemoy 1952, 236–38), and as such is the obvious reference in which to find the Karaites' rationale in codifying this verse. In general, Basyatchi is noted in Karaite historiography as one of the "distinguished ideologues" of the Karaite reformist movement who advocated both loosening the stringencies of Karaite observance and establishing closer ties to Rabbanite halakhah (Ankori 1966). Bashyazi first establishes that the literal meaning of the verse should "clearly be read exactly as it appears: one must not boil a kid together with its mother's milk" (Bashyazi 1870, 228, translated from Hebrew in Nemoy 1952, 266). Referring to the principle *'Oto ve-'et bno*, mentioned above, he explains that in the case of "not cooking a kid in its mother's milk," the rule has been extended by analogy to include not only domestic animals but wild animals as well. This extension of categories is possible, says Bashyazi, because of the belief that all regulations "are intended to apply to the general, not to the particular, since the general is better known than the special." He proceeds to establish other comparable unions, based on *'Iqar va-ferach*, that would be forbidden, such as *chibbur*, joining, as well as slaughtering, boiling, and eating. He summarizes: "It is forbidden to eat an animal's meat with milk obtained from its mother, i.e., mixed with the milk; but it is permitted to eat meat mixed with milk definitely known not to belong to the mother. This applies to both domestic and wild animals" (Nemoy 1952, 266–67).

Nikomodio's *Keter Torah* (Aaron ben Eliyahu 1972 [1866]) adds yet another dimension to the Karaite legal debate over this verse while alluding to existing, yet unaccepted, directions in Karaite interpretation. Initially, he vehemently rejected the possibility of associating etymologically the offspring (*gdi*) with the offering of the choice fruit (*meged*). Based primarily on a literal reading of the text, Nikomodio emphasizes that the motivation behind the verse stems from the concern for pity and mercy on behalf of the offspring. Raising the possibility that the practice of cooking meat in milk was not uncommon, he then attempts to justify such a habit based on his assertion that the *gdi* (the young goat) is dry—meaning its meat is tough—thereby necessitating the cooking environment of the moist milk (in order to appreciate the full texture of the debate see Aaron ben Eliyahu [1866] 1972, 79–80). Nonetheless, he concludes by emphasizing the primary role of the mother and mother's milk in this interdiction.

Carrying the True Tradition[10]

Judah ben Elijah Hadassi gives a detailed explanation of the dietary prohibition (Nemoy 1952, 377). Having contextualized the three different occasions on which the prohibition is mentioned in the Torah, he explains the justification against cooking a kid in its mother's milk during the first seven days following its birth. On the three principles of Karaite *kashrut*, Hadassi states, "One who transgresses the first principle (the mother with the young) actively annihilates [he uses four active verbs, each referring to total destruction] the root and its offspring from God's creation. He attributes cruelty to the transgression of the second principle; and, with regard to the third, Hadassi makes a key assertion: "because it [the *gdi*, the kid] is a branch, the milk of its mother, and a bit of flesh from its mother's body" ("*ve-hu' ktsat basar mi-guf 'imo*") (Hadassi 1836, 91).[11]

Already al-Qirqisani emphasizes in *Kitab al-'Anwar wal-Maraqib*, "*Fa-'asqatu qawlāt 'imo*," and they dropped the word "its mother." Emphasizing the primary connection of the mother to her milk results in an extended conception of the physical female body that includes, according to Hadassi, the offspring. In fact, the only extension beyond the mother's body that Hadassi can permit is limited to the offspring. In his conclusion, Hadassi maintains the restriction "do not cook a kid in its mother's milk: anything in its mother's milk." With the pronoun suffix of *'imo* referring to the mother's offspring, and *chalev 'imo* (its mother's milk) a precise reference to a breast-feeding entity, Hadassi's "anything" can only be that which is conditioned by a need for its mother's breast milk. Shlomo Hatroki's commentary *'Apirion 'Asah Lo* reinforces this interpretation by briefly referring to "the meat which has milk ... but not the meat of chicken and fish which have no milk" (Hatroki 1960, 25). The prohibition against slaughtering an animal together with its offspring has now established, Hadassi explicates, that the mother, for a limited time after giving birth, is the extended category. The synecdochic relations with the mother do not allow any separation. *It, the kid, is her*. But more than that, as Hadassi returns to this concept, he concludes that, in fact, the mother, her milk, and her offspring are the same: "God pitied [the kid] so it will not be cooked with some of its mother's flesh, which is the milk which raises and feeds it" (ibid.).

Nikomodio's *Keter Torah* puts it in these terms: "And maybe one can argue that the youngest is not available [edible] until it grows a little so that it will no longer have need for his mother, and if one refers to *gdi* only, then what is the reason for [mentioning] 'its mother'?" (Aaron ben Eliyahu 1972 [1866], 79–80). Later he states, "The reason that it mentions that it [the offspring] has need for his mother is because he is so small. But what is the reasoning for mentioning 'its mother's milk'—Unless one explains that it is because the text wished to prohibit *only meat that has mother's milk*" (emphasis added) (ibid., 80). Nikomodio adds to Hadassi's metonymic mother-kid paradigm a human concern: namely, the young animal's dependency upon its mother. For Hadassi, indeed, there is no separation between the mother's body and the mother's milk because the milk is a continuation of her physiology. Like the milk, the kid is considered a part of that body, eliminating any distance, one might assume, between the three (mother-milk-kid). The metonymic space around the female body is thus constructed by her reproductive capacities. Philosophically, the boundaries between mother and her offspring are blurred in favor of creating a single body that refuses distinction. Unlike the articulation of milk as an independent drink, mother's milk, according to this reading, can exist only in relation to the breast and the baby animal, which is fed by it. The discursive aspect of the milk as a speech act is manifested through its communication to the next generation. Mother's milk embodies this exclusive bond.[12]

If the Rabbanite reading of the verse became *do not cook a kid in milk,* extending the category of milk to include all dairy products, and the kid to include all meat, then the Karaite understanding of this prohibition remains close to the mother and the significance of her role. For Karaites, the verse *do not cook a kid in its mother's milk* became "do not cook a kid with its mother."

Na'imah's Narrative

Karaite folklore concerning mother and child is relatively uncommon. Among those narratives that do exist, few focus on social or religious transgression. As seen in the following narrative, the limited economy of mother's milk reveals the depth at which the ideology of motherhood and its textual reference to the dietary law is embedded in contemporary Karaite women's consciousness. While this economy determines the exclusivity of mother's milk and its privileged place in the discourse of motherhood, the text should be read as an intertext to the Karaite reading of the verse, "Do not cook a kid in its mother's milk." If one sees the nursing baby as analogous to the *gdi*, the animal offspring, then the mother's milk and its inseparability from the baby's mouth overrule all other concerns. This limited usage of milk does not allow the breast milk to become human food—even if the mother needs it to survive.

Na'imah tells this story: "A long, long time ago, there was one who was *al-wālidah,* a woman who gave birth, she had a baby. And that woman was baking bread. And she saw that the bread was very hard, so she took it out, sliced it and she squeezed milk from her breast onto the bread and wanted to eat it." Naʿimah pauses, lingering.

RUTH: Did she eat it?

NAʿIMAH: Yes. She put the bread, put the milk on it and ate. [*A dramatic pause.*] *Ya Rabbina!* [Oh, our God], *lāʿan* [cursed] is the milk if the mother will pour and drink it! Our God forbade the mother to drink the milk. Even if the baby does not want to eat and [if] you would say: "I will taste it," you will find it always salty and say: "Oh, I will try from the other breast." It is forbidden.

This one-episode narrative draws on the practice of women's domestic activities: a nursing woman preparing her own food, namely bread. The inedibility of the hard bread, along with the presumed availability of the breast milk, compounded by hunger, compels the mother to commit an act of taboo violation.

Bread production and milk production are juxtaposed in this narrative as two competing creative forces: bread baking—an activity ascribed to women resulting in human food—and milk production—an activity of the woman's body (often ascribed to God) resulting in baby's food.[13]

Bread is a metaphor for the creative power of women in Middle Eastern cultures, and women baking bread is a common motif in the folklore of the region (Delaney 1988, 75–93).[14] In Naʿimah's account, the practical need for a bread softener threatens to strip the milk of its cultural meaning, robbing its nourishing property and reducing it to a mere fluid. And thus milk and bread, wet and dry, emerge as important oppositions, leading in their extremes to life and death (Dundes 1980). They become a theme that highlights the primacy and resourcefulness of the mother's breast as a life-giving substance, even though and maybe because the usage of this substance is unavailable to anyone other than the baby. Milk is not made available, even to a thirsty mother. Psychoanalytically, feeding herself will mean that she is threatening to turn into her own mother and to regress, a regression that would lead to a rejection of the child. Once circularity replaces linearity, the future falls back to the past. Delaney's reading of bread as a symbol of promulgation, alluding to the raising of yeast (and children) (Delaney 1988), recalls the Karaite's attitude toward fermentation. Brought into conflict with the usage of the milk, it highlights milk as the ultimate unfermented food.

Mieke Bal, inspired by Shoshana Felman's study of seduction, reads the narrative of violence against women in the Book of Judges in order to examine the status of text as speech, and especially of language as violence. As a result, she persuasively demonstrates that "the story is not told; it is done" (Bal 1988, 27). Felman points out that the interesting challenge to truth implied in fire is that there is no resolution as to whether it is a thing or an event. The same can be said of the sword-in-action, the instrument of "rupture," the breaking off of the relations, and of "coupure," the cutting: penetrating and dividing (Bal 1988, 22).

In line with Bal's articulation of the (s)word (Bal 1988, 1–32), I wish to further argue that like the (s)word, milk in the Karaite's narrative adheres to an ambiguous space between "thing" and "event." Na'imah's story reveals an ambiguity toward the nature of the milk. As noted earlier, milk is just one of the several fluids of the female body; yet in its exclusive "performative act" (Searle 1969, 18) between the female body and the child, milk as an "event" reaffirms its meaning as the predicate of the post-delivery mother-baby bond. Milk effectively restates the conceptual framework that is exclusive to the creation of this bond. Therefore, the end of Na'imah's story indicates that Karaite culture cannot tolerate any ambiguity toward the milk. The narrative's position against the contiguity of signifiers of milk and bread further stresses the signifying bond between mother and child, even at the price of the female's subjectivity and the utterance of the curse.[15]

By demanding that the milk be exclusively reserved for the baby, Karaite society extends its control over reproduction in order to guarantee the existence of future generations and cultural continuity. The desire of the mother is, therefore, a counterforce of creation and communal production. Unlike the prohibition "do not cook a kid in its mother's milk," this narrative is not so much a prohibition against mixing substances as it is one against separating the mother from her breast milk, or the mother's breast milk from the baby. Exclusive access to mother's milk is granted to the baby. To echo Hadassi, milk, which is metonymic to the mother's body, and the baby, are inseparable.

Othmar Keel's approach in his study of ancient Near Eastern iconography focuses on the depiction of the mother animal suckling her offspring. He surmises that these images were considered at the time as expressions of divine fertility and abundance. Rather than being subjects of ritual sacrifice, therefore, these animals would have been accessible symbols of the idealized mother-child bond. This emotional and spiritual representation of animals and their sexuality would have inspired—as much as been inspired by—humans' hope for a similar divine blessing (Keel 1980, 142–43). Keel's appreciation for the representation of a mother with her child at her breast is consistent with Philo; he also argues along the same lines as Karaite scholars for the respect of the mother, the life force of the offspring, as opposed to severing the bond between them, which means death for the offspring. Keel and Philo implicitly state that the transition from the animal world to the human world is subtle, relying on a shared assumption of motherhood.

Because of this subtlety, "mother's milk" in each of the three biblical verses is a reference that must be understood in its ambiguity as an allusion to *both* human and animal. Karaites do not accept the reference as simply limited to animals because motherhood in Karaite culture is invested with an idealized institutional meaning. The attachment to the human mother, which informs the Karaite reading of this verse, compelled them to read "mother" literally and to ensure the mother's presence in the verse's practical application. Rather than eliminating the mother in favor of a generic category of milk, and rather than eliminating *gdi* in favor of a generic category of meat, Karaites persist in their reading of this verse as a special case that is specific to a biologically related pair. The Karaite dietary restriction, in this context, entails protecting the mother and her offspring by prohibiting cooking, seething, or eating them together. In essence, this will protect their symbolic unity.

By way of *niddah*, the value of the milk and breast feeding, the fluids of the body, and the mother-daughter teaching all constitute the vocabulary of the discourse of maintaining as kosher the social body and its reproduction. Koshering the female body is integrally connected to the cultural mechanism behind the reading of the dietary laws. This is where the appropriation of the maternal body takes on its human appearance in the women's narrative of purity.

A brief look at the Rabbanite scholarship devoted to this prohibition presents a fascinating picture of the politics of (mis)reading the "other." In general, the Karaites are represented in a dark light, often referred to by such incomplete, obscure, and dubious terms as "anonymous Karaite" (cf. Haran 1979, 25). One reference to an anonymous, seventeenth-century Karaite's textual evidence is dismissive: "another one [Karaite], . . . who is lacking in sense," as quoted by Ibn Ezra. Abarbanel and Luzzatto later applied this epithet "explicitly" to the Karaites (in Haran 1979, 29). Even though these attributions hardly constitute a serious critique of the Karaite legal system, nonetheless they reflect the extent to which Rabbanites were appalled by the Karaite's permissive practice of mixing milk and meat. Such comments reflect Rabbanites' desire to undermine the credibility of the Karaite legal system by focusing on trivial, irrelevant aspects of the Karaite argument, such as the semantic proximity of the *gdi* (goat) with the *meged* (oil), or the association of this prohibition with the cultic Temple sacrifice of firstborn animals (Haran 1979, 28 nn. 15–16). These issues are contested even within Karaite scholarship, and do not form the core of Karaite logic behind the prohibition. This negative portrayal conflicts strikingly with the fact that historically many of the Rabbanite scholars were in fact not so far apart from the core Karaite humanitarian, ethical position. Philo's exegesis, for example, stresses the cruelty of mixing mother's milk with its offspring, alluding specifically to the presence of the "mother's milk" and incorporating the same principles of analogy used by Karaites in their discussion of slaughtering the animal and its young on the same day.[16] Medieval Rabbanite scholars such as Clement of Alexandria, Ibn Ezra, and Rashbam, and more recent ones such as Ginsberg (1982), Haran (1979), and Milgrom (1990), preferred and thus further pursue Philo's perspective.

Some Rabbanite interpretations of this prohibition, which later became historical convention, moved beyond the mother-offspring paradigm and in fact viewed milk as a substance independent from mother's milk. Maimonides, for example, held that this prohibition should be explained within the same context as the laws condemning idolatry because of its proximity to them within Exodus (Exodus 23:17, 34:23).[17] He concludes, accordingly, that the practice of cooking a goat in its mother's milk had its origin in Canaanite cultic rites (Maimonides 1910, 3:48). Still within this framework, other scholars, such as Samuel Bochart (1663) and John Spencer (1685), have attributed the prohibition to magic (Haran 1979) or to superstitions based on principles of sympathetic magic (Frazer 1919, 360–77). The recent discovery of thirteenth-century B.C.E. Ugaritic texts at Ras Shamra, Syria, could indeed further support Maimonides' influential view. However, scholars' discomfort over the possibility of deciphering these fragmented and damaged tablets has led them to question any relationship between the Ugaritic texts and the biblical prohibition. Jacob Milgrom, who, like many others before him, also resolved to abandon the cultic theory, concludes his list of objections by saying, "and a key word of the biblical prohibition, 'mother,' is not there [on the tablet]" (Milgrom 1990, 146; also in Haran 1979; Gaster 1969). While for Milgrom the absence of the mother from the text is obvious, that was not the case to "virtually every interpreter" who accepted the textual reconstruction. It is possible that the understanding of the Ugaritic text was informed by traditional Rabbanite practice, which, as mentioned, omitted the mother and mother's milk in interpreting the verse and focused instead on the Talmudic augmentation that constructed the complete separation between the two categories of meat and milk. This partially explains how such a defective understanding ultimately prevailed. In fact, "it became a dogma of scholarship that Maimonides' intuition concerning the practice as a pagan rite was correct" (Milgrom 1990, 145; also see Carmichael 1976; Haran 1979, 26).[18]

Several of these explanations draw on real-life conditions, attempting to breathe life into the verse. While Milgrom wonders about the time goats were weaned in relation to their birthing season, Haran questions the very possibility of seething meat in milk, because "milk tends to boil over" (Haran 1979, 30).[19] Haran pays close attention to the difference in Arabic between *laban* or *leben* (yogurt) and *halēb* (unfermented milk), claiming that Bedouins have traditionally preferred milk that is sour or has at least "somewhat fermented and also cooled off," a drink similar to kefir. Elaborating on the practical conditions that led to the consumption of sour milk in the ancient Near East, he suggests that "since neither the climate, nor the basic, non-modern living conditions have changed, it is reasonable to assume that . . . only sour milk was drunk and that the Bible also takes this fact for granted" (ibid., 31). Haran's bias toward a kind of ecological determinism regarding Karaites is evident in his attempt to find some relevant, authentic proof, relying on nineteenth-century travelers' accounts as much as on contemporary Bedouin practices. Moreover, the disregard for the mother's milk, even for scholars like Haran who make explicit reference to its inclusion, seems to be consistent. Comparing ancient Israelite dietary practices with those of "Bedouin," "Persians," "Arabs," and "nomads in the vicinity of Crimean Peninsula" reveals the overtly presentist Orientalist representation of the non-Israelite Other, and in the case of gender difference, the distortion of the mother's relevance to the prohibition. Milk, in this context, emerges as a generic fluid, dissociated from its source.

In the attempt to guarantee full separation between *gdi* and mother's milk, the Rabbanites extended the categories. As Hadassi had already recognized in his own time, the Rabbanite interdiction was extended from *lo tevashel gdi ba-chalev 'imo* (Do not cook a kid in its mother's milk) to *lo tevashel gdi ba-chalev* (Do not cook a kid in milk). Ironically, the metaphorization of mother's milk was emphasized to such a degree that the mother disappeared entirely. The Rabbanite reading goes beyond the mother-son relationship paradigm to institute a prototypical dichotomy in which *gdi* stands for meat, and *chalev 'imo*, its mother's milk, for dairy products. Over time, the experience of this dietary prohibition has become a constitutive of a strict binary opposition of meat and milk.

Karaite reading, in contrast, insists on remaining close to the mother's body. Thus, "mother's milk" is a substance produced during the first seven days of the offspring's life. The language of the prohibition draws attention to the potential threat of the mother's milk becoming not a nurturing substance but an environment in which the offspring might be seethed, cooked, or simmered. The Karaite reading of *gdi* as anything, that is, any offspring in its first seven days of life, shifts the attention to the dependency of the offspring on its mother's milk. That contravenes any possibility of the milk becoming an environment of cooking or death. As we have seen, according to the Karaites the semiotic space of the milk is metonymic. Unambiguous contiguity between the whole body (the meat) and the milk is "implicated" as they are "enfolded within" each other. In fact, they are simultaneously outside and inside each other; meat and milk constitute, each in its turn, the interiority of the other (cf. Felman 1982, 8–9). Felman, in characterizing the relationship between literature and psychology, writes that they "compromise, each in its turn, the interiority of the other" (ibid., 8–9). However, although I was inspired by her pithy characterization, in the context of Karaites' construction of the relationship between the body (meat) and milk, the relationship is not one of compromise but rather one of mututal constitution or mutual constitutiveness.

The ethnography of woman's bodily experience reveals that breast milk is an event that commits maternity to the next generation, making mother and child intrinsically inseparable. Initially, for seven days the mother and her offspring are unavailable for human consumption whether together or separately. After this limited period, mother and offspring, humanized and pitied, can still never be brought together for slaughtering, cooking, seething, or eating. The prohibition highlights the dialectic of unity and separation; it is only by virtue of the maternal bond that mother and offspring alike are inedible. Beyond these precisely defined relations, Karaites have permitted the mixing of meat and milk in cooking and eating.

Mother's milk in Karaite culture, metonymic and limited in temporal performance, becomes a metaphor of time in which the temporal element is as important as the spatial juxtaposition of meat and milk. It identifies the quality of the dependency of the baby on its mother's milk in terms of age. But even beyond the first seven days, *gdi* refers to its status as "progeny." Just as sperm has been valorized in Jewish patriarchal culture as a statement of time, tying etymological connections between masculinity, memory, and history,[20] mother's milk, in Karaite culture, has become *the* affirmation of motherhood, making a strong case for survival and future generations.[21] Defending this link, Na'imah's story reaffirms the admonition against a separation of milk not from the meat, but from the breast; for Karaites, milk does not exist in isolation. The very fact that Na'imah told this story suggests that such a practical possibility—as inconceivable as it may seem—goes against the very essence of milk in Karaite culture. Mother's milk presupposes the baby's mouth always at the breast. Through this intimate practice, mother's milk whispers the tunes of Karaite identity. Karaite ideology incorporates motherhood and the maternal role, and has deepened the textual mother-child paradigm in its most primary manifestation. Motherhood within the identity politics of the Karaites as a marginalized minority sect, where Karaite identity relies exclusively on patrilineal bloodlines to the exclusion of conversion or intermarriage, is the primary institution that promises continuity and legitimacy, even at the price of the mother being reduced to her breast.

The prohibition "Do not cook a kid in its mother's milk" is not a separation taboo but rather an ideologically mandated interference in the promise of continuity that the maternal body offers. Rather than demanding that the symbolic yield its place to the emancipated, semiotic *jouissance* of the maternal body, such a shift restates the new ideological place of motherhood in the culture. This shift redefines the maternal body along the lines of the political position provided by the Karaites in contradistinction to the Rabbanites: a foreclosure of the maternal body not as an open-ended discursive agent but as a suspended site of patriarchy that is incorporated into the culture. A step against excess, this foreclosure recapitulates the ideological, ethical, and political centrality of the mother in Karaite culture and organizes the selective locations of her offspring and her milk. The possibility of an arbitrary and perhaps irrational reading of the prohibition against cooking a kid in its mother's milk is thereby refuted; mercy and other necessary indispensable metonymic connections in the conception of Karaite order are invoked instead.

If, as Kristeva has articulated perceptively, the main force behind Judeo-Christian monotheism is the "cathexis of maternal function," one useful way of understanding the Karaite's return to the mother is as an attempt to explicitly correct the rupture of the mother from the text as much as from the child. One could claim that the Karaite reading of this verse differs from the Rabbanite in extent more than in essence. The Karaite correction is, therefore, against over-reading, against excess in general, and against the repudiation of the mother in particular. Metaphorization for Rabbanite Jews promises an extended space. For the *niddah*, this space was translated into an extra seven days of separation, guaranteeing that sexual intercourse will resume only after the menses end. The metaphoric space around both *niddah* and the dietary laws is strictly encoded to prevent any possibility of transgression.

If reading is the founding difference at the core of Karaite culture, then the text becomes a vehicle that drives home an ideological position, one in which women must bear the existential burden of what is perceived as "natural" or supported by the Bible. Patriarchal authority infuses motherhood with religious and sacred meaning that is legitimized by the text. Motherhood therefore exists not in opposition to paternalistic social agencies but as an ideal, complementary agency that enables and ensures the generational stability of Karaite culture.

Conclusion

> Where a text is identical with truth or dogma, where it is supposed to be "the true language" in all its literalness and without the mediation of meaning, this text is unconditionally translatable. . . . For to some degree all great texts contain their potential translation between the lines; this is true to the highest degree of sacred writing. The interlinear version of the Scriptures is the prototype or ideal of all translation.
> Walter Benjamin, "The Task of the Translator"

Each chapter of this book has in some way explored the relationship between text and everyday life and between a literal approach to texts and its translation into bodily praxis. In particular, I have paid close attention to the cultural efforts, strategies, and tactics that are used to maintain a specific ideology and memory of reading. Together with internal cultural methods of reading and interpretation, the historical politics of difference and differentiation, and the wider cultural scheme of power and domination, text and body signify and function as a twofold referential system. It simultaneously sustains and challenges Karaites' ideas about culture and biology, knowledge and memory, experience and narratives.

The ethnography of the Egyptian Karaites in the San Francisco Bay Area demonstrates that the Karaites today grapple daily with articulating, negotiating, and asserting textual, religious, ethnic, and gender differences in California, even as the memory of the Jewish Karaite quarters in Cairo or Alexandria continues to loom large in their minds. But how are Karaites' peculiar difference and their identity as readers best articulated? "Ethno-reading," as I have shown, approaches Karaites from the position of its reading subject, building on the idea that indeed, to read as a Karaite is an ideological act of differentiation. With its emphasis on the literal and "naked" meaning of the language, ethno-reading explains the core of Karaite coexistence with the Bible. By taking into consideration the multiple positions of Karaites as readers and the ways they perceive themselves being read through the eyes of others—for Karaites strive to introduce their culture accurately within an embedded historical context—we can begin to recognize a multilevel Karaite representation of cultural legitimacy and legitimization.

Ethno-reading alludes to the way Karaites translate their sacred text into bodily ritual and the way this ritual becomes, once again, a language. Karaite reading is a productive intellectual and halakhic process; it is a dynamic, creative process that addresses both the text and its interpretive practices, as well as the readers, their multicultural contexts, and ideological positions. As such, it promises the continual centrality of the text in secular modern life. For instance, the use of "personal" Torahs to prepare Karaite children for their bar mitzvahs and the performance of Torah recitation reinforces another layer in the process of becoming a reading subject. Producing tapes with Karaite prayers and melodies in Israel for the young Karaites in California is still another.

More specifically, this book has elaborated on the Karaite consciousness of cleanliness within a transitional moment of their life in Northern California. Such an effort, inevitably, struggles to reconcile two ideas: first, that (internalized) impurity is an imposed category in a patriarchal and hegemonic culture; and second, that their exclusion nonetheless provides Karaites with an authentic site for cultural representation (Culler 1999, 338).[1] My representation of Karaites, therefore, is engaged in expanding the ethnographic possibilities of translating a minority culture into an intelligible, coherent, and authoritative description, and aims to take into account specific disparate aspects of Karaite identity: being Jewish and Karaite, Egyptian and American, female and woman. Approaching Karaites within the wider historical context of asymmetrical power relations, both as a colonized group and as a minority within a hierarchy of other minorities, demonstrates that within Karaite culture—and this is the case especially among today's Bay Area Karaites—the female body has become one of the last strategic sites in the politics of "koshering" and legitimizing Karaite identity.

The female body is inscribed with minority subjectivity; it constitutes a nexus of Karaite politics, poetics, and aesthetics of difference. The discursive strategy concerning the subjects of purity and impurity—the *niddah* in particular—embodies the text and the law, as well as Karaite collective memory and history; while it endorses the details of Karaite legal authority, it involves other political and cultural aspects of everyday life. As an internal method of deciphering the sacred text, Karaite reading reasserts the community's origins and its ideology as a counter-minority group within the Jewish nation. Being at the core of Karaite formation and differentiation, reading *niddah* is more than a subversive political manifesto; it has become an indispensable source of Karaite identity that secures Karaite continuity and connectivity. In its historical development, reading—and reading *niddah* in particular—promises the very survival of the community.

Indeed, the Karaite female body, or the Karaite-woman, becomes a cultural archive of narratives, decoding the history and memory of both women's and Karaite traditions. Animated as it is by the legal text, the *Kara'it*'s maternal genealogy, and personal biography, the female body shoulders the cultural projections of pleasure and desire as much as anxiety and mourning. In fact, as the chapters of this book demonstrate collectively, the Karaite-woman provides the true and accurate scale for counting, or the mode of measure through which females are included in—or excluded from—public life (through prayers or participation in community events) or private life (through sex or interaction with other family members). Counting reaffirms textual realities, engenders dichotomies related to childbearing, and protects the flow of milk by resolving conflicts with menstrual blood. In this connection, as Na'imah's "extended Bible" conveys, the Bible is similar to the female body in that both generate multiple discursive possibilities.

Such an approach, however, presupposes that the Bible is the ultimate Karaite text. Even as community members continue to allude to their culture as textual and to themselves as readers, the notion of reading is further substantiated and materialized by newly invented formats and practices around reading. In the interhalakhic, interethnic relationship of Karaites with Rabbanites and others, reading is at the center of ethnic and religious differences. It is a response to different political climates and cultural environments. Perceived as complete and finished, the Bible provides meaning that is accessible and immediate. In this tight historical relationship between the Bible and the culture, one could argue that as much as the text has invented its community, the community has invented its text.

Reading, therefore, constitutes an overarching concept of Karaite life and its representation; women's culture provides a situated reading focused on the female body. As such, Karaites' concept of reading corresponds to different geographical and bodily locations at different historical moments. Together, these different cultural variants constitute the process of "reading as a Karaite." Within a variety of Karaite diasporas, reading as a methodology is informed differently by each location; to read as a Karaite in Egypt in the early 1920s cannot tell the same story as to read as a Karaite in present-day Ramleh (Israel) much less in the San Francisco Bay Area.

Conclusion

Maintaining pure Torah, pure blood, and pure body entails acts of purification—daily intertexts of evolving traditions that translate the act of reading into minute tactics whose outward ripples help to maintain the purity of the community as a whole. On a larger cultural scale, koshering becomes a metaphor for inclusion and an internal pretext and condition for the practice of speaking about the self. Still, it is crucial to remember that a distinct Karaite voice emerges in its plurality: the *niddah* narrates a story about Karaite reading in a collective voice. While the practice of *niddah* is intimate and private, the reading of *niddah* attains meaning through collective participation. Historically, the reading of *niddah* was shaped and imagined through the institutionalization of mother-daughter teaching, the secretive language of menstruation, and the janusian visibility-invisibility of language and body. As such, the *niddah* as an identity reaches much further into the general culture than the Levitical proper noun designating an individual woman; it synchronically and diachronically connects chains of women's traditions that tell about Karaite "religious correctness" as part of the whole narrative of the pure Karaite body, male and female.

Even in the case when contemporary Karaites underplay reading differences, as the recent situation in Israel indicates, Rabbi Halevi's assertion in one of his lectures to Israeli scholars is revealing. Addressing the problem of the misrepresentation of Karaite's history, Halevi concludes that only Karaites should speak *their* truth, presenting words in the name of its speakers (*dvarim she-ne'emru be-shem 'omram*). He highlights the crucial need for speaking for oneself, contending that, "We [Karaites] say, and this is a conclusion to all the questions that were asked, we say, any interpretation, any halakhah or any oral tradition, be it the Mishnah, or the Talmud, be it explicit or implicit, be it written by [Saadia], Maimonides, or any other Rabbanite scholar—this exegesis, if it is supported by the Scripture, emerging from within it, and it does not contradict it—this interpretation is accepted by us without any question" (Halevi 1988a).

Text, therefore, articulates the epistemological apparatus of the sex-gender system and its institutions, be it motherhood, *niddah*, the mother tongue, the maternal body, or the mother's presence in securing the flow of milk in breast feeding. It is precisely because of the specific nature of Karaite reading and its internal modeling after literal and analogous meaning that a certain consistency in other domains of Karaite life (such as dietary habits or the Passover celebration) is permitted. As such, reading mimics the experience and interpretation of life, going back and forth from the text to its reader and from the reader back to the text. Ironically, the Karaites' adoption of a melancholic posture is an attempt to heal the historical rupture through the symbolic preservation of the text in its entirety. Ultimately, the most productive aspect in this reading is the dynamic process of referentiality to the accumulated textual canon—real and fictive, imagined and concrete—allowing Naʻimah and other women to rewrite their commentary back into the tradition, according to their own understanding.

An ethno-reading of the *niddah* strips Karaite women of their cultural defenses and casts an inquisitive light on their bodily fluids and breasts. We peer at their personal hygiene and analyze their humble seat at the corner(ed) table. And yet, it is precisely the dialectical position of this exposure that allows her clean, kosher body to emerge. Even though the study of the *niddah* is a study of a contaminated site, it nevertheless depicts both a real, concrete persona and an imagined one—a surreal, at times grotesque womanhood, exaggerated and amplified. To a certain extent, such an anxious and dramatized representation of the Karaite woman is eased by the contextual framework that reading provides. Karaites' "signs of intimacy" encapsulate a narrative of bodily representation that corresponds with the Karaite model of "naked reading": hers is an illuminated and transparent body, as are its "pages" and their articulated meaning.

Such a literal reading looks for immediate materials, approximating the notion of truth and its process of signification. A literal reading may aim to hold on to both the exact and the analogous, but it is also referential. Thus, such a reading both revisits Karaite origins *and* engages the mother, emphatically bringing her back into the text, albeit as another patriarchal institution. *Niddah* is an important part of this institution. Indirectly, it engages other bodily fluids, especially breast milk, as the ultimate precursors in the broader production of Karaite genealogy. Motherhood as a patriarchal institution corresponds to the polarity of women's different bodily postures and stages in reproduction. "Reading," as an allegory of a community that imagines and constructs itself through the Scriptures, becomes the enduring voice that connects the Karaites' story and Karaite history from one generation to another.

According to the Karaite body politics of everyday life, purity of body enables an accurate reading of texts; it is equal to a truthful meaning of texts. The purity and impurity of bodies and objects is also extratextual. A Karaite religious teacher once asked an anthropology colleague of mine in a matter-of-fact manner, "*Mah ha-matsav shelakh?*" (How is your situation/condition?). He went on to explain that "it is not shameful [to be menstruating or to ask about it]. It's natural. If you have it we should wash the chair afterwards."[2] *Niddah* as a situation of the social body has been accepted and normalized. Articulating *niddah* as a situation not only corresponds with the immediate, cyclical condition of the body, it is also part of the greater body politics of Karaite culture and its representation. The body as situation, as Judith Butler asserts, participates in the wider political project called "gender" and "ethnicity." The body operates as a locus of cultural meaning both received and invented, a process of both interpretation and innovation (or choice) within power relations and hierarchies (Butler 1987, 133–34).

Reading metaphorically in a sociopolitical climate of asymmetrical power relations, distortions, and misrepresentations can become reductive. Like stereotypes and other cultural constructs that are symptoms of fixed, static categorizations, a reading that privileges metaphors can warp any representation of reality, in the sense of actual, everyday life. A metaphoric reading of Karaite culture would add layers of stain onto the female body; therefore, enlisting the literal offers a way to scrape away the dirt and impurity deposited with the accumulation of derivative meanings. Against the horror of the bleeding body, its shadow and its humiliated presence, its dirt and defilement, a situated, literal reading works to recuperate and restore textual meanings in light of new realities. For Karaite women, ethno-reading scripts a performance that enables them to reckon, however ambivalently, with their impurity. For all Karaites, a literal and situated reading performs the text, thereby animating their co-existence with the Bible and simultaneously reasserting their legitimate presence within the Jewish nation.

NOTES

Preface

1. In Weinberger's recent compiled Hebrew collection *Jewish Poet in Muslim Egypt* (2000).
2. Initial translation by Nemoy (1952), with my emendations.
3. See also Weinberger (2000, 12) on the root *b'r*, another poem.
4. I follow convention and use "Rabbanite" as distinct from "Karaite." For more on Karaite ethnography and folklore, see Fahn 1928; Zajackowski 1961; Kashani 1978; Colligan 1980; Algamil 1981, 1985; Semi 1984, 1990, 1991, 1994; al-Qudsī 1987; and Hirshberg 1987. On Karaite law see Corinaldi 1984; Revel 1971 [1913]; Faraj 1970 [1935]; Zohar 1987, 1988. *Pe'amim,* an Israeli journal in cultural studies of Oriental Jewry, published three special issues on Karaite studies; see *Pe'amim* vols. 32 (1987), 89 (2001), and 90 (2002).
5. On the construction of Karaites as "Others" in Israeli society, see Virginia Dominguez (1989, 153–88).
6. All names were changed in order to protect the confidentiality of the members of the community.
7. Fieldwork was carried out between 1988 and 1991 under a Koret Foundation Fellowship in Jewish Studies and Chancellor's Predoctoral Fellowship at the University of California, Berkeley. Frequent follow-up visits, supported by grants from the University of Utah and the Frankel Center, University of Michigan, were undertaken until August 1994, and I still maintain contact with the community.
8. Colligan, an American anthropologist, reports that on several occasions she was explicitly asked whether she had her period, so that the host would know to wash the chair on which she was sitting (Sumi Colligan, personal communication, April 1992). In Rabbanite tradition the status of *niddah* has been transformed so that it applies only to sexual marital relations (Biale 1984, 147–74). The Karaites maintain the all-encompassing social aspect of her impurity. I refer to Colligan again in the conclusion.

Introduction

The American Karaite quoted in the epigraph to this chapter reflects, in the same conversation, "Maybe if it was in a regular water it would help the integrity of the water. The biggest mistake it was that we did not settle in Israel, trying to stay away from troubles."

1. The English transliteration should be *Qara'im qor'im*, from the root *qr'*, but the consonant *k* is consistent with the way Karaites write their name in English.
2. Few individual Karaites remained in Egypt. See Dabbah's report on the Israeli Karaite delegation to Egypt in April 1980 (Algamil 1985, 273–318).
3. The founding leader of the community is a computer programmer by profession who assumed the role of acting rabbi.
4. *Ha'atakah mishtalshelet* directly preserves the quality of exact transmission, explicated the term *ha'atakah*, which means "copying" or "duplicating."
5. See discussion in Polliack (1997, 23–36 and 23n. 1).
6. The historical Karaite/Rabbanite paradigm is an essential component to the understanding of Karaism. For a detailed comparison between Karaites and Rabbanites see al-Qudsī's Appendix A (1987, 315–28).
7. Personal communication, Stanford University, April 1992.
8. Beinin's recent chapter on Karaites in Egypt and in the Bay Area illustrates this point, and is consistent with other representations of Karaites by Rabbanite scholars. Beinin's definitions of "ethnographer," "Jew," and "translator" are overly narrow and oversimplified and bespeak his unreflexive position as a Rabbanite (Beinin 1998, 179–203). The negative responses that Beinin's book provoked among many Karaites demonstrate Karaites' deep awareness (and sensitivity) to issues of representation.
9. The connection between *begged* and *boged*, clothing and fidelity, is already established in the very expression "*begged bogdim*," which means high treason and is traced back to at least the twelfth century. See *Sefer Zohar* 1951, *Ra'aya Mehaimna* vol. 3, p. 175a.
10. The Torah itself is treated like a body: the scrolls are dressed and adorned with silver or gold crowns that cover both rollers. In cases when deemed ritually disqualified, or nonkosher, the Torah is dressed in a white linen shroud and buried in a special ceremony. The treasure found in the Geniza of the old Cairo synagogue, for example, contained old Jewish and Karaite documents and ritual objects dating from the mid-eighth through fifteenth centuries.
11. The Israeli Karaite Court (an internal Karaite authority) ruled (1964–65) that a woman could divorce her husband if he "hit his wife with heavy blows and forced her to agree to have sexual relations with him on the Eve of the Shabbat ... or while menstruating" (Corinaldi 1984, 88). On having sexual relations with a menstruating woman the court reasserts that the issue "has been absolutely forbidden in our holy Torah." The court emphasizes that even if the husband only wanted or attempted to have sex but did not actually do it, the wife still can ask to divorce him.
12. The term is attributed to Rabbi David Ibn Zimra, the sixteenth-century scholar and leader of Egyptian Jewry (Asaf 1936, 214).
13. In general, even Karaite men are uncomfortable talking about menstruation. In

academic circles the discomfort that the subject raised among men in particular was often transformed into a lack of appreciation, and an underestimation, of its centrality in contemporary Karaite culture.

14. I am using the term "koshering" although it is somehow problematic and was not used explicitly by Karaites. "Koshering" is a Rabbanite category of cleanliness that has emerged from specific practice and ritual. It is useful because it emerged from the issues surrounding purity and impurity.

Chapter 1

Epigraph quoted in Nemoy 1972–73, 116–17.

1. See chapter 3 of al-Qudsī 2002, 97–189, "Comments on Al-Gamil's Book *The Karaite Jewry in Egypt in Modern Times*."
2. Al-Qudsī (2002) corrects the works of five authors (both Karaites and Rabbanites) who published chapters or books during the period 1979–98. It is beyond the scope of this book to detail the emotional investment that led to the publication of *Just for the Record* and the bitter exchanges between these writers. I should mention, though, that the book reveals some of the behind-the-scenes attempts to write Karaite history; al-Qudsī presents us with the actual photocopies of the corrected material, underlying wrong dates and handwriting on top of erased lines, as well as providing documents, pictures, and other important correspondence and records to support his claims. His motivation for correcting these works, is, in part, due to his conviction that history is irrefutably equal to truth (2002, 1).
3. On the subtitle of his book, *The Death of William Gooch: A History's Anthropology*, Dening explains, "By the ambivalence that apostrophes create, *A History's Anthropology* comprises at the one time the anthropology of history, historical anthropology, and anthropological history. But not the history of anthropology!" (Dening 1995, 13).
4. Admittedly, Karaites are constructed as heresy. As such, the scholarly attention that they received is limited to a certain degree of tolerance to heresy in the culture. But the ambivalence toward Karaites and the tremendous curiosity that they evoke can be understood as both a desire to control, through some kind of voyeurism, cultural acts of resistance and subversion.
5. Roughly, this narrative begins in Genesis with the Patriarchs, proceeding to Moses, to the cultic priestly religion in Jerusalem, and then to rabbinic commentary following the destruction of the Temple in 70 C.E. Subsequently, it moves from the Babylonian Talmud to the Geonim and to Spain, migrating after the Inquisition into Ashkenazi Europe and culminating with the Enlightenment.
6. See the critique of Mahler (1949, 28–45), "A Critical Overview of Approaches Toward Karaites."
7. About Salmon Ben Jeroham, Nemoy concludes: "Certainly, Salmon had no genuine poetic gift; his quatrains are the fruit of his considerable learning in biblical, Karaite and Rabbanite lore rather than the product of inspiration. Yet, his style is, on the whole, fluent and easily understood, and the epistle makes interesting and informative reading." On Moses Dar'i, for example, he comments, "It is no

reflection upon his literary merit to state the simple fact that with all his accomplishments he did not attain the lyric heights and stylistic brilliance of the best poets among his Rabbanite predecessors in Spain" (Nemoy 1952, 133).

8. The late Rina Drori's work on the emergence of Jewish-Arabic contacts at the beginning of the tenth century is an innovative literary approach that examines the interactions of both Arabic and Hebrew literary traditions, and canonic and noncanonic literary models, within intertextual historical developments.

9. In the field of ethnology, ethnographic writing was developed as early as the sixteenth century in relation to "primitive," "savage," "traditional," or "popular" orality that it established as its other (de Certeau 1988, xxvi).

10. "And God said: Behold, I will rip the kingdom (apart)" (I Kings 11:31).

11. The exilarch was the chief scholar of the Jewish community and was responsible for internal Jewish affairs, acting as representative before the Persian and later Muslim rulers from the second to the eleventh century.

12. Published by Schechter Salomon, *Fragments of the Book of Commandments by Anan* (Cambridge, 1910) and Harkavi 1969 [1903].

13. According to Ben-Sasson and in contrast to Mahler, al-Nahawandi's work suggests that the Karaite society of his time consisted of middle-class merchants, slave owners, and artisans (Ben-Sasson 1950, 50–55).

14. See also Polliack 1997, 23–36; Nemoy 1952, xvi–xvii; and Wieder 1962, 53–94.

15. His books *Kitab al-'Anwar wal-Maraqib* (The Book of Lights and Watchtowers) and *Kitab al-Riyad wal-Ḥada'iq* (The Book of Gardens and Parks) are monumental commentaries, and, like all his work, indicate his profound knowledge in the fields of law, history, science, astronomy, and philology. See also Ben-Shamai 1978, 1982; and the al-Qirqisani center's Web site, which promotes recent Karaite studies (http://www.karaitejudaism.com/qirqisani/).

16. Saadia's position today is so uncontested and prominent in Jewish historiography that often scholars attribute his *Tafsir* (the translation of the Bible into Arabic) as the first, even though it is historically established that the Karaites began translating the Bible at least a century before. Even informed scholars such as Ammiel Alcalay or Ross Brann make similar attributions (see, e.g., Alcalay 1993, 156).

17. His work includes *Sefer Milchamot ha-Shem* (The Book of the Wars of the Lord) in rhymed quatrains, as well as commentaries on many books in the Bible, including Job, Psalms, Esther, and perhaps even the Pentateuch and Isaiah (Nemoy 1952, 71n. 3).

18. Sahl ben Masliah is also the author of *Sefer Ha-miswot* (The Book of Precepts) in Arabic, of which only the introduction has been published. He wrote famous Hebrew missionizing epistles (Nemoy 1952, 110).

19. Aaron ben Eliyahu wrote three important books: *'Ets Chayim* (Tree of Life), a philosophy of religion (1346), *Gan 'Eden* (The Garden of Eden), a legal treatise (1354), and *Keter Torah* (The Crown of Torah), a commentary of the Pentateuch (1362).

20. Karaites were admitted into Poland by his brother, King John Albert. In 1503 they were permitted to return to Lithuania.

21. Detailed population counts of the local Karaites survived from the middle sixteenth to the late eighteenth centuries, helping to trace the changes and developments of the different Karaite communities.

22. Firkovitch's personality and the controversial historiography that he attempted to rewrite are the subject of recent studies that are being published with the newly available Leningrad collection. See, for example, Shapira's 2002 monograph devoted to the Istanbul crises (1830–32).
23. More on the Karaites under Nazi rule can be found in Green 1978, 1979; Semi 1990.
24. During the early 1930s Karaites changed the title of the Karaite association to fit into the mainstream Egyptian public. In order to dissociate themselves from the Rabbanite Jews, they highlighted their Israelite/Israeli identity as the people of Moses. Their formal name became "The Organization of Israeli Karaites in Egypt." As Colligan points out, "Israeli" in both Hebrew and Arabic can also be read as "Israelite," and thus alludes to Karaites beyond the immediate, contemporary politics of Zionism (Colligan 1980, 38–40).
25. They were permitted to return to Jerusalem once Salah al-Din recaptured the city in 1187 (al-Qudsī 1987, 5). Al-Din redeemed the codex of Ben Asher (otherwise known as the Aleppo codex, which is still the oldest Masoretic copy of the Bible) and returned it the Karaites (al-Qudsī 1987, 5).
26. In a letter of Ovadia of Bartenura from Jerusalem. See also David 1988, 23–34.
27. This is in response to a recent attempt to depict Karaites as Arab-Jews. If Karaites imagine themselves as both Jewish and Egyptians, it comes as little surprise that referring to them as "Arab Jews" or "as Arabized ... emphasizing the Arab element of Egyptian Karaite culture" (Joel Beinin, quoted in al-Qudsī 2002, 220) raised Karaite hackles.

Chapter 2

1. Praying without shoes on a prayer rug or mat (*sajjadah* in Arabic) was a reason for the accusation of Muslim influence on the Karaites. See for example "Question and a Responsum by Rabbi Shmu'el Wilyisid (1640)" in Asaf's appendix (1936, 248–51).
2. In 1990 the Karaites purchased an existing building in San Francisco, which they converted into a synagogue ("Editorial" 1991, 9). In October 1991, the first High Holiday services celebrated the inauguration of the building. See also the series of articles introducing Karaites to the Bay Area Rabbanites by Tamar Kaufman, in the *Northern California Jewish Bulletin* (1991a, 1991b, 1992).
3. Until the second half of the thirteenth century there were three Karaite prayer books available, which were then codified. They eventually merged into a single text, the present Karaite prayer book that contains biblical quotations, hymns, prayers, and ceremonies for daily and festival services, as well as for marriage, death, and other life-cycle events (see Nemoy 1952, 271–74; on various examples from the Karaite liturgy see 274–321).
4. On Karaite reading the *parashat ha-shavu'a* see Kashani 1978, 47. On the music tradition see Hofman 1971, 783–85, and Hirshberg 1987, 1994.
5. Fund raising in education was used in the lottery system in Cairo. Early at the beginning of the century and until the Israeli-Arab war of 1948, *Nasib al-Madrasah* (School Lottery) was a successful Karaite communal enterprise that supported education (al-Qudsī 1987, 102–4).

6. For Colligan, the Karaite claims of pure blood and pure Torah are key interpretive symbols in the ideology of the contemporary Israeli Karaite community (1980, 169–85). The notion of blood purity gave rise to several biological/genetic studies. In 1968 (at Hadassah Hospital, Jerusalem) a blood (genetic) test was performed on sixty-three Egyptian-Karaite families, which Bashan refers to in his "Interview of the Week with the Elder, Emanual Masouda, the Head of the Karaite Community of Israel" (*Ma'ariv*, May 26, 1961, 10 [Hebrew]; cf. Colligan 1980, 171–72). Another study of a small inbred Iraqi-Karaite isolate was conducted by E. Goldschmidt, K. Fried, A. G. Steinberg, and T. Cohen (1976, 243–52). The presence of several unique gene frequencies for blood group and isoenzyme markers, not observed among other Jewish groups, are explained by isolation and genetic drift that occurs in a very small community. Of 136 individual Karaites, 98 (72 percent) of at least six years of age who were known to have lived in Hit, a city in Iraq, since the tenth century were examined. In Iraq this group maintained a highly inbred existence but intermarried with Karaites from Egypt after immigrating to Israel in 1951. Ironically, during the Second World War the Germans used the concept of "pure blood" in order to "diagnose" the identity of the Karaites. See Friedman 1960; Spector 1986; Green 1978, 1979; and Semi 1990.
7. See also Faraj 1970 (1935), 36.
8. The Karaite naming system draws heavily on the Bible, especially in the case of male first names. For a discussion of the lists of names that appear in Karaite documents and on the environmental influences on Karaite names, see Brinner 1982.
9. In Egypt, Algamil mentions that until recently, reporting the birth of a son to the Karaite religious authorities was mandatory, whereas the birth of a girl often went unreported (1985, 170).
10. On the subject of Rabbanite-Karaite intermarriage, see Asaf (1936, 208–51, esp. 209–18), and the debate between Zvi Zohar (1987, 21–39) and Shochetman (1988, 29–46), as well as Zohar's response (1988, 47–50). For legal aspects, see Corinaldi (1984, 101–42).
11. Semi's description is outstanding, as it is not situated in a discussion about reproduction or women. The article is an updated general account of the different communities of Karaites in Europe.
12. Even in Israel, the contemporary Karaite community is evolving away from the strictures of *Toharat ha-Mishpachah* (family purity), a fact that explains the need for educational initiatives like Halevi's book.
13. Other feminist anthropologists attest to such a lack of representation or to its low status. See Delaney 1991.
14. I do not mention language shifts in the transcript. All translations from Hebrew and Arabic are mine unless otherwise indicated.
15. This situation is not uniquely Karaite. In Brazil, for example, a woman would refer to her life, saying, "I live with one (child) inside and one outside" (Linda-Anne Rebhun, personal communication).
16. An interval of two and a half to three years is what Saad Gadalla considers the "ideal birth interval" among rural Egyptian communities (Gadalla 1978, 79–82).
17. In Arabic the verb *tgibi*, "give" or "bring," is used to designate giving birth.
18. Dabbah alludes to the problematic relationships of several Karaite co-wives, still

living in Cairo, in 1980. According to Corinaldi (1984), men who are sexually ill equipped (impotent, hermaphrodite) are prohibited from marriage. Women after ten years of marriage with no children could be divorced by their husbands.
19. Women are mentioned in Fahn's two-volume collection (1928), and in Egypt, in Algamil two volumes, 1981 and 1985. Some indirect references to women's life can be found in *Al-Kalim* (literally, the male speaker) and later in *ha-Dover*, the Karaite monthly issued by the Israeli community. It should be mentioned that in *ha-Dover*, even issues concerning women's beauty and cosmetics are written about by men.
20. This note appears several times with reference to different women (Dabbah 1985, 277–78).
21. In colloquial Arabic, *jinn* means "demon."
22. Shmuel Figit's (1977) and Haberman's (1947) collections of Eastern European Karaite folktales do not depict a much better picture of womanhood. In the background of most narratives, the Karaite woman is the domestic, obedient wife. If she fails to act out this role, she is, as the title of one tale indicates, "A Woman of Strife" who has infinite demands and brings on herself, and on those engaged with her, only evil.
23. Although Dabbah's biased report presupposes that those who had remained in Cairo after 1948 were forced to leave, those individuals who did not seem to have led a full life in Egypt, among them several Karaites (mostly men), Jews in the free professions, and several Jews who had intermarried with Muslims.
24. In Egyptian Arabic *zghrir* means both "young in age" and "small in size."
25. Murad Faraj indicates that the suitable age for marriage according to the civil law (in Egypt, 1935) is at least eighteen for a man and seventeen for a woman (Faraj 1970 [1935], 13).

Chapter 3

1. Throughout the book of Leviticus, the semantic separation is maintained between the menstruating woman and the bodily condition, *niddah*. Therefore, in Leviticus *niddah* always appears attached to the feminine pronoun suffix, as in *niddatah* (her *niddah*). In later biblical books, *niddah* appears with no pronominal suffix and identifies the woman with the physical condition of her body.
2. Typically, in Rabbanite Judaism, only the *niddah*'s husband knows about her period; the secret is revealed only for practical reasons, as it determines the timetable of the couple's sexual life.
3. Until recently, the subject of menstruation has been excluded from Israeli public discourse. Yehudit Hendel's collection of short fiction *Kesef Katan* (1988) was among the earliest works dealing with this subject. In her short story, the female prisoner is writing with her own blood on the prison cell walls: "Like a bleeding animal whose blood is coming out of her body dirty." See also Wasserfall (1992, 309–27) on *niddah* among Moroccan immigrants to Israel, as well as Yanay and Rapoport (1997) on the relation between menstruation and nationalism in Israel. In 1996, Yael Tsadok's radio show "*Kol Ha-'Ishah*" (The Woman's Voice) was a pioneering feminist attempt to discuss the subject of menstruation publicly, and resulted in lively, emotional arguments even among the participants.

In Rabbinic Hebrew the reference for a woman's period is *'oreah*, a singular masculine noun denoting "a guest," "wanderer," or "traveler" (Bereshit Rabbah 18, 16; Nedarim 64), and probably is derived from *'orach* (a path, way, manner of life) as in *'orah nashim* (the way of women). *Veset*, the modern Hebrew term most common in formal language for "period," is derived from the verb meaning "to regulate," "control," or "govern." Teenage girls circumvent the term *veset* by using instead the phrase *Varda soreget garbayim* (*Varda* [a female proper name] knits socks), because the Hebrew letters "v", "s", and "g" compose the acronym *veseg*, which subverts *veset*. In addition, *Varda* has a double reference to the color red, as it is derived from *varod* (pink) and *vered* (a rose). In colloquial language, a common reference among women is the reflexive verb "*hitcharbanti*" or its passive form "*mechurbenet*" (menstruating), derived from the root h.r.b.n, slang for to "get messed up" or "to get fouled up." Another common expression in Hebrew is the verb "*kibalti*" (I received), which is a short form of "*kibalti veset*" (I received the period).

4. Texts that deal at length with bodily secretions are common in the midrashic and Talmudic literature.
5. Only the back cover of the book reveals that "Fatna A. Sabbah" is a pseudonym. Writing on women's silence under a pseudonym is in itself an ironic gesture that underscores the social taboo (see Sabbah 1984).
6. At an early stage of my work, I composed a lengthy questionnaire exclusively devoted to menstruation. A second questionnaire, which I sent to all the women in the community, referred to various aspects of female life. Only a few women responded to these questionnaires.
7. This is, in fact, not consistent with the perception of American women, who remark that menstruation is a subject about which they feel uncomfortable. A similar response has been echoed in studies of menstruation in other cultures. On menstruation among American women, see Weideger (1976, 8) and Martin (1987). Even American feminists were ambivalent about the representation of menstruation in American culture. Whereas one opinion called upon women to celebrate and highlight the experience as part of their life cycle, another tried to silence it in order to minimize sexual differences, such as menstruation (see, e.g., Weideger 1976; Delaney, Lupton, and Toth 1976; Lander 1988; Buckley and Gottlieb 1988, 1–50).
8. This occurs in many Hebrew expressions, common in folklore, slang, and popular culture. In other cultures, such as the United States, Mexico, or China, the period is a figurative visitor, personified with a common female name, as in "Sue is coming this week" (see Laws 1990).

Chapter 4

1. "Becoming," in de Beauvoir's sense (1973, 301); see also Butler 1990.
2. Whereas recent attempts to approach Rabbinic Judaism through the body/text paradigm are increasing in number (see, e.g., Eilberg-Schwartz 1990, 1991; Biale et al. 1992; D. Boyarin 1993), ethnographies on the subject are still rare (Goldberg 1987).
3. See Delaney 1991 and her notion of "Islam embodied."

4. Brenner and Neumann's 1990 film, *The Last Marranos*, provides an excellent example of women's ability to maintain oral tradition secretly. The film shows that as long as religion was practiced secretly, it was entirely in the hands of the women; once it was out in public, it was institutionalized around and monopolized by male authority. Since the time of the Inquisition, female Marranos preserved Jewish prayers and customs, such as baking unleavened bread for Passover, reciting the story of the Exodus, or praying for "Adonai" ("God," one of the few Hebrew words left in the Marranos' vocabulary). Once the Marrano young men established connection with Israel in the late seventies, the power structure shifted into patriarchal (imported and native) authority (Brenner and Neumann, *The Last Marranos* 1990).
5. Islamic law recognized the central role of a mother in raising and educating children. In the case of divorce, the mother has automatic custody of girls up to the age of twelve and of boys up to the age of nine (Mikhail 1979, 20).
6. On women as primary caretakers and their specific role in girls' psychological development in Western culture, see Chodorow 1974, Gilligan 1982, and Rosaldo 1974.
7. Rahel Wasserfall makes the same point, indicating that the observance of *niddah* for the Moroccan immigrant women in Israel means being both female and Jewish (1992).

Chapter 5

1. The situation is different in Rabbanite Judaism. Especially on the High Holidays and Yom Kippur, a menstruating woman may "enter the synagogue like other women, for otherwise it would cause her great sorrow to remain outside while everyone else congregates" in the synagogue (commentary of Rema [Moses Isserles], cf. Biale 1984, 168). The rules of separation that do exist are, as stated by Rashi, to prevent any possibility of intimacy and sexual intercourse between husband and wife (ibid., 162). Rachel Biale's explanation asserts, "The destruction of the two Temples . . . removed the concrete locus and justification of the laws of impurity. This historical change made way for the ascendancy of the second context and meaning of the laws of *niddah* in the Bible: the sexual prohibitions" (Biale 1984, 147).
2. In the Bible, the word *sopher* refers exclusively to a scribe. H. Mack Horton discusses the significance of a similar "etymological phenomenon" in other languages, alluding to the fact that in Japanese the word *yomu* refers to both oral counting and oral telling. Horton gives parallel constructions in other Western languages, such as *tellan* in Old English, which means both "to tell" and "to narrate," or *compter*, "to count," and *conter*, "to tell a story," in French, which are from the Latin root "computare" (Horton 1992, 156–57). Horton adds to this list a less persuasive example of the Hebrew verb *hagah*. Although less commonly used than *saphar*, *hagah* makes clear that this connection is established on more than one linguistic occasion (in English, for example, one can add other verbs such as "count" and "recount").
3. This passage first appeared in Mann 1972, 2: 171–73 and later in Ankori 1959, 292–93, especially chapter 7. Also in Nemoy 1952.

4. The subject of observing the holidays on different dates was introduced early on to Karaite children in Israeli schools. Being a minority within the majority of Rabbanite children and teachers, they feel excluded from mainstream culture, or as they said, "We feel cut off. Everyone celebrates the holidays together, except for us" (Ichilov and Stern 1978, 27).
5. This contrasts with the fixed Rabbanite calendar, in which a date may fall out on one of only four days of the week.
6. One of the controversial halakhic questions dealt with the boundaries of the days. See Erder 1988, chapter 4; Halevi 1988b, 26–34.
7. The last sentence is a quote from Ben-Ze'ev's *Proselytes and Proselytizing Past and Present*. Boris Tukan studied the calendrical terminology used by the Karaites of Eastern Europe in order to trace cultural influences. His comparative study reveals influences of Hebrew, Turkic, and other local dialects (Tukan 1987, 60–66).
8. "If a woman has an issue and her issue in her flesh be blood, she shall be put apart seven days" (Leviticus 16, 19).
9. Halevi's *Toharat ha-Mishpachah* (1981) mentions, after Leviticus, under the subtitle "The impurity of the *zavah* and the difference between *niddah* and *zavah*," that the *niddah* purifies on the eighth day: "When she [the *zavah*] becomes clean of her discharge, she shall count off seven days, and after that she shall be clean" (Leviticus 15:28). Defining the latter, Halevi states: "The *zavah* is she who will find blood of any kind during many days, out of her *niddah* days, or [whose blood] continued to flow at the end of the *niddah* either continuously or with intervals." (Halevi 1981, 16–17).
10. Determining the duration of the menstrual cycle preoccupied many legal authorities, and varies considerably. The strict Iranian rules, for example, state that "the length of menstruation is not less than 3 days or more than 10 days and if it is slightly less than 3 days it is not menstrual blood" (Khomeini 1984, 55).
11. Snowden and Christian's cross-cultural study of patterns and perceptions of menstruation reports that most women bleed between three and four days (48 percent) or between five and six days (35 percent). Residence (urban or rural) and literacy appear to have an effect on the reported length of the period (Snowden and Christian 1983, 95). Weideger quotes L. Israel's medical experience stating that "bleeding periods of from 3 to 7 days duration fall within physiological limits" (cf. Weideger 1976, 32).
12. Leviticus continues: "And in the eighth day the flesh of his foreskin shall be circumcised. And she shall then continue in the blood of her purifying three and thirty days; she shall touch no hallowed thing, nor come into the sanctuary, until the days of her purifying be fulfilled. But if she bears a maid child, then she shall be unclean two weeks [*shvu'ayim*] as in her separation; and she shall continue in the blood of her purifying threescore and six days. And when the days of her purifying are fulfilled, for a son, or for a daughter, she shall bring a lamb of the first year for a burnt offering and a young pigeon, or a turtledove, for a sin offering, unto the door of the tabernacle of the congregation, unto the priest: Who shall offer it before the Lord, and make an atonement for her; and she shall be cleansed from the issue of her blood. This is the law for her that hath borne a male or a female" (Leviticus 12:2–7). For comparative notes with other halakhic systems regarding the origin of this prohibition, see Revel 1971 (1913), 42; Fin-

kelstein 1938–39, 184; and Corinaldi 1984.
13. According to Rabbi Halevi's guide, a Caesarean section is considered a normal delivery in terms of impurity (Halevi 1982, 130–31).
14. Although men also expressed their dissatisfaction during this incident, I refer mainly to women because they were the main participants in resolving it.
15. Leviticus 12:6–8. After the destruction of the Temple, the Karaite *yoledah*, as in the case of the *niddah*, could either fast for one day, give charity or alms, or light candles in the synagogue. See Halevi 1982, 129.
16. Other scholars discuss the forty/eighty gender differences in Leviticus 12. See Eilberg-Schwartz 1990, 190–91 and Biale 1984, 151–52.
17. As Kristeva theorizes, "I agree that it [circumcision] concerns an alliance with the God of the chosen people; but what the male is separated from, the other that circumcision carves out on his very sex, is the other sex, impure, defiled. By repeating the natural scar of the umbilical cord at the location of sex, by duplicating and thus displacing through ritual the preeminent separation, which is that from the mother, Judaism seems to insist in symbolic fashion—the very opposite of what is 'natural'—that the identity of the speaking being (with his God) is based on the separation of the son from the mother. Symbolic identity presupposes the violent difference of the sexes" (Kristeva 1982, 100).
18. The Bible uses the Hebrew dual form *shvu'ayim* (two weeks, a fortnight) for the longer bleeding duration of the *niddah*, and thus helps to create a sense of doubling.

Chapter 6

1. Belief in demons is common in the Middle East, especially in the female demon, the *'ifrit*. Invisible, residing in dark, humid, unsettled places, she is depicted as a constant threat in the folk imagination. The supernatural space is not totally isolated, since it interferes in people's lives and is believed to be provoked by certain acts. Ahron, as I mentioned in chapter 3, made a clear reference to his several encounters with the *'ifrit*. On demonology in Egypt and the Middle East, see Boddy 1989.
2. See, for example, Gross (1980) and Douglas (1966).
3. Foucault's *heterotopias* are "counter-sites" in which all other cultural sites are "simultaneously represented, contested, and inverted." Accordingly, "places of this kind are outside of all places, even though it may be possible to indicate their location in reality. Because these places are absolutely different from all the sites that they reflect and speak about, I shall call them, by way of contrast to utopias, heterotopias" (Foucault 1986, 24).
4. By "materialization" I follow Elizabeth Grosz: "Materialism, a non-reductive (discourse), which rather than mere brute physicality, also includes the materiality of discourse, as well as psychical drives and unconscious processes. The subject is produced as such by social and institutional practices and techniques, by *the inscription of social meaning, and by the attribution of psychical significance to body parts and organs*. The interlocking of bodies and signifying systems is the precondition both of an ordered, relatively stable identity for the subject and of the smooth, regulated production of discourses and stable meanings" (my emphasis;

Grosz 1989, 81–82).
5. Nadia's son has since remarried. In general, divorce is uncommon among Karaites. I encountered only two Karaite women in the Bay Area who are divorced.
6. Although Nadia's lengthy description of her educational background reveals her exceptional vigor, it still depicts a feeling common among women of missing the opportunity to obtain higher education or, in the best of cases, of having had to struggle to attain the little education they have. Because medicine was taught in English, which was not Nadia's first language, she wanted to study in France. After applying and being accepted to the medical school at Montpellier, her family reconsidered and decided not to allow Nadia to go abroad by herself. As a result she remained in Cairo, where she studied philosophy.
7. Delaney 1988, 1991; Paige and Paige 1981.
8. For more on the extent to which women are prohibited from touching objects during menstruation see Buckley and Gottlieb 1988, 6.
9. Mira's arrangement with her sisters-in-law to share the responsibility for taking care of her mother-in-law was exceptional.
10. Lailah was the least comfortable of all my informants discussing her menstrual period. In fact, Lailah referred to it merely as "*zeh*," a pronoun that literally means "this" or "that," but is commonly used in spoken modern Hebrew as "it." She was nervous about personal interviews and changed our appointments several times. Though Lailah refused to be recorded, she agreed to my writing down our conversation.
11. The first Karaite Passover Seder in which I participated was in 1988, with the Pessah family. The service was videotaped and complemented by several interviews with members of the family. In 1989 and 1990 I spent the holiday with another Karaite family that figures centrally in this book.
12. Unlike Rabbanites, who celebrate two Seders outside of Israel, Karaites celebrate only one.
13. The following is a partial list of prohibited foods taken from the last page of the Karaite Passover Haggadah: yogurt, cheeses, pasta, yeast, baking powder, baking soda, chocolate, processed meats, corn oil, all sodas and soft drinks, wines, and hard liquors. The Karaites categorize all fermented food as nonkosher for Passover.
14. Wine made of raisin, usually acidified, was fairly common in Cairo as a "more acceptable" alcoholic drink for the Muslims. Eliyahu Ashtor (Strauss) (1944) attributed the business of this wine, called *Nabbid*, to the non-Muslims. Ashtor mentions a street in the Jewish neighborhood in Cairo called "*al-Nabbadin*" (those who serve Nabbid) (Strauss-Ashtor 1944, 188).
15. Little has been written about the Karaite Passover. Yoram Erder used the controversial halakic Karaite exegesis of Passover (the time of the Paschal Sacrifice) as a departure point for speaking on the origins of early Karaism, its history, and development (Erder 1988). See also Semi's anthropological study (1984, in Italian). For Rabbanite Passover see Fredman's anthropological study (1981) and Boxer's halakhic, textual interpretation (1984).
16. The Pessah lamb is one of the three main substances of the ritual, going back to Exodus 12:22. Sophia recalls how in Egypt her father used to buy lamb and distribute it to the poor.

17. "And the Lord spake unto Moses, saying, Speak unto the children of Israel, saying, If any man of you or of your posterity shall be unclean by reason of a dead body, or be in a journey afar off, yet he shall keep the Passover unto the Lord. The fourteenth day of the second month at even they shall keep it, and eat it [the paschal sacrifice] with unleavened bread and bitter herbs" (Numbers 9:9–11).
18. A year later Susana's period again coincided with Passover; I had already decided to sit with her at the side table. As it turned out, however, Susana and her husband, much to the the disappointment of the other participants, did not attend. Susana made a last minute phone call and said she did not feel well and preferred to stay home. It was obvious that the two women hosting the Seder were not pleased that she begged off at the last minute.
19. Being compared to a dog is a common disparaging expression in both Arabic and Hebrew. A whole vocabulary is derived from this dehumanized sociology of dogs. Insulting expressions such as *kalb*, dog; *kalba*, a female dog, a bitch; or *maklūb* (passive participle), "possessed," "crazed," are common in colloquial language.
20. The Arabic language distinguishes between two kinds of shadow. The first, *zhill*, means the shadow of an everyday object, shelter, or umbrella (*mazall*). The second is *khayāl*, "disembodied spirit, ghost, imagination, phantom, apparition" (Hans Wehr, *Arabic-English Dictionary* [1976]).
21. The belief that the dough will not rise if handled by a menstruating woman appears also in South Wales. See Buckley and Gottlieb 1988, 154.
22. On the High Holidays Karaites met at individual houses. Not only did this make the holidays intimate and domestic, but also the festive meals, served at the end of the day, or the fast on Yom Kippur, were a natural continuation of the religious ceremony.
23. Traditionally Karaites (like Rabbanites) refrain from driving on Yom Kippur. American modern life has created long commutes to the religious gathering, and as a result, Karaites now drive during the holidays when and if necessary.
24. Joëlle Allouche-Benayoun reports the same approach among Algerian Jewish women who later immigrated to Paris (Allouche-Benayoun 1999, 198–216).
25. Snow and Johnson's 1977 study of the relations between menstrual folk beliefs and behavior during menstruation among multiethnic low-income populations is illuminating in this regard. The correlation within such populations of bodily cleanliness and health status was manifested in the fact that "many women reported what clinicians would doubtless view as an overdependence on douching" (1977, 2738). Snow and Johnson conclude by citing Neumann and DeCherney's study "Douching and Pelvic Inflammatory Disease" (*New England Journal of Medicine* 295 [14]: 789 [1976]), demonstrating that vigorous douching has in fact been associated with pelvic inflammatory disease.
26. The *mikveh* in Rabbanite Judaism, for example, traditionally signified an immense communal and institutional endorsement of purity that goes beyond the intimate rite of immersion in water. As such, it amplifies the woman's transitional status and subjects her to its scrutiny. Through her close supervision, the *mikveh* attendant becomes the guardian of this authority (Sered, Kaplan, and Cooper 1999, 145–65). The *mikveh* is the place that receives the *niddah* in her impurity and ensures her return back to the community clean and sexually available. As such, it is a place of containment; it holds the water and accepts the woman's symbolic

impurity without itself becoming defiled. Yet within these contours, the *mikveh* resolves the infinite struggle of life and death; in its secluded space it relieves the drama of the open body.

27. This is the way the Karaite halakhah refers to the impurity of the dead person. See Aderet Eliyahu, chapter 19, "*Seder Tum'ah ve-Taharah*" (Bashyachi 1870 [1530]).

28. Restricting the use of water during menstruation varies in different cultures. Some cultures allow bathing but not washing, while others forbid washing during the whole period. Vieda Skultans mentions the restriction on bathing among South Welsh women (1988, 143–44). Three-eighths (37.5 percent) of the women in Snow and Johnson's (1977) study believe that menstruating women should avoid water and cold air because of the vulnerability of the open uterus to cold or disease.

29. In English the term "douche" refers to a stream of water directed to wash especially the female genital zone.

30. A dead body is ritually washed with a wet pad, which is repeatedly replaced until the washing is completed.

31. There is no doubt among scholars that Maimonides is referring here to the Karaites as the heretic.

32. Whereas mixed Karaite-Rabbanite marriages have been documented, pointing to the immense male-female connection between the two, little has been written about the interaction between Karaite and Rabbanite women. In that sense, Cohen, in the tradition of Maimonides, discounts the extent of Karaites' influence on Rabbinic Egyptian women, and on the cross-ethnic interaction between them. His attempt to understand the practice of "sprinkling" within linear, historical development does not take into consideration women's reality.

33. Delaney commented on the needs of an assisting woman in Turkish villages, while bathing the bride due to the lack of bathing facilities and water scarcity (Delaney 1991, 128–29).

34. Even in houses without modern showers, the woman stands using a hand-held nozzle, while the movement of the washing water descends; the movement is from the top down.

Chapter 7

1. Midwifery was the first step in a woman's career in Egypt; see Mikhail (1979, 47–64). Eugenie Massouda, for example, known by her married name Geni Ovadia, was a famous Karaite midwife in Cairo who married a gynecologist. Currently living in Providence, Rhode Island, she is a practicing nurse. She mentioned to me that from 1919 on, midwives in Cairo were educated in professional schools for women. On Doctor Zalel, an important Karaite woman physician who was also a midwife, see Dabbah (1985, 298–300).

2. *Childbirth crisis* and *childbirth revolution* are terms widely used by feminists to refer to recent challenges to long-standing medically managed hospital-based childbirth (Rich 1976; Davis-Floyd and Sargent 1997). Emily Martin (1987) discusses the influence of technology on women's body perception in Western culture. Analyzing the metaphorical vocabulary of the discourse of the body, she draws an analogy between the production of goods (the dual meaning of the

word *labor*, for example) and the reproduction of babies. Among the phenomena that result from the medical co-optation of child delivery, she refers to the fragmentation of birth and the encouragement of the split between body and self.
3. Jewish Rabbanite midwives in Egypt used to deliver Karaite babies "even on Shabbat, or especially on Shabbat," because Karaite Jews, unlike Rabbanites, do not follow the rule that "the duty of saving a life overrides the Shabbat laws." This role often put strains on the relationship between Rabbanites and Karaites (Asaf 1936, 227), since it forced Rabbinates to become the "Shabbat goy" of the Karaites (the term refers to a Gentile who does any work forbidden to Jews on the Shabbat, such as turning lights on or off in the synagogue and Jewish houses).
4. On the male-dominant role in the medical sector in Arab countries and its relationship to contemporary women's health issues, see Haddad 1988, 93–97.
5. The Karaites believe in the literal expression of the evil eye, or the "bad eye," or "sick eye," as articulated in the story of the man whose eye was so "bad" that he went to the eye doctor in order to "fix" it. Belief in the evil eye is common among Karaites and appears in their folklore and in several of my interviews (Tsoffar 1995; Fahn 1928, 207–9). Whereas in some cultures the "evil eye" is ascribed to individuals with abnormal attributes, the Karaites believe that the evil eye acts in an involuntary, uncontrolled manner, whether the subject wills it or not, and is sometimes even self-inflicted.
6. Egyptian Arabic distinguishes between two different kinds of milk, *halēb* and *laban*. *Halēb* is unfermented fresh milk, and *laban* or *leben* is sour milk or kefir (Haran 1979, 30–31). This distinction is based historically on the way in which milk was preserved and on the time it took to sour it. Algamil recalls his own vivid memory of the cow that used to accompany the milk vendor while passing from one household to another in preindustrial Egypt, pointing to the fact that the milk was sold fresh and warm from the animal's body (Algamil 1985). The distinction between mother's milk, *chalav*, or *hlīb* (with its immediate reference to the institution of breast feeding and maternal discourse), and any other milk available for consumption became apparent.
7. It is interesting to compare milk in this regard to semen. Semen in Karaite literature is regarded as a limited resource. Some cultures tie linguistically milk and semen. Throughout Spain, for example, milk, "leche," is also a metaphor of masculinity, as it also means "semen" as a reference to "male sexual fluid" (Brandes 1980, 82–84). In Sri Lanka, milk, like semen, is a transformation of the blood (McGilvray 1982, 61–62). See also Laqueur 1990, especially chapter 2.
8. In Northern Sudan, Janice Boddy finds that all white food is believed to increase the invigoration of the blood. In a broader sense, white food relates to the preference for a white complexion, as in rituals of brightening the face or painting it with white, light colors (Boddy 1989, 61–66).
9. In Leviticus 12:1–8, the impurity of the *yoledah* is placed amidst a wider discussion on purity and impurity. Leviticus chapter 11 is devoted to dietary laws and the abomination of animals, and chapter 13 discusses the impurity of the body, especially in cases of skin disease like leprosy. In chapter 12 the association of the *yoledah* to the *niddah* locates her impurity within the wider Levitical context of blood impurities. For comparative notes with other halakhic systems regarding the origin of this prohibition, see Revel 1971 [1913], 42; Finkelstein 1938–39,

184; and Corinaldi 1984.
10. Rabbanites established that a woman would count seven days after her blood had stopped, and then conclude the cycle with a visit to the *mikveh*, the public ritual bath.
11. I am not sure to what extent one can easily assume the attribution of Hebrew grammatical formulations in the Karaite context; however, because Karaite Hebrew is the language of prayer, the point is worth making.
12. Fluids carry updated information concerning different processes in the body at any given time. Thus, it is not surprising that in Western medicine, illness and health are diagnosed by the condition of urine and blood.
13. Mary Douglas finds the danger of pressing on external boundaries the first of four kinds of physical and social pollution. The second is "danger from transgressing on external lines of the system," the third is "danger in the margins of the lines." The fourth is "danger from internal contradiction" (Douglas 1966, 122).
14. Na'imah is referring to the *hammam baladi (sha'abi)*, the native restroom, common in Egypt and throughout the Middle East. It is basically a hole in the ground where, while squatting, one puts one's feet on both sides and urinates. She also at times uses the French euphemism *les cabinets*, a lavatory, or water closet, as in the phrases "*ne'mal kabine(t),*" or "*nrūh el-kabine(t).*" The expressions are typical of the secretive language of females and mean "Let's go to the W.C. (water closet)" or "Let's go to the bathroom."
15. Here I use folklore as including oral as well as textual data. Following Alan Dundes's wider definition, I refer to any sociocultural production by multiple authors and of multiple distributions (Dundes 1965, 1–3).
16. I agree that coded language relies in part on being a discourse of familiarity, as suggested by Bourdieu. This type of discourse "leaves unsaid all that goes without saying: the informant's remarks. . . ." Bourdieu elaborates: "Insofar as it is an outsider oriented discourse it tends to exclude all direct references to particular cases. . . . Because the native is that much less inclined to slip into the language of familiarity to the extent that his questioner strikes him as unfamiliar with the universe of reference implied by the discourse . . . , it is understandable that anthropologists should so often forget the distance between learned reconstruction of the native world and the native experience of that world, an experience which finds expression only in the silence, ellipses, and lacunae of the language of familiarity" (Bourdieu 1977, 18). Yet kara'iyots' narrative is characteristic of women's discourse, which used innately narrow, limited language that is particular in its references to the female body.
17. In Persian literature there is an extensive use of the theme of blood and milk, especially in mystical poetry. As the following Rumi line says: "An interval was needed in order that the blood might turn to milk" (Jalal Al-Din 1960, 222). Milk and blood as antithetical substances are found in different versions in folklore. Cow's milk in the domestic sphere is considered as vulnerable to menstruation as mother's milk—the Thongwa, for example, believe that a menstruating woman could not go near the *kraal* or look at the cattle, and among the Banyoro the menstruating woman was permitted to milk only from old cows (Leach 1949).
18. A good example of the folk equivalency of urine with water is the expression in English "passing water" (a euphemism for urinating), and the expression in Rab-

binic Hebrew *mayim 'achronim* (last water, which refers to urine as the end-phase of the bodily water cycle).
19. In the folklore of different cultures urine is considered a life force used in sympathetic magic to produce fertilizers that will induce rain. The Masai (of Kenya and Tanganyika), for example, use cow's urine (instead of water) when washing milk vessels to impart a peculiar odor (Leach 1949, 725). Karaites, like other Middle Easterners, use urine as a disinfecting acid that repels insects when rubbed on the skin.
20. Even though the period comes back after six months, usually fertility continues to be low. In the interviews, women referred to the freedom that breast feeding allowed them.
21. A similar inversion takes place in the Sudan, where it is said that the presence of a menstruating woman may easily provoke any kind of bleeding—including menstruation and hemorrhoids—in a breast-feeding woman (Boddy 1989).

Chapter 8

1. Emphasis added. The guide, written by Hakohen in Egypt, is a good summary of Karaite laws concerning slaughtering. The publisher specifies that "the intention of this booklet is to explain the matter of slaughtering according to its written orders, laws and ordeals in the written Torah in Sinai by Moses, Our Teacher, father and head of the prophets (peace be upon him) as the human mind derives following the correct *pshat*, which comes out of the written Torah with no tendency to incline to the right or to the left pursuing external words [foreign ideas]" (1958).
2. For example, Halevi's *Toharat ha-Mishpachah* lists all rules concerning purity but does not mention this prohibition.
3. For the Karaites, counting of seven days is an important measure. A mother cow can only be slaughtered seven days after she has given birth. Similarly, a kid (*gdi*) can only be slaughtered seven days after its birth. The milk of the mother cow is also prohibited for the first seven days.
4. The word "chicken" differs. In Hebrew, unlike in English, there are two words: *tarnegolet* designates the living bird and *'of* the edible meat.
5. Other prohibitions against mixing substances include *sha'atnez* (mixing wool with linen), or *kil'ei ha-kerem* (mixing grapes with wheat or barley).
6. Early on, Anan introduced the prohibition regarding intercourse with a pregnant woman (Harkavy 1969 [1903], 60). The reason given is the waste of the seed. Today, Karaites allow intercourse during pregnancy.
7. Among other scholars of Karaism, Mann perceives the Karaite permission of eating fowl together with milk as a contradiction to other dietary and slaughtering prohibitions such as the slaughtering of a pregnant animal. Documents from the Cairo *genizah* shed more light on these relations: "As regards the dietary laws the Karaites, on the one hand, permitted the eating of fowl together with milk but prohibited, on the other hand, the tail-fat of animals, the slaughtering of a pregnant animal, the [kidneys] and the large lobe of the liver" (Mann 1972, 2:54).
According to Kashani (1978, 12), Anan prohibited mixing beef, but not fowl, with milk. The explanation: the Bible does not say not to cook a fowl but a *gdi*, re-

ferring to a kid (see Kashani 1978, 25, on the charges of Ibn Kammunah against the Rabbanites). Also see Nemoy (1972–73, 114): "The prohibition contained in the Bible (Exod. 23:19, 34:26; Deut. 14:21) of boiling a kid in its mother's milk is also accepted by the Karaites as forbidding the consumption of the meat of the cattle (not of fowl) with milk or butter; they do not, however, accept the additional restrictions enacted by the rabbis. Karaites permit the consumption of the meat of those animals only that are enumerated in the Bible, and reject the criteria for permitted mammals and birds as formulated in the Talmud. Many Karaite scholars hold that ever since the destruction of the Temple, any consumption of meat is prohibited" (Nemoy 1971, 780).

8. The Karaites reversed the order, by way of analogy (syllogism) and claimed that the meat of the mother and the milk of the child will not be consumed. Still, it remains unclear what is meant by the milk of the child (the offspring) or the milk of the father.

9. "If a bird's nest chance to be before thee in the way in any tree, or on the ground, whether they be young ones, or eggs, and the dam sitting upon the young, or upon the eggs, thou shalt not take the *'em*, the dam, with the young" (Deut. 22:6).

10. "Who said that they are the ones carrying the true tradition?" The quote is from al-Qirqisani (1939–43, 1213), referring to the Rabbanites.

11. Compare Genesis 2:23, "And Adam said, this is now bone of my bones, and flesh of my flesh: she shall be called Woman, because she was taken out of Man. Therefore, shall a man leave his father and his mother, and shall cleave unto his wife, and they shall be one flesh" (*Vayomer ha-'adam, Zot ha-pa'am 'etsem me-'atsamai u-vasar mi-bsari . . . ve-davak be-'ishto ve-hayu le-vasar echad*). Hadassi, and further on, Nikomodio, writing in Hebrew, uses masculine—or default—pronouns.

12. Although I do not elaborate in this chapter, milk was appropriated as a national—masculinist—symbol in the Zionist discourse as a corollary to the utopian depiction of Israel as a "land flowing with milk and honey." See Tsoffar 2005a; 2005b.

13. In contrast, in Jewish tradition the creation of *lehem* (bread) is attributed to God, as shown in the ceremonial blessing *Hamotsi'*, recited by both Karaites and Rabbanites prior to every meal (see D. Boyarin 1993, 90–94, about the death penalty).

14. In Jewish Rabbanite culture specifically, women are instructed to prepare the Shabbat bread and fulfill the *mitzvah* of *hafrashat challah*, the dough offering, by setting aside and burning a small part of the dough in commemoration of the pre-exilic time when the priest would have received a share of the bread (D. Boyarin 1993, 90).

15. As described by Julia Kristeva, milk is a "medium that is common to mother and child, a food that does not separate but binds" (Kristeva 1982, 105). She discusses milk in the context of the milk/meat prohibition in which cow milk stands for a wider category of (dairy) food.

16. On Philo's influence on Karaites see Revel 1971 (1913).

17. Maimonides (*Guide to the Perplexed* 3:48) treats this prohibition as he does other taboos, maintaining that its purpose is "to train us in the mastery of our appetites, desire and pleasure." As a physician, he also argues for the health and mental benefits of the prohibition, paying attention to the fact that "meat boiled in milk is undoubtedly gross food, and makes a person feel overfull."

18. Milgrom (1990) gives several examples of those who hold accordingly. Milgrom's approach seems to support Philo's (and Karaites') explanation as he himself, by attempting to explain the Rabbanites' rationale, questions rhetorically: "Is it so far-fetched for the rabbis to have deduced that all meat (not just of a kid) and all milk (not only that of the mother) may not be served together? Their interpretation is clearly an old one" (Milgrom 1990, 153n. 6).
19. Haran emphasizes that even today, boiling in milk (referred to specifically as "its mother's milk), while having no ritual significance, is a common way of preparing a kid or a lamb among Arabs.
20. *Zakhar,* masculine, and *zikkaron,* memory; see Yerushalmi 1982, Funkenstein 1991, Zerubavel 1995.
21. This is where milk and semen are biologically similar.

Conclusion

1. Note, for example, Bill Germano's definition of "Cultural Studies" as an interdisciplinary, trans-disciplinary, counter-disciplinary study that "operates in the tension between its tendencies to embrace both a broad, anthropological and a more narrowly conception of culture" (cited in Culler 1999, 336).
2. Sumi Colligan, personal communication, April 1992. See also note 8 to the preface of this volume.

BIBLIOGRAPHY

Aaron ben Eliyahu (Nikomodio). 1972 [1866]. *Keter Torah* [The Crown of the Torah]. Ed. J. Savuskan. Gozlow: Ramleh, Israel.

Abaza, Mona. 2001. "Shopping Malls, Consumer Culture and the Reshaping of Public Space in Egypt." *Theory, Culture and Society* 18 (5): 97–122.

Abu-Lughod, Lila. 1986. *Veiled Sentiments: Honor and Poetry in a Bedouin Society*. Berkeley: University of California Press.

Adler, Rachel. 1973. "Tumah and Taharah: Ends and Beginnings." In *The Jewish Catalog: A Do It Yourself Kit*, ed. Richard Siegel, Michael Strassfeld, and Sharon Strassfeld, 167–71. Philadelphia: Jewish Publication Society.

———. 1983. "In Your Blood, Live: Re-Visions of a Theology of Purity." *Tikkun* 8 (1): 38–41.

Alcalay, Ammiel. 1993. *After Jews and Arabs*. Minneapolis: University of Minnesota Press.

Algamil, Yosef Ben Ovadia. 1979. *Toldot ha-Yahadut ha-Kara'it: Korot Chayei ha-Kehilah ha-Kara'it ba-Galut uve-'Erets-Yiśra'el* [The History of the Karaite Jewry: Life and Times of the Karaite Community in Exile and In Israel]. Vol. 1. Ramleh: Ha-Mo'etsah ha-'Artsit shel ha-Yehudim ha-Kara'im be-Yiśra'el.

———. 1981. *Toledot ha-Yahadut ha-Kara'it* [The History of the Karaite Jewry]. Vol. 2. Ramleh: Ha-Mo'etsah ha-'Artsit la-Yehudim ha-Kara'im be-Yiśra'el.

———. 1985. *Ha-Yahadut ha-Kara'it be-Mitsrayim ba-'Et ha-Chadashah* [Karaite Jewry in Egypt in Modern Time]. Ramleh: Ha-Mo'etsah ha-'Artsit la-Yehudim ha-Kara'im be-Yiśra'el.

———. 1987. "Chakham Toviah Simhah Babovitch" [The Last Karaite Hakham in Egypt]. *Pe'amim* 32: 40–59.

———. 1988. "*Ha-Yahadut ha-Kara'it be-Mitsrayim 1517–1918*" [The Karaite Jews in Egypt 1517–1918]. In *Toldot Yehudei Mitsrayim ba-Tekufah ha-'Otomanit 1517–1914* [The Jews in Ottoman Egypt 1517–1914], ed. Jacob Landau, 513–56. Jerusalem: Misgav Yerushalayim.

———. 1997a. *Pirkei Tuvia Ben Simchah Levi-Babovitch* [Tuvia Ben Simhah Levi-Babovitch]. Vol. 1, Introduction. Ramleh: Ha-Merkaz le-Cheker ha-Yahadut ha-Kara'it.

———. 1997b. *Pirkei Tuvia Ben Simchah Levi-Babovitch* [Tuvia Ben Simchah Levi-Babovitch]. Vol. 2, Sources. Ramleh: Ha-Merkaz le-Cheker ha-Yahadut ha-Kara'it.
Algamil, Yosef Ben Ovadia, and Levi Hayim Ben Yitshak. 1981. *Dod Mordechai*. Ramleh: Chevrat ha-Tslachah li-Vnei Mikra'.
Allouche-Benayoun, Joëlle. 1999. "The Rites of Water for the Jewish Women of Algeria: Representation and Meaning." In *Women and Water: Menstruation in Jewish Life and Law*, ed. Rahel Wasserfall, 198–216. Hanover, N.H.: Brandeis University Press.
Al-Qirqisani, Ya'qub. 1939–43. *Kitab al-'Anwar wal-Maraqib* [Book of Lights and Watchtowers]. Ed. Leon Nemoy. New York: Alexander Kohut Memorial Foundation.
Al-Qirqisani Center for the Promotion of Karaite Studies. http://www.karaitejudaism.com/qirqisani.
Al-Qudsī, Murād. 1987. *The Karaite Jews of Egypt, 1882–1986*. New York: Wilprint.
———. 2002. *Just for the Record in the History of the Karaite Jews of Egypt in Modern Times*. New York: Wilprint.
Ankori, Zvi. 1959. *Karaite in Byzantium: The Formative Years 970–1100*. New York: Columbia University Press.
———. 1966. *Beit Bashyatchi ve-Takanotav* [House of Bashyatchi and Its Reforms]. Ramleh: Hotsa'at 'Adat ha-Yehudim ha-Kara'im be-Yiśra'el.
Asad, Talal. 1973. Introduction to *Anthropology and the Colonial Encounter*, ed. Talal Asad. New York: Humanities Press.
———. 1984. "The Concept of Cultural Translation in British Social Anthropology." In *Writing Culture: The Poetics and Politics of Ethnography*, ed. James Clifford and George Marcus, 141–64. Berkeley: University of California Press.
Asaf, Simhah. 1936. *The History of the Middle Eastern Karaites. Tsiyon* 1/2: 208–51.
Assmann, Jan. 1997. *Moses the Egyptian: The Memory of Egypt in Western Monotheism*. Cambridge: Harvard University Press.
Astren, Fred. 2004. *Karaite Judaism and Historical Understanding*. Columbia: University of South Carolina Press.
Bakhtin, Mikhail. 1968. *Rabelais and His World*. Cambridge: MIT Press.
———. 1981. *The Dialogic Imagination*. Austin: University of Texas Press.
Bal, Mieke. 1985. *Narratology: Introduction to the Theory of Narrative*. Toronto: University of Toronto Press.
———. 1987. *Lethal Love: Feminist Literary Readings of Biblical Stories*. Bloomington: Indiana University Press.
———. 1988. "The Rape of Narrative and the Narrative of Rape: Speech Acts and Body Language in Judges." In *Literature and the Body*, ed. Elaine Scarry, 1–32. Baltimore: Johns Hopkins University Press.
Baron, Salo. 1957. "Karaite Schism." In *A Social and Religious History of the Jews* 5: 209–85. Philadelphia: Jewish Publication Society.
Barthes, Roland. 1972. "Wine and Milk." In *Mythologies*, 58–61. Trans. Annette Lavers. New York: Hill and Wang.
Bashyatchi, Eliyahu. 1870 [1530]. *Aderet Eliyahu* [The Mantle of Elijah]. Odessa.
Beauvoir, Simone. 1973. *The Second Sex*. Trans. E. M. Parshley. New York: Vintage.
Beinin, Joel. 1988. *The Dispersion of Egyptian Jewry: Culture, Politics, and the Formation of a Modern Diaspora*. Berkeley: University of California Press.

Benjamin, Walter. 1968. *Illuminations: Essays and Reflections.* Trans. Harry Zohn. New York: Schocken.
Ben-Sasson, H. Hillel. 1950. "*Rishonei ha-Kara'im: Kavim le-Mishnatam ha-Chevratit*" [The First Karaites: The Trend of Their Social Conception]. *Tsyion* 15: 42–55.
Ben-Shamai, Haggai. 1978. "The Doctrines of Religious Thought of Abū Yūsuf Ya'qūb al-Qirqisānī and Yefet ben 'Elī" [in Hebrew]. Ph.D. diss., Hebrew University, Jerusalem.
———. 1982. "Hebrew in Arabic Script: Qirqisani's View." In *Studies in Judaica, Karaitica and Islamica Presented to Leon Nemoy on his Eightieth Birthday*, ed. Haggai Ben-Shamai, 115–26. Ramat Gan: Bar Ilan University.
———. 1984. "The Attitude of Some Early Karaites toward Islam." In *Studies in Medieval History and Literature*, ed. I. Twersky, 2:3–40. Cambridge: Harvard University Press.
Bettelheim, Bruno. 1971. *Symbolic Wounds: Puberty Rites and the Envious Male.* New York: Collier.
Bhabha, Homi. 1994. "The Other Question." In *The Location of Culture.* New York: Routledge.
Biale, David. 1982. "The God with Breasts: *El Shadai* in the Bible." *History of Religions* 21 (3): 240–56.
———. 1992. *Eros and the Jews: From Biblical Israel to Contemporary America.* New York: Basic.
Biale, David, et al., eds. 1992. *From Intercourse to Discourse: Control of Sexuality in Rabbinic Literature.* San Anselmo, Calif.: Center for Hermeneutical Studies.
Biale, Rachel. 1984. *Woman in Jewish Law: An Exploration of Women's Issues in Halakhic Sources.* New York: Schocken.
Birnbaum, Philip. 1971. Introduction to *Karaites Studies*, v–xiii. New York: Hermon.
Boddy, Janice. 1989. *Wombs and Alien Spirits: Women, Men, and the Zar Cult in Northern Sudan.* Madison: University of Wisconsin Press.
Bóid, Ruairidh. 1989. *Principles of Samaritan Halacha: Studies in Judaism in Late Antiquity.* Leiden: Brill.
Bordo, Susan. 1986. "The Cartesian Masculinization of Thought." *Signs* 11 (3): 439–56.
———. 1989. "The Body and the Reproduction of Femininity: A Feminist Appropriation of Foucault." In *Gender/Body/Knowledge: Feminist Reconstructions of Being and Knowing*, ed. Alison Jaggar and Susan Bordo, 13–33. New Brunswick, N.J.: Rutgers University Press.
Bourdieu, Pierre. 1977. *Outline of a Theory of Practice.* Trans. Richard Nice. New York: Cambridge University Press.
Boxer, Baruch. 1984. *The Origins of the Seder.* Berkeley: University of California Press.
Boyarin, Daniel. 1992. "Placing Reading: Ancient Israel and Medieval Europe." In *The Ethnography of Reading*, ed. Jonathan Boyarin, 10–37. Berkeley: University of California Press.
———. 1993. *Carnal Israel: Reading Sex in Talmudic Culture.* Vol. 25 of "The New Historicism: Studies in Cultural Poetics," ed. Stephen Greenblatt. Berkeley: University of California Press.
Boyarin, Jonathan, ed. 1992. *The Ethnography of Reading.* Berkeley: University of California Press.

Brandes, Stanley. 1980. *Metaphors of Masculinity: Sex and Status in Andalusian Folklore.* Philadelphia: University of Pennsylvania Press.

———. 1985. *Forty the Age and the Symbol.* Knoxville: University of Tennessee Press.

Brenner, Frederic, and Stan Neumann. 1990. *The Last Marranos.* 65 minutes, color (16mm/video), Portuguese with English subtitles.

Briggs, Charles. 1996. "The Politics of Discursive Authority in Research on the Invention of Tradition." *Cultural Anthropology* 11 (4): 345–469.

Brinner, William M. 1982. "The Egyptian Karaite Community in the Late Nineteenth Century." In *Studies in Judaica, Karaitica and Islamica Presented to Leon Nemoy on his Eightieth Birthday,* ed. S. Brunswick, 127–44. Ramat Gan: Bar Ilan University Press.

———. 1987. "Karaism and Judaism: A Question of Identity." Paper presented at the Tenth Annual Jewish American Studies Conference, Cambridge, December 15–17.

———. 1989. "Karaites of Christendom—Karaites of Islam." In *The Islamic World: From Classical to Modern Times (Essays in Honor of Bernard Lewis),* ed. C. E. Bosworth, Charles Issawi, Roger Savory, and A. L. Udovitch, 55–73. Princeton: Darwin.

Buckley, Thomas, and Alma Gottlieb. 1988. *Blood Magic: The Anthropology of Menstruation.* Berkeley: University of California Press.

Butler, Judith. 1987. "Variation on Sex and Gender." In *Feminism as Critique,* ed. Seyla Benhabib and Drucilla Cornell, 128–42. Minneapolis: University of Minnesota Press.

———. 1990. *Gender Trouble.* New York: Routledge.

———. 1993. *Bodies That Matter.* New York: Routledge.

Bynum, Caroline Walker. 1987. *Holy Feast and Holy Fast: The Religious Significance of Food to Medieval Women.* Berkeley: University of California Press.

Cahn, Zvi. 1937. *The Rise of the Karaite Sect: A New Light on the Halakah and the Origins of the Karaites.* New York: M. Tausner.

Carmichael, Calum M. 1976. "On Separating Life and Death: An Explanation of Some Biblical Laws." *Harvard Theological Review* 69: 1–7.

Chaouachi, Kamal. 2003. "Le narguilé: Analyse socio-anthropologique. Culture, convivialité, histoire et tabacologie d'un mode d'usage populaire du tabac." Ph.D. diss., Université Paris X.

Chodorow, Nancy. 1974. "Family Structure and Feminine Personality." In *Women, Culture and Society,* ed. Michelle Zimbalist Rosaldo and Louise Lamphere, 43–66. Stanford: Stanford University Press.

———. 1978. *The Reproduction of Mothering: Psychoanalysis and the Sociology of Gender.* Berkeley: University of California Press.

Chow, Rey. 1995. *Primitive Passions: Visuality, Sexuality, Ethnography, and Contemporary Chinese Cinema.* New York: Columbia University Press.

Clifford, James. 1984. "Introduction: Partial Truths." In *Writing Culture: The Poetics and Politics of Ethnography,* ed. James Clifford and George Marcus, 1–26. Berkeley: University of California Press.

———. 1997. *Routes: Travel and Translation in the Late Twentieth Century.* Cambridge: Harvard University Press.

Clifford, James, and George Marcus. 1986. "On Ethnographic Allegory." In *Writing Culture: The Poetics and Politics of Ethnography.* Berkeley: University of California Press.

Cohen, Shaye J.D. 1999. "Purity, Piety, and Polemic: Medieval Rabbinic Denunciations of 'Incorrect' Purification Practices." In *Women and Water: Menstruation in Jewish Life and Law,* ed. Rahel Wasserfall, 82–100. Hanover, N.H.: Brandeis University Press.

Colligan, Sumi Elaine. 1980. "Religion, Nationalism and Ethnicity in Israel: The Case of the Karaite Jews." Ph.D. diss., Princeton University.

———. 2001. "The Ethnographer's Body as Text and Context: Revisiting and Revisioning the Body through Anthropology and Disability Studies." *Disability Studies Quarterly* 21 (3): 113–24.

Cook, Leslie A. 1999. "Body Language: Women's Rituals of Purification in the Bible and Mishnah." In *Women and Water: Menstruation in Jewish Life and Law,* ed. Rahel R. Wasserfall, 40–59. Hanover, N.H.: Brandeis University Press.

Corinaldi, Michael. 1984. *Ha-Ma'amad ha'-Ishi shel ha-Kara'im* [The Personal Status of the Karaites]. Jerusalem: Reuven Mas.

Culler, Jonathan. 1982. *On Deconstruction: Theory and Criticism after Structuralism.* Ithaca: Cornell University Press.

———. 1990. "Rubbish Theory." In *Framing the Sign: Criticism and Its Institutions,* 168–82. New York: Blackwell.

———. 1999. "What Is Cultural Studies?" In *The Practices of Cultural Analysis: Exposing Interdisciplinary Interpretation,* ed. Mieke Bal, 335–47. Stanford: Stanford University Press.

Culpepper, Emily. 1979. "Exploring Menstrual Attitudes." In *Women Look at Biology Looking at Women: A Collection of Feminist Critiques,* ed. Ruth Hubbard, Mary Sue Henifin, and Barbarb Fried, 135–62. Boston: G. K. Hall.

Dabbah, Eliyahu. 1985. "Bikur Mishlachat Kehilah Kdoshah mi-Yiśra'el le-Mitsrayim be-Pessah 1980" [A Visit of the Delegation of the Jewish Karaite Community to Egypt during Passover 1980]. In *Ha-Yahadut ha-Kara'it be-Mitsrayim ba-'Et ha-Chadashah* [Karaite Jewry in Egypt in Modern Time], ed. Yosef Ben Ovadia Algamil, 274–318. Ramleh: Ha-Mo'etsah ha-'Artsit la-Yehudim ha-Kara'im be-Yiśra'el.

Davis, Natalie Zemon. 1981. "The Sacred and the Body Social in Sixteenth-Century Lyon." *Past and Present* 90: 40–70.

———. 1986. "Boundaries and the Sense of Self in Sixteenth-Century France." In *Reconstructing Individualism: Autonomy, Individuality, and the Self in Western Thought,* ed. Thomas C. Heller et al., 53–63, 332–36. Stanford: Stanford University Press.

———. 1989 "The Sacred and the Body Social in Sixteenth-Century Lyon." *Past and Present* 90: 40–70.

Davis-Floyd, Robbie, and Carolyn F. Sargent. 1997. "The Anthropology of Birth." In *Childbirth and Authoritative Knowledge,* 1–51. Berkeley: University of California Press.

Deinarda, Ephrayim. 1880. "Masa' ba-Chatsi ha-'Ei Krim" [Travels in Crimea]. Warsaw: Alexander Ginz.

De Certeau, Michael. 1984. *The Practice of Everyday Life.* Trans. Steven Rendall. Berkeley: University of California Press.

———. 1988. *The Writing of History.* New York: Columbia University Press.

Delaney, Carol. 1988. "Mortal Flow: Menstruation in Turkish Village Society." In *Blood Magic,* ed. Thomas Buckley and Alma Gottlieb, 75–93. Berkeley: University of California Press.

———. 1991. *The Seed and the Soil: Gender and Cosmology in Turkish Village Society.* Berkeley: University of California Press.
Delaney, Janice, Mary Jane Lupton, and Emily Toth. 1976. *The Curse: A Cultural History of Menstruation.* New York: Dutton.
Deleuze, Gilles, and Felix Guattari. 1986. "What Is Minor Literature." In *Kafka: Towards a Minor Literature,* 16–27. Trans. Dana Polan. Minneapolis: University of Minnesota Press.
Dening, Greg. 1995. *The Death of William Gooch: A History's Anthropology.* Honolulu: University of Hawaii Press.
Denny, Frederick. 1985. *An Introduction to Islam.* New York: Macmillan.
Derrida, Jacques. 1978. "Structure, Sign, and Play in the Discourse of the Human Sciences." In *Writing and Difference.* Trans. Alan Bass. Chicago: University of Chicago Press.
DiMaggio, Paul. 1979. "Review Essay: On Pierre Bourdieu." *American Journal of Sociology* 84 (6): 1460–74.
Dominguez, Virginia. 1989. *People as Subject, People as Object: Selfhood and Peoplehood in Contemporary Israel.* Madison: University of Wisconsin Press.
Douglas, Mary. 1966. *Purity and Danger: An Analysis of Concepts of Pollution and Taboo.* London: Routledge and Kegan Paul.
———. 1970. *Natural Symbols: Exploration in Cosmology.* London: Barrie and Rocklife.
———. 1975. *Implicit Meanings: Selected Essays in Anthropology.* London: Routledge and Kegan Paul.
Drori, Rina. 2000. *Models and Contacts: Arabic Literature and Its Impact on Medieval Jewish Culture.* Leiden: Brill.
Drori, Rina, and Polliack, Meira. 2003. *A Guide to Karaite Studies: The History and Literary Sources of Medieval and Modern Karaite Judaism.* Leiden: Brill.
Dundes, Alan. 1965. "What Is Folklore?" In *The Study of Folklore,* 1–3. Englewood Cliffs, N.J.: Prentice-Hall.
———. 1978. "The Number Three in American Culture." In *Essays in Folkloristics,* 265–76. New Delhi: Folklore Institute.
———. 1980. "Wet and Dry, the Evil Eye: An Essay in Indo-European and Semitic Worldview." In *Interpreting Folklore,* 93–133. Bloomington: Indiana University Press.
Durkheim, Émile. 1961 [1915]. *The Elementary Forms of the Religious Life.* Trans. J. W. Swain. New York: Collier.
"Editorial: Karaites Find a Home." 1991. *Northern California Jewish Bulletin.* October 4, p. 20.
Eilberg-Schwartz, Howard. 1990. *The Savage in Judaism.* Bloomington: Indiana University Press.
———. 1991. "People of the Body: The Problem of the Body for the People of the Book." *Journal of The History of Sexuality* 2 (1): 1–24.
———, ed. 1992. *People of the Body: Jews and Judaism from an Embodied Perspective.* Albany: State University of New York Press.
Eliade, Mircea. 1957. *The Sacred and the Profane.* New York: Harper and Row.
El-Saadawi, Nawal. 1988. *Memoirs of a Woman Doctor.* Trans. Catherine Cobham. London: Saqi.
Erder, Yoram. 1988. "The Origins of the Early Karaism and Outlines of Its Develop-

ment in the Light of the Controversies over the Time of the Paschal Sacrifice." Ph.D. diss., Tel Aviv University.

Ernster, Virginia. 1975. "American Menstrual Expression." *Sex Roles* 1: 3–13.

Fabian, Johannes. 1992. "Keep Listening: Ethnography and Reading." In *The Ethnography of Reading*, ed. Jonathan Boyarin, 80–97. Berkeley: University of California Press.

———. 2000. *Out of Our Minds: Reason and Madness in the Exploration of Central Africa.* Berkeley: University of California Press.

Fahn, Reuben. 1928. *Kitvei Reuben Fahn* [Reuben Fahn's Writings]. 2 vols. Lwów, Poland: Va'ad Ha-Yovel.

Faraj, Murad. 1970 [1935]. *Sefer ha-Ma'amad ha-'Ishi* [The Book of Personal Status]. Ramleh: Ha-Yehudim ha-Kara'im be-Yiśra'el, Ha-Mo'etsah ha-Datit.

Faur, José. 1997. "Basic Concepts in Rabbinic Hermeneutics." *Shofar* 16 (1): 1–12.

Felman, Shoshana. 1982. Introduction. In *Literature and Psychoanalysis: The Question of Reading, Otherwise*, ed. Shoshana Felman. Baltimore: Johns Hopkins University Press.

Ferguson, Russell. 1990. "Introduction: Invisible Center." In *Out There: Marginalization and Contemporary Cultures*, ed. Russell Ferguson, Martha Cever, Trinh T. Minh-ha, and Cornel West, 9–14. Cambridge: MIT Press.

Figit, Shmuel ben Shmaryahu. 1977. *Sefer Davar Dabur* [Tales and Fables]. Ramleh: Ha-Yehudim ha-Kara'im be-Yiśra'el, Ha-Mo'etsah ha-Datit.

Finkelstein, Louis. 1938–39. "The Resistance of Rejected Customs in Palestine." *Jewish Quarterly Review* 29: 179–86.

Fonrobert, Charlotte Elisheva. 2000. *Menstrual Purity: Rabbinic and Christian Reconstructions of Gender.* Palo Alto, CA: Stanford University Press.

Foster, George. 1972. "Peasant Society and the Image of Limited Good." In *Reading in Anthropology*, ed. Jesse Jennings and E. Adamson Hoebel, 324–34. New York: McGraw-Hill.

Foucault, Michel. 1972. *The Archaeology of Knowledge and the Discourse of Language.* New York: Pantheon.

———. 1977. "Intellectuals and Power." In *Language, Counter-Memory, Practice*, 205–17. Ithaca: Cornell University Press.

———. 1978. *History of Sexuality. Vol. 1: An Introduction.* New York: Pantheon.

———. 1985. *History of Sexuality. Vol. 2: The Use of Pleasure.* New York: Pantheon.

———. 1986. "Of Other Spaces." *Diacritics* 16: 22–27.

Frank, Daniel. 1988. "Karaism." http://www.muslimphilosophy.com/ip/rep/J052.htm.

———. 1990. "The Study of Medieval Karaism, 1959–1989, A Bibliographical Essay." *Bulletin of Judeo-Greek Studies* 6: 15–22.

Frazer, J. G. 1919. *Folk-Lore in the Old Testament*, Vol. 3. London: Macmillan.

Fredman, Ruth. 1981. *The Passover Seder: Afikoman in Exile.* Philadelphia: University of Pennsylvania Press.

Freund, Roman. 1991. *Karaites and Dejudaization: A Historical Overview of an Endogenous and Exogenous Paradigm.* Stockholm Studies in Comparative Religion. Stockholm: Almqvist and Wiksell International, Acta Universitatis Stockholmiensis.

Friedman, Philip. 1960. "The Karaites under Nazi Rule." In *On the Track of Tyranny: Essays Presented by the Wiener Library to Leonard G. Montefiore, on the Occasion of*

His Seventieth Birthday, ed. Max Beloff, 97–123. London: Valentine.

Friemann, A., Seeligmann, S., Zeithin, W., and M. Grunwald. 1911. "Bibliographie der hygienischen Literatur der Juden." In *Die Hygiene der Juden. Im Anschluss an der Internationale Hygiene-Asstellung*, 18–29.

Funkenstein, Amos. 1991. *Perception of Jewish History from the Antiquity to the Present*. Tel Aviv: 'Am 'Oved.

Gadalla, Saad. 1978. *Is There Hope? Fertility and Family Planning in a Rural Egyptian Community*. Chapel Hill: Carolina Population Center, University of North Carolina.

Gallagher, Catherine, and Thomas Laqueur. 1987. Introduction to *The Making of the Modern Body*, vii–xv. Berkeley: University of California Press.

Gaster, Theodore F. 1969. *Myth, Legend and Custom in the Old Testament*. New York: Harper and Row.

Geertz, Clifford. 1973. *The Interpretation of Culture*. New York: Basic.

Geller, Jay. 1992. "'A Glance at the Nose': Freud's Inscription of Jewish Difference." *American Imago* 49 (4): 427–44.

———. 1996. "The Aromatic of Jewish Difference: or, Benjamin's Allegory of Aura." In *Jews and Other Differences*, ed. Jonathan Boyarin and Daniel Boyarin, 203–56. Minneapolis: University of Minnesota Press.

Gilligan, Carol. 1982. *In a Different Voice*. Cambridge: Harvard University Press.

Gilman, Sander L. 1992a. "The Jewish Body: A Foot-Note." In *People of the Body: Jews and Judaism from an Embodied Perspective*, ed. Howard Eilberg-Schwartz, 223–41. Albany: State University of New York Press.

———. 1992b. *The Visibility of the Jew in the Diaspora: Body Imagery and Its Cultural Context*. Syracuse: Syracuse University Press.

Ginsberg, Harold Louis. 1982. *The Isralian Heritage of Judaism*. New York: Jewish Theological Seminary of America.

Ginzberg, Louis. 1976. *An Unknown Jewish Sect*. New York: Jewish Theological Seminary of America.

Girard, René. 1977. *Violence and the Sacred*. Trans. Patrick Gregory. Baltimore: Johns Hopkins University Press.

Goitein, Shelomoh Dov. 1954. "A Caliph's Decree in Favor of the Rabbinite Jews of Palestine" (from the Genizah Collection in the University Library, Cambridge). *Journal of Jewish Studies* 5: 118–25.

———. 1964. "Passover with the Last Karaites in Jerusalem." In *The Book of Holidays*, ed. Yom Tov Levinski, 2: 402–4. Tel Aviv: Dvir.

———. 1967. *A Mediterranean Society: The Jewish Communities of the Arab World as Portrayed in the Documents of the Cairo Geniza*. Berkeley: University of California Press.

Goldberg, Harvey. 1987. "Torah and Children: Symbolic Aspects of the Reproduction of Jews and Judaism." In *Judaism Viewed from Within and from Without*, 107–30. Albany: State University of New York Press.

Goldschmidt, E., K. Fried, A. G. Steinberg, and T. Cohen. 1976. "The Karaite Community of Iraq in Israel: A Genetic Study." *American Journal of Human Genetics* 28: 243–52.

Good, Mary-Jo DelVecchio. 1980. "Of Blood and Babies: The Relationship of Popular Islamic Physiology to Fertility." *Social Science and Medicine* 14B (3): 147–56.

Gordon, Nehemia. 2004. "The Karaite Korner." http://www.karaite-korner.org/main.shtml.
Gottlieb, Alma. 1988. "Menstrual Cosmology among the Beng of Ivory Coast." In *Blood Magic*, ed. Thomas Buckley and Alma Gottlieb, 55–74. Berkeley: University of California Press.
Green, W. P. 1978. "The Nazi Racial Policy toward the Karaites." *Soviet Jewish Affairs* 8 (2): 36–44.
———. 1979. "The Fate of Oriental Jews in Vichy France." *Wiener Library Bulletin* 32 (49): 40–50.
Gross, Rita. 1980. "Menstruation and Childbirth as Ritual and Religious Experience among Native Australians." In *Unspoken Worlds: Women's Religious Lives*, ed. N. Falk, 277–92. San Francisco: Harper and Row.
Grosz, Elizabeth. 1989. *Sexual Subversions: Three French Feminists*. Sydney: Allen and Unwin.
———. 1994. *Volatile Bodies: Toward a Corporeal Feminism*. Bloomington: Indiana University Press.
———. 1995. *Space, Time, and Perversion*. New York: Routledge.
Haberman, A. M. 1947. *Mi-Sipurei Ha-Karaim*. Merchaviah: Sifriyat ha-Po'alim.
Hadassi, Judah b. Eliyahu. 1836. *'Eshkol Ha-Kofer* [Cluster of Henna]. Göslöw-Eupat'oria.
Haddad, May. 1988. "Women and Health in the Arab World." In *Women in the Arab World*, ed. Nahid Toubia, 93–97. London: Zed.
Hakohen, Hachakham Shmu'el. 1958. *'Inyan ha-Shchitah* [Concerning Slaughtering]. Ramleh: Mar Shlomo Ben Avraham Marzuk.
Halevi, Hayim. 1981. *Toharat ha-Mishpachah be-Yiśra'el* [Family Purity in Israel]. Ramleh: Ha-Yehudim ha-Kara'im be-Yiśra'el, Ha-Mo'etsah ha-Datit.
———. 1988a. "The Karaite Jews." Lecture co-sponsored by the Departments of Near Eastern Studies and Comparative Literature, University of California, Berkeley, January 27.
———. 1988b. *Sefer ha-Chinukh Ma'ayan Chayim* [The Book of Teaching: The Spring of Life]. Tel Aviv: Niv.
Hall, Edward. 1963. "A System for the Notation of Proxemic Behavior." *American Anthropologist* 65: 1003–26.
Handelman, Susan A. 1982. *The Slayers of Moses: The Emergence of Rabbinic Interpretation in Modern Literary Theory*. Albany: State University of New York Press.
Haran, Menachem. 1979. "Seething a Kid in Its Mother's Milk." *Journal of Jewish Studies* 30: 23–35.
Harkavy, Abraham. 1969 [1903]. *Zikaron la-Rishonim* [Studien und Mittheilungen]. Vol. 8. *Anan ben David, ha-Sarid veha-Palit mi-Sifrei ha-Mitsvot ha-Rishonim li-Vene ha-Mikra'* [Anan's book of commandments]. St. Petersburg. Reprint, Jerusalem: Makor.
Harrell, Barbara. 1981. "Lactation and Menstruation in Cultural Perspective." *American Anthropologist* 83: 796–823.
Hatroki, Shlomo. 1960. *Sefer 'Apirion 'Asah Lo*. Tel Aviv: Chevrat ha-Hatslachah li-Vnei Mikra'.
Helman, Boruch K. 1979. "The Karaite Jews of Cairo." *Hadassah Magazine* (March), 4–9.

Hendel, Yehudit. 1988. *Kesef Katan* [Small Change]. Jerusalem: Keter.
Hirshberg, Jehoash. 1987. "Musikah ke-Gorem be-Likud ha-Kehilah ha-Kara'it be-San Fransisko" [Music as a Unifying Factor in the Karaite Community of San Francisco]. *Pe'amim* 32: 66–81.

———. 1994. "Reconstruction and Self-Inspection in a Displaced Community." http://www.music.ed.ac.uk/colloquia/conferences/esem/hir.html.

Hobsbawm, Eric. 1983. "Introduction: Inventing Traditions." In *The Invention of Tradition,* ed. Eric Hobsbawm and Terence Ranger, 1–14. Cambridge: Cambridge University Press.
Hoffman, Shlomo. 1971. "Karaites." *Encyclopedia Judaica,* 10: 761–86. Jerusalem: Keter House.
Holyoak, Keith James, and Paul Thagard. 1995. *Mental Leaps: Analogy in Creative Thought.* Cambridge: MIT Press.
Horton, H. Mack. 1992. "Japanese Spirit and Chinese Learning: Scribes and Storytellers in Pre-Modern Japan." In *The Ethnography of Reading,* ed. Jonathan Boyarin, 156–79. Berkeley: University of California Press.
Hubert, Henri, and Marcel Mauss. 1967. *Sacrifice: Its Nature and Function.* Trans. W. D. Halls. Chicago: University of Chicago Press.
Hurston, Zora Neale. 1976. "Folklore Field Notes from Zora Neale Hurston." *Black Scholar* 7: 41–42.
Ibn Ezra, Abraham. 1977. *Perushei Ha-Torah le-Rabenu Avraham Ibn 'Ezra.* Jerusalem: Mosad Ha-Rav Kuk.
Ichilov, Orit, and Yehudith Stern. 1978. "Patterns of Ethnic Separation among the Karaites in Israel." *Ethnic Groups* 2 (1): 17–34.
Indurkhya, Bipin. 1992. *Metaphor and Cognition.* London: Kluwer.
Inhorn, Marcia Claire. 1991. "Umm Il-Ghayyib, Mother of the Missing One: A Sociomedical Study of Infertility in Alexandria, Egypt." Ph.D. diss., University of California, Berkeley.

———. 1996. *Infertility and Patriarchy.* Philadelphia: University of Pennsylvania Press.

"An Interview with our New President." 1994. *KJA Bulletin* 10 (2): 18–19.
Irigaray, Luce. 1985. "The Mechanics of Fluids." In *This Sex Which Is Not One,* 106–18. Ithaca: Cornell University Press.

———. 1991. "Volume without Contours." In *The Irigaray Reader,* ed. and trans. Margaret Whitford, 53–67. Cambridge: Basil Blackwell.

Itzhak, N. 1973. *Ha-ma'amad ha-'Ishi shel ha-Kara'im* [The Personal Status of the Karaites]. Master's thesis, Tel Aviv University.
Jabès, Edmond. 1993. *The Book of Margins.* Trans. Rosemarie Waldrop. Chicago: University of Chicago Press.
Johnson, Barbara. 1980. *The Critical Difference.* Baltimore: Johns Hopkins University Press.
Jong, Walter. 1989. *Orality and Literacy: The Technologizing of the Word.* London: Methuen.
Jordan, Brigitte. 1993. *Birth in Four Cultures: A Cross-Cultural Investigation of Childbirth in Yucatan, Holland, Sweden and the United States.* 4th ed. Prospect Heights, Ohio: Waveland.

———. 1997. "Authoritative Knowledge and Its Construction." In *Childbirth and Authoritative Knowledge: Cross-Cultural Perspectives,* ed. Robbie Davis-Floyd and

Carolyn Sargent, 55–79. Berkeley: University of California Press.
Joseph, Suad. 1994. "Brother/Sister Relationship: Connectivity, Love, and Power in the Reproduction of Patriarchy in Lebanon." *American Ethnologist* 21 (1): 50–73.
Kashani, Reuven. 1978. *Ha-Kara'im: Korot, Masorot u-Minhagim* [The Karaites: History, Tradition and Customs]. Jerusalem: n.p.
Katriel, Tamar. 1997. *Performing the Past: A Study of Israeli Settlement Museums*. Mahwah, N.J.: Lawrence Erlbaum Associates.
Kaufman, Tamar. 1991a. "Karaites Battle Neighbors in Bid to Buy 1st Synagogue." *Northern California Jewish Bulletin*, October 4, pp. 1, 8.
———. 1991b. "Karaites Get Go-Ahead on 1st Synagogue." *Northern California Jewish Bulletin*, November 8, p. 9.
———. 1992. "Why Is This Seder Different from Others?" *Northern California Jewish Bulletin*, April 17, pp. 1, 52.
Keel, Othmar. 1980. *Das Böcklein in Der Milch seiner Mutter und Verwandtes*. Göttingen: Vandenhoeck and Ruprecht.
Khan, Geoffrey. 1990. *The Karaite Bible Manuscripts from the Cairo Genizah*. Cambridge: Cambridge University Press.
———. 2000a. *The Early Karaite Tradition of Hebrew Grammatical Thought*. Leiden: Brill.
———, ed. 2000b. *Early Karaite Grammatical Texts*. Masoretic Studies, no. 9. Atlanta: Society of Biblical Literature.
———, ed. 2001. *Exegesis and Grammar in Medieval Karaite Texts*. Oxford: Oxford University Press.
Khomeini, Ayatollah. 1984. *A Clarification of Questions. An Unabridged Translation of Resaleh Towzih al-Masael*. Trans. J. Borujerdi. Boulder: Westview.
Kittler, Friedrich. 1990. *Discourse Networks 1800/1900*. Trans. Michael Metteer with Chris Cullens. Stanford: Stanford University Press.
Kizilov, Mikhail. 2003. "Karaites and Karaism: Recent Developments." The CESNUR International Conference, Center for Religious Studies and Research at Vilnius University, and New Religious Research and Information Center Vilnius, Lithuania, April 9–12. http://www.cesnur.org/2003/vil2003_kizilov.htm.
Kraïmer, Gudrun. 1989. *The Jews in Modern Egypt, 1914–1952*. Seattle: University of Washington Press.
Kridli, Suha Al-Oballi. 2002. "Health Beliefs and Practices among Arab Women." *American Journal of Maternal Child Nursing* 27 (3): 178–82.
Kristeva, Julia. 1981. "Women's Time." In *Feminist Theory: A Critique of Ideology*, ed. Nannerl Keohane, Michelle Rosaldo, and Barbara Gelpi, 31–53. Chicago: University of Chicago Press.
———. 1982. *Powers of Horror: An Essay on Abjection*. Trans. Leon S. Roudiez. New York: Columbia University Press.
———. 1986. *The Kristeva Reader*. Ed. Toril Moi. New York: Columbia University Press.
Kuper, Hilda. 1972. "The Language of Sites in the Politics of Space." *American Anthropologist* 74: 411–25.
Landau, Jacob. 1988. *Toldot Yehudei Mitsrayim ba-Tekufah ha-'Otomanit 1517–1914* [The Jews in Ottoman Egypt 1517–1914]. Jerusalem: Misgav Yerushalayim.
Lander, Louise. 1988. *Images of Bleeding: Menstruation as Ideology*. New York: Orlando.

Laqueur, Thomas. 1986. "Orgasm, Generation and the Politics of Reproductive Biology." *Representation* 14 (April): 1–41.

———. 1990. *Making Sex: Body and Gender from the Greeks to Freud.* Cambridge: Harvard University Press.

Lasker, Daniel. 2001. "Ha-kara'i ke-''Acher' Yehudi" [The Karaite as Jewish "Other"]. *Pe'amim* 89 (Autumn): 97–106.

Laskier, Michael M. 1992. *The Jews of Egypt, 1920–1970: In the Midst of Zionism: Anti-Semitism and the Middle East Conflict.* New York: New York University Press.

Laws, Sophie. 1990. *Issues of Blood: The Politics of Menstruation.* London: Macmillan.

Leach, Edmund. 1979. "Two Essays Concerning the Symbolic Representation of Time." In *Reader in Comparative Religion,* ed. William Lessa and Evon Vogt, 221–29. New York: Harper and Row.

Leach, Maria, ed. 1949. *Standard Dictionary of Folklore, Mythology, and Legend.* New York: Funk and Wagnalls.

Littman, Michael. 1988. "The Jewish Family in Egypt." In *The Jews in Ottoman Egypt (1517–1914),* 217–44. Jerusalem: Misgav Yerushalayim.

Lubin, Orly. 2003. *'Ishah Koret 'Ishah* [Women Reading Women]. Haifa / Or Yehudah: Haifa University / Zmorah-Bittan.

Maccoby, Hyam. 1996. "Holiness and Purity: The Holy People in Leviticus and Ezra-Nehemiah." In *Reading Leviticus: A Conversation with Mary Douglas,* ed. John F. A. Sawyer. Sheffield: Sheffield Academic Press.

MacCormack, Carol, ed. 1982. *Ethnography of Fertility and Birth.* London: Academic Press.

Mahler, Raphael. 1949. *Ha-Kara'im* [The Karaites]. Merchaviah: Sifriyat ha-Po'alim.

Maimonides (Moses ben Maimon). 1910. *The Guide of the Perplexed.* New York: Dutton.

Mann, Jacob. 1971. "Anan's Liturgy and His Half-Yearly Cycle of the Reading of the Law." In *Karaite Studies,* ed. Philip Birnbaum, 283–318. New York: Hermon.

———. 1972. *Texts and Studies in Jewish History and Literature.* 2 vols. New York: Ktav.

Marcus, Julie. 1984. "Islam, Women and Pollution in Turkey." *Journal of the Anthropological Association of Oxford* 15 (3): 204–18.

Margold, Jane. 1993. "The Politics of Silence: Class and Political Consciousness among Filipino Labor Migrants." Ph.D. diss., University of California, Berkeley.

Martin, Emily. 1987. *The Woman in the Body: A Cultural Analysis of Reproduction.* Boston: Beacon.

McGilvray, Dennis. 1982. "Sexual Power and Fertility in Sri Lanka: Batticaloa Tamils and Moors." In *Ethnography of Fertility and Birth,* ed. Carol MacCormack, 15. London: Academic Press.

Meiselman, Moshe. 1978. *Woman in Jewish Law.* New York: Ktav.

Mendes-Flohr, Paul. 1995. *The Jew in the Modern World.* Oxford: Oxford University Press.

Messick, Brinkley. 1993. *The Calligraphic State: Textual Domination and History in a Muslim Society.* Berkeley: University of California Press.

Meyer, Michael. 1987. *Ideas of Jewish History.* Detroit: Wayne State University Press.

Mikhail, Mona. 1979. *Images of Arab Women: Fact and Fiction.* Washington, D.C.: Three Continents.

Milgrom, Jacob. 1990. "Milk and Meat: Unlikely Bedfellows." In *By Study and Also by Faith, Essays in Honor of Hugh W. Nibley*, ed. John Lundquist and Stephen Ricks, 1: 144–54. Salt Lake City: Deseret Book Company.
Miller, Philip E. 1993. *Karaite Separatism in Nineteenth-Century Russia: Joseph Solomon Lutski's Epistle of Israel's Deliverance*. Cincinnati: Hebrew Union College Press.
Minai, Naila. 1981. *Women in Islam: Tradition and Transition in the Middle East*. London: John Murray.
Mitchell, Timothy. 1988. *Colonizing Egypt*. Berkeley: University of California Press.
Montgomery, Rita E. 1974. "A Cross-Cultural Study of Menstruation, Menstrual Taboos, and Related Social Variables." *Ethos* 2 (2): 137–70.
Mopsik, Charles. 1989. "The Body of Engenderment in the Hebrew Bible, the Rabbinic Tradition and the Kabbalah." In *Fragments for a History of the Human Body, Part One*, ed. Michel Feher, Ramona Naddaff, and Nadia Tazi, 48–73. New York: Urzone.
Mulvey, Laura. 1988. "Visual Pleasure and Narrative Cinema." In *Feminism and Film Theory*, ed. Constance Penley, 57–68. New York: Routledge.
Nemoy, Leon. 1952. *Karaite Anthology*. New Haven: Yale University Press.
———. 1971. "Karaites." *Encyclopedia Judaica* 10:763–84. Jerusalem: Keter House.
———. 1972–73. "Ibn Kammunah's Treatise on the Difference between the Rabbanites and the Karaites, A Modern Egyptian-Karaite Digest of the Duties and Rights of Husband and Wife." *Jewish Quarterly Review* 63: 97–135.
———. 1976. "Question Sermon to the Karaites." Reprint from *Proceeding of the American Academy for Jewish Research*, vol. 42.
———. 1980. "A Modern Karaite Arabic Poet (Murad Farag)." *Jewish Quarterly Review*, n.s., 74: 63–87.
Niranjana, Tejaswini. 1992. *Siting Translation: History, Post-Structuralism, and the Colonial Context*. Berkeley: University of California Press.
Olszowy-Schlanger, Judith. 1988. *Karaite Marriage Documents from the Cairo Geniza: Legal Tradition and Community Life in Mediaeval Egypt and Palestine*. Leiden: Brill.
Ortner, Sherry. 1978. *Sherpas through Their Rituals*. Cambridge: Cambridge University Press.
Ortner, Sherry B., and Harriet Whitehead. 1981. *Sexual Meaning: The Cultural Construction of Gender and Sexuality*. Cambridge: Cambridge University Press.
Paige, Karen Ericksen, and Jeffrey M. Paige. 1981. *The Politics of Reproductive Ritual*. Berkeley: University of California Press.
Pessah, Joe. 1983. "Preface: The Haggadah of Passover." In *Haggadah shel Pessah* [Passover Haggadah], 1. Daly City, California: Karaite Jews of America.
Pessah, Maurice. 1994. "President Message." *KJA Bulletin* 10 (2): 3–4.
Polliack, Meira. 1997. *The Karaite Tradition of Arabic Bible Translation: A Linguistic and Exegetical Study of Karaite Translation of the Pentateuch from the Tenth to Eleventh Centuries*. Leiden: Brill.
Polliack, Meira, ed. 2003. *Karaite Judaism: A Guide to Its History and Literary Sources*. Leiden: Brill.
Revel, B. 1971 [1913]. "The Karaite Halakhah and Its Relations to Sadducean, Samaritan and Philonian Halakhah." In *Karaite Studies*, ed. Philip Birnbaum, 1–88. New York: Hermon.

Rich, Adrienne. 1976. *Of Woman Born: Motherhood as Experience and Institution.* New York: Norton.
Rosaldo, Michelle Zimbalist. 1974. "Woman, Culture, and Society: A Theoretical Overview." In *Woman, Culture and Society,* ed. Michelle Rosaldo and Louise Lamphere, 17–42. Stanford: Stanford University Press.
Rumi, Jalal Al-Din. 1960. *Mathnawi of Rumi.* Book 2. Trans. Raymond A. Nicholson. Memorial Series. London: E. J. W. Gibb.
Ryan, Mary. 1960. *Women in Public: Between Banners and Ballots, 1825–1880.* Baltimore: Johns Hopkins University Press.
Sabbah, Fatna A. 1984. *Woman in the Muslim Unconscious.* New York: Pergamon.
Said, Edward. 1978. *Orientalism.* New York: Vintage.
Scarry, Elaine. 1985. *The Body in Pain.* New York: Oxford University Press.
———, ed. 1988. *Literature and the Body.* Baltimore: Johns Hopkins University Press.
Schechter, Solomon. 1910. *Documents of Jewish Sectaries, vol. 2: Fragments of the Book of the Commandments by Anan.* Cambridge: Cambridge University Press.
Scheper-Hughes, Nancy, and Margaret Lock. 1987. "The Mindful Body: A Prolegomenon to Future Work in Medical Anthropology." *Medical Anthropology Quarterly* 1: 6–41.
Schur, Nathan. 1992. *The Karaite History.* New York: Peter Lang.
———. 1995a. *The Karaite Encyclopedia.* New York: Peter Lang.
———. 1995b. "The Karaite Encyclopedia." Internet version. http://www.turkiye.net/sota/karatur.html.
———. 2003. *Toldot ha-Kara'im* [The History of Karaites]. Jerusalem: Mosad Bialik.
Searle, John. 1969. *Speech Acts: An Essay in the Philosophy of Language.* London: Cambridge University Press.
Sefer Zohar. 1951. *Ra'aya Mehaimna* [The Faithful Shepherd], vol. 3, pp. 175a (361). Margaliyot: Mosad Ha-Rav Kuk.
Semi, Emanuela Trevisan. 1984. *Gli Ebrei Caraiti Tra Ethnia e Religione* [The Karaite Jews between Ethnicity and Religion]. Rome: Carucci.
———. 1990. "The Image of the Karaites in Nazi and Vichy France Documents." *Jewish Journal of Sociology* 32: 81–93.
———. 1991. "A Brief Survey of Present Day Karaite Communities in Europe." *Jewish Journal of Sociology* 33: 97–106.
———. 1994. "The Crimean Karaites as Seen by the French Jews in the Second Half of the Nineteenth Century." In *Proceedings of the Eleventh World Congress of Jewish Studies* 3: 9–16.
Sered, Susan Starr, Romi Kaplan, and Samuel Cooper. 1999. "Talking about Miqveh Parties, or Discourses of Gender, Hierarchy, and Social Control." In *Women and Water: Menstruation in Jewish Life and Law,* ed. Rahel R. Wasserfall, 145–65. Hanover, N.H.: Brandeis University Press.
Shamir, Shimon, ed. 1987. Preface to *The Jews of Egypt: A Mediterranean Society in Modern Times,* xiii–ix. Boulder: Westview.
Shapira, Dan. 2003. *Avraham Firkowicz in Istanbul, 1830–1832: Paving the Way for Turkic Nationalism.* Ankara: Karam.
Shochetman, Eliav. 1988. "Li-Sh'elat Heter ha-Chitun 'im ha-Kara'im bi-Fsikatam shel Chakhmei Mitsrayim" [On the Question of Permission to Intermarry with Karaites in the Ruling of Egyptian Rabbis]. *Pe'amim* 34: 29–46.

Shostak, Marjorie. 1983. *Nisa: The Life and Words of a !Kung Woman.* New York: Vintage.
Silverman, Kaja. 1988. *The Acoustic Mirror: The Female Voice in Psychoanalysis and Cinema.* Bloomington: Indiana University Press.
Skultans, Vieda. 1988. "Menstrual Symbolism in South Wales." In *Blood Magic: The Anthropology of Menstruation,* ed. Thomas Buckley and Alma Gottlieb, 137–60. Berkeley: University of California Press.
Slyomovics, Susan. 1998. *The Object of Memory: Arab and Jew Narrate the Palestinian Village.* Philadelphia: University of Pennsylvania Press.
Snow, Loudell F., and Shirley M. Johnson. 1977. "Modern Day Menstrual Folklore: Some Clinical Implications." *Journal of the American Medical Association* 237 (25): 2736–39.
Snowden, Robert, and Barbara Christian. 1983. *Patterns and Perceptions of Menstruation.* New York: St. Martin's.
Soler, Jean. 1979. "The Dietary Prohibitions of the Hebrews." *New York Review of Books,* June 14, 24–30.
Somekh, Sasson. 1987. "Participation of Egyptian Jews in Modern Arabic Culture and the Case of Murad Faraj." In *The Jews of Egypt: A Mediterranean Society in Modern Times,* ed. Shimon Shamir, 130–40. Boulder: Westview.
Spector, Shmuel. 1986. "Ha-Kara'im be-'Eropah shebi-Shlitat ha-Natsim bi-r'i Mismakhim Germaniyim" [The Karaites in Europe under the Nazi Rule in German documents]. *Pe'amim* 29: 90–108.
Stock, Brian. 1992. Afterword to *The Ethnography of Reading,* ed. Jonathan Boyarin, 270–75. Berkeley: University of California Press.
Strauss-Ashtor, E. 1944. "History of the Jews in Egypt and Syria (Volumes I–III) under the Rule of the Mamluks." Jerusalem: Mosad Ha-Rav Kuk.
Street, Brian. 1984. *Literacy in Theory and Practice.* New York: Cambridge University Press.
Swidler, Leonard. 1976. "Impure Menstruous Women." In *Women in Judaism: The Status of Women in Formative Judaism,* 130–39. Metuchen, N.J.: Scarecrow.
Szyszman, Simon. 1980. *Le Karaïsme.* Lausanne: L'Age D'Homme.
Thompson, E. P. 1968 [1963]. *The Making of the English Working Class.* Harmondsworth: Penguin.
Troki, Solomon. 1745 [1960]. *'Apiryon 'Asah Lo: 'Al Chalukat ha-Kara'im.* Tel Aviv: Hevrat ha-Hatslachah li-Vnei Mikra'.
Tsoffar, Ruth. 1995. "Reading *it,* Naming *it,* and Talking *it:* The Karaite *Niddah,* '*Adah,* and the Language of Menstruation." In *Folklore Interpreted: Essays in Honor of Alan Dundes,* ed. Regina Bendix and Rosemary Levi Zumwalt, 375–400. New York: Garland.
———. 2004. "Beads for Babies: Karaite Fertility Practices." Unpublished manuscript.
———. 2005a. "From the Literal to the Metaphoric and Back Again: 'A Land Flowing with Milk and Honey.'" Unpublished manuscript, Brown Bag Series, Center of Middle Eastern and North African Studies (CMENAS), University of Michigan, March 25.
———. 2005b. "Cannibal Ideology: Sexuality, Ethnicity, and Colonialism in Hebrew Cultures." Unpublished book manuscript.
Tukan, Boris. 1987. "The Karaite Calendar and Holidays." *Pe'amim* 32: 60–66.

Turner, Bryan. 1984. *The Body and Society*. London: Basil Blackwell.
Turner, Victor. 1979. "Betwixt and Between: The Liminal Period in Rites de Passage." In *Reader in Comparative Religion*, ed. William Lessa and Evon Vogt, 234–43. New York: Harper and Row.
Wasserfall, Rahel R., ed. 1992. "Menstruation and Identity: The Meaning of Niddah for Moroccan Women Immigrants to Israel." In *People of the Body: Jews and Judaism from an Embodied Perspective*, ed. Howard Eilberg-Schwartz, 309–27. Albany: State University of New York Press.
———. 1999. "Introduction: Menstrual Blood into Jewish Blood." In *Women and Water: Menstruation in Jewish Life and Law*, 1–18. Hanover, N.H.: Brandeis University Press.
Watson, O. M., and E. D. Grave. 1966. "Quantitative Research in Proxemic Behavior." *American Anthropologist* 68: 971–85.
Weideger, Paula. 1976. *Menstruation and Menopause: The Physiology and Psychology, the Myth and the Reality*. New York: Random House.
Weinberger, Leon. 2000. *Jewish Poet in Muslim Egypt: Moses Dar'i's Hebrew Collection*. Leiden: Brill.
White, Hayden. 1973. *Tropics of Discourse: Essays in Cultural Criticism*. Baltimore: Johns Hopkins University Press.
———. 1987. *The Content of the Form: Narrative Discourse and Historical Representation*. Baltimore: Johns Hopkins University Press.
Wieder, Naphtali. 1962. *The Judean Scroll and Karaism*. London: East and West Library.
Woolf, Virginia. 1928. *A Room of One's Own*. Middlesex: Penguin.
Wright, Gwendolyn, and Paul Rabinow. 1982. "Spatialization of Power: A Discussion of the Work of Michel Foucault." *Skyline* (March): 14–20.
Yanay, Niza, and Tamar Rapoport. 1999. "Ritual Impurity and Religious Discourse on Women and Nationality." In *Women's Studies International Forum* 20 (5–6): 651–63.
Yerushalmi, Yosef Hayim. 1989. *Zakhor: Jewish History and Jewish Memory*. New York: Schocken.
Zajaczkowski, Ananiasz. 1961. *Karaism in Poland: History, Language, Folklore, Science*. Paris: La Haye.
Zerubavel, Eviatar. 1981. *Hidden Rhythms: Schedules and Calendars in Social Life*. Chicago: University of Chicago Press.
———. 1985. *The Seven Day Cycle: The History and Meaning of the Week*. New York: Free Press.
———. 1991. *The Fine Line: Making Distinctions in Everyday Life*. New York: Free Press.
Zerubavel, Yael. 1995. *Recovered Roots: Collective Memory and the Making of Israeli National Tradition*. Chicago: University of Chicago Press.
Zohar, Zvi. 1987. "Bein Nikur le-'Ahavah: Nisu'im bein Kara'im le-Rabanim 'al pi Chakhmei Yiśra'el be-Mitsrayim ba-Me'ah ha-'Esrim" [Between Alienation and Brotherhood: Karaite-Rabbinite Intermarriage according to Egyptian Jewish Scholars in the Twentieth Century]. *Pe'amim* 32: 21–39.
———. 1988. "Teguvah" [Response]. *Pe'amim* 34: 47–50.

INDEX

Aaron ben Elijah, 38–39
Abarbanel, Isaac, 187
'Abd al-Jabbar, 38
'Abd al-Malik, 35
Abel, Joe, 25
abortion, 58
Abu Isa al-Isfahani, Ishak Ben Ya'kub Obadiah, 35
'ādah, contemporary reference to menstruation, 77, 79, 84–85
Afendopolo, Caleb ben Eliyahu, 39
'ahl el-kitab, 7
'alay al-ḥamra, 85–86
'aleeha al-'ādah, 85
Aleppo codex, 203n. 25
al-Fayyumi, Saadia ben Joseph (Saadia Gaon), 37, 38, 109, 202n. 16
Algamil, Yosef, 25, 28, 45, 46
Ali, Muhammad, 43
Al-Kalim, 47, 205n. 19
al-Kumisi, Daniel, 37
al-Maghribi, Samuel ben Moses, 43
al-Murshid (The Guide), 43
al-Nahawandi, Benjamin, 33, 36, 202n. 13
al-Qirqisani, Abu Yusuf Ya'qub: *Kitab al-'Anwar wal-Maraqib,* 37, 183
al-Qudsī (El-Kodsi), Murād, 10, 28, 44, 45; *Just for the Record in the History of the Karaite Jews in Egypt in Modern Times,* 25, 201n. 2; *The Karaite Communities in Poland, Lithuania, Russia and Crimea,* 46; *The Karaite Jews of Egypt 1882–1986,* 46
'am ha-sefer, 7
analogy. See *hekesh* (analogy)
Anan ben David, 155, 180; arrival in Cairo, 41; as Karaite father, 33; Karaite ideological doctrine, 36; *nidduy 'olam,* 16; prohibition regarding intercourse with a pregnant woman, 215n. 6; *Sefer Hamitzvot* (The Book of Precepts), 7, 15, 35–36
Ananites (*'Ananim*), 15, 35
Ankori, Zvi, 29, 36, 108
"anthro-historical" approach, 27
Ashdod, 47
Asher, Ben, 203n. 25
Astren, Fred, 30
Avelei Zion (the Mourners of Zion), 36, 38

Babi Yar, 41
Babovitch, Tubiah Simhah Levi, 40, 41, 45, 46
Babylonian Talmud, 35
Bachelard, Gaston, 171
Bakhtin, Mikhail, 166–67, 173
Bal, Mieke, 172, 180, 185
barley (*abib*), 108
bar mitzvah, 109–12, 149, 194

235

Baron, Salo, 29
Barthes, Roland, 171
basar be-chalav, 178, 180. See also milk-meat taboo
Bashyazi, Eliyahu ben Moses: *Aderet Eliyahu* (The Mantle of Eliyahu), 39, 182
bathing, defined, 155
bat mitzvah, 96, 112
Bay Area Karaite community, 2–6, 139; changes in menstrual prohibitions, 110, 131–32; efforts to incorporate children in the reading of the Torah, 111–12; restrictions on *wāidah*, 117–23; Shabbat, 51–55
Beauvoir, Simone de, 89, 128
Beinin, Joel, 200n. 8
Ben-Gurion, David, 48
Benjamin, Walter, 14; "The Task of the Translator," 193
Benjaminites, 36
Ben-Shamai, Haggai, 30
Biale, Rachel, 120–21, 207n. 1
Bible: as "discursive authority," 160; literal interpretation, 7–8; as a "total discourse," 6; translation into Arabic, 38
birth control, 58
blood: as antithetical substance to milk, 214n. 17; pure, 56, 196, 204n. 6; quantifying, 113, 114. See also *dam asil; dam tahor*
Bnei Mikra', 6, 36
bo'alei niddot, 17, 18
Bochart, Samuel, 188
Boddy, Janice, 167, 213n. 8
bodily fluids, European models of the cultural economy of, 171–72
body: as a closed unit, 168; grotesque, discourse of, 166–67; incorporation into ideology of reading, 11, 122, 176, 197; Karaite construction of, 58; pure, 67, 196; as a self-regulatory system, 172; Torah as, 200n. 10. See also woman, Karaite, body of
Boethusians, 33
Bourdieu, Pierre, 214n. 16

Brandes, Stanley, 121
bread making, as metaphor for creation and procreation, 146, 185
breast feeding, 58, 61, 164. See also mother's milk
breast-feeding woman. See *wālidah/yoledah*
Brill, E. J.: "Études sur le Judaïsme Médiéval, 30
Brinner, William, 30, 42
brit milah (male circumcision) 56, 57, 149. See also circumcision
Buckley, Thomas, 16
Butler, Judith, 198
Byzantine Empire, Ottoman conquest, 40

Caesarean section, 209n. 13
Cahn, Zvi: *The Rise of the Karaite Sect*, 51
Cairo, as junction of Karaite life and history between Europe and the Middle East, 41–42
Cairo Genizah, 29, 30, 35, 43, 155
calendar: Karaite, 9, 106–9; and purity/impurity issues, 113; Rabbanite, 107, 109; role in identity politics between minorities, 107–9; symbolic power with regard to unity of people of Israel, 108
Catherine II, 40
Certeau, Michel de: *The Practice of Everyday Life*, 10, 105, 127; *The Writing of History*, 27
Chevrat Hatslachah Li-vnei Mikra', 47
childbirth: blurs distinction between the woman who gives birth and she who is herself being born into motherhood, 164; and impurity, 117–23; and Karaite culture, 58; medical co-optation of, 162, 212n. 2
childbirth crisis/resolution, 212n. 2
child-rearing practices, 58
Chow, Rey, 12
Christian, Barbara, 208n. 11
circumcision, 56, 58, 120, 209n. 17. See also *brit milah*
class, and positions toward infertility and

patriarchy, 63
cleaning, vocabulary of, 98
Clement of Alexandria, 188
Clifford, James, 139
collective memory, 10
Colligan, Sumi, 48, 199n. 8
colonialism, 44
concentration camps, in Egypt, 138
counting: conceptual metaphor that guards women from impurity, 106, 114; and identity politics between minorities in Israel, 107–9; personal narratives of, 113–17; quantified blood, 114; seven and forty as units of significance, 122; of seven days, 215n. 3
Crimea, 39, 40

Dabbah, Eliyahu, 64–65
dam asil, 159
dam tahor (pure blood), 56. *See also* blood
Dar'i, Moses Ben Abraham, 139, 176, vii–ix
David Ibn Zimra, 200n. 12
degel 'adom (red flag), 86–87
"dejudaization," 40–41
Delaney, Carol, 167
Deleuze, Gilles, 7
Dening, Greg: *The Death of William Gooch: A History's Anthropology*, 27, 32, 201n. 3
dhimmī, 42, 43
"Diasporic Asceticism," 36
dietary laws: as a means of cutting a people off from others, 180; Rabbanite vs. Karaite, 177–78. *See also* Karaite dietary laws
divorce, 200n. 11, 210n. 5
domestic space, divided according to symbolic hierarchy of cleanliness, 151
douching, 155, 211n. 25
Douglas, Mary: *Purity and Danger*, 16, 115, 167, 175, 179, 214n. 13
Dover Bnei Mikra', 47, 205n. 19
Drori, Rina, 30, 202n. 8
Dubnow, Simon, 29

Eastern European Karaites, 26, 42
'eb (shame), 81
'edah (community), 54
Egypt: as ambivalent site of nostalgia, 139; Ayyubid dynasty, 43
Egyptian folk culture, dog in, 143. *See also* folk beliefs; evil eye
Egyptian Karaites: immigration to Israel in 1948, 45–47; imprisonment of men who supported Zionism, 134, 138; substitution of term *niddah* for other Arabic terms and expressions, 77
Eliyahu, Aaron ben, 202n. 19
El-Saadawi, Nawal, 94
endogamy, 49
engenderment, ideology of, 57–58
Essenes, 33
Ethiopian Jews, 48
ethnicity, politics of, 48
ethnographic writing, 202n. 9
ethnography: as an autonomous discourse, 19; crisis of, 12; as a project of translation, 12; as a "travel encounter," 139–40
ethno-reading, 2, 12, 13–14, 22, 193–94
evil eye, 162, 213n. 5. *See also* folk beliefs
exilarch, 35, 202n. 11
exogamy, 49

Faraj Lisha', Murad, 44–45
fasting, 133
Felman, Shoshana, 185, 190
female body. *See* woman, Karaite, body of
feminist studies, 125–26
fermented food, prohibition against, 136, 185, 210n. 13
Festival of Weeks (Shavu'ot), 108
Firkovitch, Abraham ben Samuel (Even Reshef), 40, 41, 203n. 22
Firkovitch Collection, St. Petersburg, 30
folk beliefs: about breast feeding, 162; about menstruating woman, 146–47, 211n. 25; ambivalent nature of, 169; as an unfavored category in Karaite history, 159; concerning mother and child, 184–86; evil eye, 162, 213n. 5;

folk beliefs (*continued*)
'*ifrit* (female demon) 80, 209n. 1; milk and blood as antithetical substances in, 214n. 17; as oral as well as textual data, 214n. 15; as textual data, 214n. 15; urine in, 215n. 19; urine's equivalency with water, 214n. 18; of women, 165
folktales, womanhood in, 205n. 22
Foster City, 51–55
Foster City Karaites. *See* Bay Area Karaite community
Foucault, Michel, 56, 209n. 3, ix; "Of Other Spaces," 125, 126
Frank, Daniel, 30
fundamentalist Islamic movement, 42
Funkenstein, Amos, 10, 26
Fustat, 42. *See also* Cairo
fūtah, 97; and change in woman's status, 91, 95, 96; coded meaning of potential uncleanliness, 96; washing, 92, 97–98

Galuthocentric nationalism, 36
Gatet li, 85
Geiger, Abraham, 29
Genesis, metaphoric week, 115–16
Geonim, 35, 177
Ginsberg, Harold Louis, 188
Goitein, Shelomoh Dov, 29, 44
Gordon, Nehemia, 109
Gottleib, Alma, 16
Graetz, Heinrich, 29
Grosz, Elizabeth, 209n. 4
grotesque body, discourse of, 166–67
Guattari, Felix, 7

Ha'ataka mishtalshelet (duplicated transmission), 7, 13, 200n. 4
Hadassi, Yehudah (Judah) ben Eliyahu (Elijah): *Eshkol ha-Kofer*, 38, 181, 183, 184, 186, 189
ha-dodah mi-Rusyah (the aunt from Russia), 86
ha-Dover, 205n. 19, 47
hakhamim (Karaite Sages), 43
Hakohen, Hackakham Shmu'el: *Concerning Slaughtering*, 177
halakhah: and Anan ben David, 35; discourages intermarriage, 67; driving on Yom Kippur, 211n. 23; end result of concern with God's truth, 13; prohibits conversion, 67; prohibits purification on Saturday, 117; rules for women that expose their condition, 76; seven days of impurity, 115–16; vocabulary of legislation, 16. *See also niddah; wālidah/yoledah*
halēb (milk), 213n. 6
Halevi, Hayim: *Ma'ayan Hayyim*, 47; on need for speaking for oneself, 196; reading of the week, 115–16; *Toharat ha-Mishpachah be-Yisra'el* (Family Purity in Israel), 58, 208n. 9
hammam baladi (sha'abi), 214n. 14
harām, 81, 84
Haran, Menachem, 188, 189, 217n. 19
Ḥarat 'Abbāsiyyah, 54
Ḥarat al-Yahūd, 60, 131
Ḥarat al-Yahūd al-Kara'iyim, 42, 54
Ḥarat al-Yahūd al-Rabbaniyin, 42
Harkavy, Abraham, 29
Hatroki, Shlomo: *Sefer 'Apirion 'Asah Lo*, 178, 183
He-Halutz, 45
hekesh (analogy), 7, 8, 35, 180, 181
Hendel, Yehudit: *Kesef Katan*, 205n. 3
herem, 177
heterotopias, 209n. 3
HIAS, 46
High Holidays, 211n. 22
Hirshberg, Jehoash, 30, 31, 49
history, 27. *See also* Karaite history
Holdheim, Samuel, 29
Horton, H. Mack, 207n. 2
Hurston, Zora Neale, 169

Ibn Ezra, Abraham, 177, 187, 188
identity, Karaite: dialectical interaction with Rabbanite Judaism, 10; only acquired through birth, 55; origins at genesis of Judaism, 56; role of Passover in, 137; three main prin-

ciples of, 37
identity politics, 42
'*ifrit* (female demon), 80, 209n. 1
impurity (*tum'ah*): childbirth and, 117–23; counting, 106, 114; difference between male and female, 118, 119–21; hierarchy of, 166; as imposed category in patriarchal and hegemonic culture, 194; Karaite female body as locus of, 22, 31, 169; Leviticus on, 115–16, 121, 163, 213n. 9; measures of, 21–22; menstruation as uncontained, 22; physical sites of, 125, 150; salience of during Passover and Yom Kippur, 133; *tum'ah mishtalshelet* (transmitted impurity), 153, 165; *tum'at ledah* (postpartum impurity), 163, 208n. 12; of urine, 172; of *wālidah,* 164; of *yoledah,* 163
infertility, 62
Inhorn, Marcia, 62
intermarriage, between Karaites and Rabbanites, 42–43
'Iqar va-ferach, 181, 182
Irigaray, Luce, 171–72
Israel: conflict with Egypt, 46; identity politics, 18, 107–9; immigration of Egyptian Karaites to, 45–47; Karaite attachment to, 36; menstruation in public discourse, 205n. 3; nationalism, 46; Sinai campaign, 134; State of, 45. *See also* Zionism
Israeli Haggadah, 136
Israeli Karaites, 46–49, 56
Izhak Ben Zvi Institute, 30

Jabès, Edmond: *The Book of Margins,* 19, vii
Japhet al-Barqamani, 43
Japhet ben 'Eli, 38
Japhet ibn Saghir, 43
Jeroboam, 33, 56
Jerusalem: capture by the crusaders, 38; center of nationalistic diasporic community, 36; intellectual and cultural center for the production of Karaite knowledge, 37; Karaite community, 47
Jeshuah ben Judah: *Sefer a-Yteser* (The Book of Desire), 38
Johnson, Shirley M., 211n. 25
Judaism, Otherness in, ix
Judeo-Tatar dialect, 39

Kaddish, 54
Kafka, Franz, 7
Karaim (Qaraim), 36, 39
Karaism, emergence of, ix
Karaite Bet Din (Courts of Law), 47, 48; in Israel, 200n. 11
Karaite dietary laws, 173–74, 175–92; attitude towards fermentation, 136, 185, 210n. 13; koshering process, 179; and the maternal discourse, 176; "mother's milk" as substance produced during first seven days of offspring's life, 189–90; during Passover, 136; permit mixing of meat with milk, 174, 176–77, 178, 180–84, 215n. 7; three principles of, 181–82, 183
Karaite-Egyptian food, 55
Karaite Exodus, 2, 134, 137–40
Karaite historiography, 28–32
Karaite history, 33–39; admission into Poland, 202n. 20; assigned to Department of Muslims and Druze in Israel, 48; community in Lithuania, 40; complete rupture from mainstream Judaism, 37; dispersion to Egypt and Byzantium, 38; forced relocation, 39; historical isolation, 55–56; intellectual center in Crimea, 40; as mourners of the destruction of the Temple, 15; origin story, 33; problematic, 25–26; question of origins during the Second World War, 41; Rabbanite and Karaite differences, 26; seventh to twentieth century settlements, 34; Tatar and Turkish rule, 39, 40; as truth, 28
Karaite Jews of America (KJA), 3–4

Index

Karaite Korner (www.karaite-korner.org), 33, 109
Karaite Passover, 134–37, 210n. 15; exaggerates unclean posture of menstruating woman, 148; Haggadah, 135–37; prohibited foods, 210n. 13; reading of, 116; salience of purity and impurity issues during, 133; Seder, 135–36, 140–45; and Shavu'ot, 108; women's preparations for, 60–61
Karaite-Rabbanite relations: and calendars, 108; Karaite attempts to differentiate themselves from Rabbanite, 40–41; Karaite dialogical relationship to Rabbanite legal discourse, 177; Karaite view of themselves in reference to the dominant Rabbanite, 19; split between, 56
Karaites: in Asia Minor, 38; constructed as heresy, 201n. 4; Eastern European, 26, 42; in Egypt, 41–46; in Europe, 39–41; in Middle East, 42
karet, 16, 17
Kashani, Reuven: *The Karaites: History, Tradition and Customs*, 109
katuv (*pshat*, literal interpretation), 7–8, 14–15, 159, 197
Kaufman, Tamar, 203n. 2
Keel, Othmar, 186
ketubbah (marriage contract), 106–7
Khan, Geoffrey, 30
Kipchak-Turkish pagans, 39
kippah, 52
Kittler, Friedrich, 90
Kizilov, Mikhail, 30
KJA Bulletin: October 1994 edition, 3–4; Passover greeting, 135; 1994 Passover issue, 47
Kohen, 54
"Kol Ha-'Ishah," 205n. 3
koshering, 179, 196, 201n. 14
Kristeva, Julia, 90, 120, 179–80, 191, 209n. 17, 216n. 15; *Powers of Horror*, 16

Laban (sour milk), 213n. 6
lactation, empowers women to exercise some agency over birth control, 173
language, abbreviated, 76
Laqueur, Thomas, 171
Lasker, Daniel, 30
Last Marranos, The, 207n. 4
legal codes: Karaite, 7; Rabbanite, Karaite dialogical relationship to, 177
lehafshit, 14
Leningrad Public Library, collection of Karaite books and manuscripts, 40
Leviticus: analogy between birth mother's impurity and the rules of the *niddah*, 121; codes of pollution, 179; constructs impurity according to the duration of bleeding, 115–16; impurity of the *yoledah*, 213n. 9; Karaite reading of, 113; Kara'iyot's commentary on, 106; on *niddah*, 16, 75–76, 205n. 1; on postpartum impurity, 163, 208n. 12; role in constituting Karaite consciousness, 20; seven days of *tum'at niddah*, 115
literature, Karaite: golden age of, 36–37; representations of Karaite women limited to motherhood, 63–64
Lod, 47
Lo tikach ha-'em 'al ha-banim, 181
Luzzatto, Moshe Chaim, 187
Lvov, 40

ma'dan 'asil (pure metal), 55
Mahler, Raphael, 29
Maimonides, 155, 188–89, 216n. 17
Mamluks, 43
Mann, Jacob, 29, 180
marginality, 167
maror, 137
marriage: *ketubbah* (marriage contract), 106–7; at a young age, 65–66
Marzuq, Moshe, 45
masturbation, 58
"maternal voice," 90
matzah: avoidance of by menstruating woman, 145; as focal point of ritual enactment of Exodus, 136, 145–46

Medini, Rabbi Hayim Hezkeyah, 17
Meir, Golda, 48
men, and menstruation discourse, 101–2
menstruating woman. See *niddah*
menstruation: among American women, 206n. 7; association with dirt in Israeli context, 18; as converse process of fermentation, 146; discourse of, 19–20, 76–88, 85, 101–2, 151, 160
Messick, Brinkley: *The Calligraphic State: Textual Domination and History in a Muslim Society*, 8
midwifery, 212n. 1
mikveh, 17, 211n. 26, 214n. 10
Milgrom, Jacob, 188, 189, 217n. 18
milk: as antithetical substance to blood in folk beliefs, 214n. 17; as a generic fluid, 188, 189; as a national symbol in Zionist discourse, 216n. 12. See also mother's milk; laban; *halēb*
milk-meat taboo, 174, 178, 180, 187–88, 215n. 7
Miller, Philip, 30
Miranjana, Tejaswini, 12
mitzvah (commandment), 119
"*mi'utim*" (religious minorities in Israel), 48
Mizrahim (Jews of Middle Eastern and North African ancestry), 18
Mopsik, Charles, 57–58
mother-daughter teaching, 31, 59, 89–103; of cleanliness, 21, 94; and reading of *niddah*, 196
motherhood: all-encompassing role, 164; indelibility of mother-child bond, 23; and position of honor within the community, 62, 65
mother's milk: as the affirmation of motherhood in Karaite culture, 190–92; as an allusion to both human and animal in Karaite culture, 187; beliefs concerning stoppage of, 162; exclusive access to granted to the baby, 185–87; as a limited good, 162, 165, 213n. 8; as substance produced during first seven days of offspring's life, 189–90; valorization of, 22; and the *yoledah/wālidah*, 163–74
"mother's mouth," 90
mourning rituals, 49
Muslim Brotherhood, 42
Mu'tazilite school, 38

Nabbid, 210n. 14
naked reading. See *pshat*
naming system, 204n. 8
Nasib al-Madrasah, 203n. 5
Nasser, Abdel, 134
National Karaite Council, 47
Nazis, attempt to define Karaites, 41
Nebat, 33
nedunyah, 64
Nemoy, Leon, 29–30, 201n. 7
nesi'im, 41
"New Moon Reports," 109. See also calendar
Nidchei Yisrael, 48
niddah, 16–20; associated with Jewish scholarship and law of Leviticus, 79; avoidance of sexual interaction and physical contact, 81; at the bar mitzvah, 149; barred from kitchen and cooking, 130–33; as Biblical term, 75–76; at the *brit*, 149; and care of objects, 97; codes of secrecy, 84–88; as collective experience, 19; contaminated space of, 145–51; culturally constructed rules for, 16; encapsulates power struggle between the Karaites and the Rabbanites, 17; inappropriate topic of conversation, 83–84; initiates the Karaite girl child into adult womanhood, 95; and invisibility of women, x; limit woman's intimacy within the world, 67; and linguistic split between the self and the body, 128; location of, 130; as "malfunctioning" body, 147; in mixed marriages, 155; narratives about first menstruation, 18, 89–103; as "Other," 151; prohibition against bathing and

niddah (continued)
    showering, 152–57, 212n. 28; prohibition against cooking or entering kitchen, 146; prohibition against kneading dough or baking, 146–47; purification ritual, 151–57; reading of, 196; refers to the social body and its socioreligious representation, 77, 80–81; at the Seder, 140–45; separation and confinement, 128–30; specifies woman's distance from the book and highlights her social inadequacy, 67; taboo against touching during, 145; and transmitted impurity, 153, 165; unclean shadow of, 145–46; uncontained impurity, 22; as a woman in a temporal bodily condition, 76; "x," 86; and Yom Kippur, 133–34
nidduy 'olam (life sentence), 16
Nietzsche, Friedrich, 10
Nikomodio: *Keter Torah*, 182, 183–84
North Africa, British and French Mandates in, 44
Northern California Jewish Bulletin, 203n. 2

Ofakim, 47
Olszowy-Schlanger, Judith, 30
Omar, pact of, 43
oral tradition: as extension of the written law, 160; and folk beliefs, 214n. 15; redefined by reading, 136; rejection of, 103
"The Organization of Israeli Karaites in Egypt," 203n. 24
'Oto ve-'et bno, 181, 182
Ottoman Empire: decline of, 44; rise of, 43

Palestine, 37
pan-Arab nationalism, 42
parashat ha-shavu'a, 53, 54, 111
pareve, 178
Passover. See Karaite Passover; Rabbanite Passover
patriarchy, 56–57, 58

patrilocality/patrilineality, 56
"people of the book" (*ahl el-kitab*), 45
Pessah, Maurice, 3
Pessah Dorot, 116
Pessah Mitsrayim, 116
Pessah sheni (Pessah Katan), 140
Pharisees, 35
Philo, 186, 188, 217n. 18
Pinsker, Simhah, 29
poetics, and history, 27
Polliack, Meira, 30
postpartum bleeding, 117, 118, 121, 170
postpartum impurity (*tum'at ledah*), 163, 208n. 12
Poznanski, Samuel Abraham, 29
prayer book, 203n. 3
pshat (naked reading), 7–8, 14–15, 159, 197
pure blood, 56, 196, 204n. 6
pure body, 67, 196
pure Torah, 56, 67, 196, 204n. 6
purification ritual, 31, 151–57
purity (*taharah*), 110, 156; burden of Karaite woman, 11, 22, 31, 58, 169; prohibited on Saturday, 117; and Shabbat, 67
qasida, viii

Rabbanite Judaism: accusations that Karaites are not "pure," 17–18; appalled by Karaite practice of mixing milk and meat, 187–88; calendar, 107, 109; dietary separation between dairy and meat products, 178; hierarchy of pollution, 175; *mikveh*, 211n. 26; monopoly of writing Karaite history, 28–30; *niddah* laws, 17, 199n. 8, 207n. 1; "people of the book," 45; prayer as an alternative to cultic ritual, 15; reciting the *Shma'*, 156–57; silencing power of, 28; view of Karaism as a deviation from normative Judaism, 29
Rabbanite Passover, 135–36
rabbinic authority, resistance to, 33, 35
rahatsah, 155
raisin wine, 136, 146

Ramleh, 47
Rashbam, 188
reading, 6–11; as an act of resistance, 7, 9; based on two aspects of identity, 6–7; body as a discursive agent, 11, 122, 176; cross-cultural, interethnic differences in reading and misreading, 119; of history, 28; and identity, 8, 12; of Leviticus, 113; literal, 14–15; naked reading (*pshat*), 7–8, 14–15, 159, 197; overarching concept of Karaite life and its representation, 1–2, 195–98; and position as an allegory of resistance, 7; post-structuralist approach to Karaite culture, 9; productive and halakhic process, 194–95; redefines oral tradition, 136; resist accumulated and layered meanings of the Bible, 15; socially embedded, 8–9; specific reading of the Bible, 36; strives to keep close to the biblical texts and narratives, 13; as a woman, 6, 9–10, 160. *See also* ethno-reading
Red Cross, 46
Renan, 47
reproduction: female responsibility over, 58–59; ideologically tied to the constraints of patriarchy, 56–59; inseparable from the maternal conception of knowledge, 103
Rosh Chodesh, 108
running water, and purification ritual, 156–57
Russell, Bertrand, 76

Saadia Gaon. *See* al-Fayyumi, Saadia ben Joseph (Saadia Gaon)
Sabbah, Fatna, 78
Sadducees (Zadokites), 33
safek mamzer, 17
sages, 7, 13, 15, 38
Sahl ben Masliah, 38, 47, 202n. 18
Salah al-Din, 43, 203n. 25
Salmon ben Jeroham, 30, 37–38, 201n. 7
Samaritans, 45
San Francisco Karaite community. *See* Bay Area Karaite community
Scarry, Elaine, 107, 113–14
Schechter, Salomon, 29
Schur, Nathan, 30
semen, as a limited resource in Karaite literature, 213n. 7. *See also* sperm
Semi, Emanuela Trevisan, 48–49, 58
Sevel ha-yerushah, 7, 55, 173. See also *halakhah*
sex: exists solely for the sake of procreation, 65; as a taboo subject among women, 66
Shabbat: in Bay Area Karaite community, 51–55; delivery of Karaite babies on, 213n. 3; and experience of community, 66–67; and issues of women's purity, 67; meal, 55; prohibition of sexual relations during, 67–74
shadow, of menstruating woman, 145–46
Shapira, Dan, 30
Shma', 156–57
Shmini Atseret, 112
shomer kashrut, 178
showering: impact on fertility, virginity, and menstrual pain, 153–54
Silverman, Kaja, 90
Simchat Torah, 5, 96, 112
Simhah Isaac ben Moses, 40
single women, marginality, 65
Six Day War, 45, 134, 137
Snow, Loudell F., 211n. 25
Snowden, Robert, 208n. 11
Soler, Jean, 179, 180
Somekh, Sasson, 45
sopher, 106
spaces: contaminated, of menstruating woman, 145–51; domestic, and hierarchy of cleanliness, 151; of silence, 126; types, 126
Spencer, John, 188
sperm, in Jewish patriarchal culture, 190. *See also* semen
Stock, Brian, 10
Sukkot, 112
Sura Academy, Iraq, 37
Suzin, Rabbi Moshe, 17

Talmud, 17, 33, 35, 176
tame'ah (impure woman), 84, 117
Temple, 36
Temple in miniature (*mikdash me'at*), 36
Temple period, purification after menstruation, 152
textual practices: and coexistence with the Bible, 6; eschew Biblical commentary, 31; folk beliefs as textual data, 214n. 15; purity of body equal to a truthful meaning of texts, 197; as reading, 8; rejection of oral tradition, 103
Toharat ha-Mishpachah (family purity), 204n. 12
Torah: of Moses, 33; treated like a body, 200n. 10; pure 56, 67, 196, 204n. 6
Torah shebe-'al peh, 134
Troki, Isaac ben Abraham: *Hizzuk Emunah*, 40
truth, preoccupation with, 159
tsarah, 62
Tukan, Boris, 208n. 7
tum'ah mishtalshelet (transmitted impurity), 153, 165
tum'at ledah (postpartum impurity), 163, 208n. 12

Ugaritic texts, 188
urination ritual, 168, 170, 172
urine: folk equivalency with water, 214n. 18; in the folklore of different cultures, 215n. 19; impurity of, 172

Vital, Rabbi Shmuel, 109

walad/yeled (child, new born), 163–64
wālidah/yoledah (mother postpartum): defensive strategy when interacting with menstruating woman, 165–74; impurity, 163; open body, 164, 166–67; prohibitions against, 119–23, 164; upper body is productive and lower body is restricted, 170; vulnerability rooted in production of milk, 162, 164, 165
washing, defined, 155

water: "cupping," 156–57; dichotomy of pure and impure, 153; use of during menstrual cycle, 152–57
Weinberger, Leon, 30
White, Hayden, 26–27, 28
wine, forbidden during Passover, 136
Wissenschaft des Judentums, 29
Withold of Lithuania, 39
woman, Karaite, body of: bodily ritual guarantees male bodily purity, 153; generates multiple discursive possibilities, 195; locus of the social forces of purity and impurity in Karaite body politics, 169; nexus of Karaite politics, poetics, and aesthetics of difference, 194; represented through its three bodily fluids, 170, 179; social representation of as "dangerous" and "uncontrollable," 126; spoken of body in euphemistic language, 85–88; textual reading of, 122. See also *niddah*; *wālidah/yoledah*
women, Karaite: commitment to child-bearing, 59, 61–62; cultural ambivalence toward, 163; *Kara'iyot*, 1, 11, 76; knowledge about preparation for menstruation, 66; life structured by issues of purity and impurity, 11, 22, 31; need to legitimate daily culture with authority of perceived Bible, 160; and reading, 9–10, 160; responsibility within the community to impart laws and tradition, 5; sex perceived as potentially dangerous or shameful, 66; single, marginality of, 65; spend most of their reproductive years either pregnant or breast feeding, 161
Woolf, Virginia: *A Room of One's Own*, 89
World War II, and devastation of Karaite community, 41
writing: and condition of otherness, viii–ix; ethnographic, 202n. 9; of Karaite history, 28–30

"x." See *niddah*

yeled, 163–64
Yemen textual practice, 8
Yerushalmi, Yosef Hayim, 26
yetzikah, 155
yoledah. See *wālidah/yoledah*
Yom Kippur: driving on, 211n. 23; and menstruation, 133–34; salience of purity and impurity issues during, 133

Yusuf ibn Nuh, Abu Yaakub, 38

Zajaczkowski, Ananiasz, 39
zavah, 115, 116, 121, 208n. 9
Zerubavel, Eviatar, 115, 121
Zerubavel, Yael, 26
Zionism, rise of, 42
Zunz, Leopold, 29

www.ingramcontent.com/pod-product-compliance
Lightning Source LLC
Chambersburg PA
CBHW071815230426
43670CB00013B/2467